PROBLEM SOLVING in
ENDODONTICS

PROBLEM SOLVING in ENDODONTICS

Prevention, Identification, and Management

third edition

James L. Gutmann, D.D.S., F.A.C.D., F.I.C.D.

Professor and Director
Graduate Endodontics
Department of Restorative Sciences
Texas A & M University System—Baylor College of Dentistry
Dallas, Texas
Diplomate, American Board of Endodontics

Thom C. Dumsha, D.D.S., M.S.

Associate Professor and Chairman
Department of Endodontics
Baltimore College of Dental Surgery
University of Maryland at Baltimore
Baltimore, Maryland
Diplomate, American Board of Endodontics

Paul E. Lovdahl, D.D.S., M.S.D.

Private Practice Limited to Endodontics
Bellingham, Washington

Eric J. Hovland, D.D.S., M.Ed., M.B.A., F.A.C.D., F.I.C.D.

Professor of Endodontics and Dean
Louisiana State University School of Dentistry
New Orleans, Louisiana
Diplomate, American Board of Endodontics

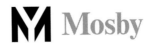

St. Louis Baltimore Boston Carlsbad Chicago Naples New York Philadelphia Portland
London Madrid Mexico City Singapore Sydney Tokyo Toronto Wiesbaden

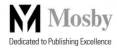
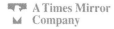

Dedicated to Publishing Excellence

A Times Mirror
Company

Vice President and Publisher: *Don Ladig*
Executive Editor: *Linda L. Duncan*
Developmental Editor: *Jo Salway and Melba Steube*
Project Manager: *Dana Peick*
Senior Production Editor: *Stavra Demetrulias*
Manuscript Editor: *Carl Masthay*
Designer: *Amy Buxton*
Manufacturing Supervisor: *Karen Boehme*

THIRD EDITION

Printed in the United States of America
Composition by Accu-color Inc.
Printing/binding by Maple-Vail Book Manufacturing Group

Mosby–Year Book, Inc.
11830 Westline Industrial Drive
St. Louis, Missouri 63146

0-8151-4044-4

96 97 98 99 00 / 9 8 7 6 5 4 3 2 1

CONTRIBUTORS

▼

Gerald N. Glickman, D.D.S., M.S., M.B.A.

Associate Professor and Director of Endodontics
Department of Cariology, Restorative Sciences, and
    Endodontics
School of Dentistry
University of Michigan
Ann Arbor, Michigan
Diplomate, American Board of Endodontics

Curtis K. Wade, D.D.S.

Private Practice Limited to Periodontics
Bellingham, Washington
Diplomate, American Board of Periodontics

*To my wife, Marylou, for her unwavering acceptance, support,
encouragement, and understanding, and to Fred Harty, a colleague,
an inspiration, and a friend who will be dearly missed.* — JLG

To MAD, TAD, and CLD for their support and love: Gotcha! — TCD

*To Dr. Gerald Harrington, my friend and mentor,
and to my parents, who made dentistry possible.* — PEL

*To my parents, who have inspired me to strive for excellence,
and to Carol, Allison, and Whitney, for their love and support.* — EJH

PREFACE

to Third Edition

▼

Since the first edition of this text was published in 1987, the value of the "problem-solving" approach to the delivery of endodontic care has been so successful that it has been claimed and adopted by many other authors. Girded with this reality, we have attempted to more clearly characterize and enhance the problem-solving concept that we initiated over 10 years ago. To accomplish this we have chosen a multifold approach.

Initially we expanded and embellished the cognitive and psychomotor problem-solving skills, which are time tested and proved and can be mastered by the competent and dedicated professional. Second, we incorporated new and valuable technological concepts. Third, we continued to emphasize the fact that the key to success in treatment is a cognizant inspection of the process that produces the finished product and identifies the causes of variations and eliminates them, as opposed to only assessment of the final product. Fourth, we highlighted and integrated the fact that the delivery of quality endodontic care must be based on a thorough understanding of its science—endodontology. Finally, what makes this text *unique* and *distinct* from all others is that we have integrated the above initiatives into a realistic clinical perspective that is guided by the standard of care and quality assurance.

To achieve these objectives it was necessary to make some significant changes to our text. Chapter 1 has been greatly expanded with regard to concepts of success and failure, standards of care, and quality assurance. These issues serve to enhance the problem-solving concept in diagnosis and treatment planning, which are the cohesive forces throughout the text. Additionally each chapter has been carefully updated and detailed with problem-based cases that highlight and emphasize the need for critical thinking and assessment. In these cases, logical data gathering, interpretation, and application are emphasized within sound treatment-planning principles, clinical techniques, and the timely delivery of care.

New and contemporary concepts in the problem-solving management of dental trauma are detailed, and expanded horizons in canal preparation and obturation are clarified. Two new chapters have been added to address challenging and often misunderstood concepts in pulpal and periodontal relationships and the restoration of endodontically treated teeth. Information in both chapters is presented in a problem-solving, clinically relevant format with a special emphasis on a scientific and biological rationale for treatment planning and management. Creative and contemporary techniques designed to manage both common and unusual problems are found in every chapter and are highlighted with many new clinical cases.

With the quality of patient oral health care being at the heart of our commitment to the dental profession, all practitioners who perform endodontic therapy for their patients are strongly encouraged to embrace and incorporate the problem-solving concept on a regular basis. In doing so, quality assurance, for all practical purposes, is guaranteed. For dental academicians, problem-solving or problem-based learning is essential to elevate the quality of the educational process and to guide the student to the appropriate levels of competence.

Our sincere thanks are extended to our developmental editors, Jo Salway and Melba Steube. Melba in particular has been a keen guiding force over the years in textbook production. Second, we would like to thank Linda Duncan, Executive Editor, for her continued belief in and support for our efforts. Third, we would like to extend a warm and generous thanks to Stavra Demetrulias for her patience, guidance, and professional expertise as our production editor. Finally, a special vote of thanks is due to all the graduate students and faculty who have enriched this edition and previous editions with their valuable clinical cases and enlightening critiques. To them we have given the charge to strive always for excellence. To you, the reader of this text, we extend the same challenge.

James L. Gutmann, D.D.S.
Thom C. Dumsha, M.S., D.D.S.
Paul E. Lovdahl, D.D.S., M.S.D.
Eric J. Hovland, D.D.S., M.Ed., M.B.A.

PREFACE

▼

to Second Edition

Since the publication of the first edition of *Problem Solving in Endodontics,* a keen awareness of this approach to diagnosis and treatment has been evident in all levels of dental education. In fact, "problem solving" has become a contemporary "buzzword" within dental curriculums and continuing education programs. With this realization, we have chosen to expand and clarify the concepts of problem solving in endodontics to meet the needs of not only the practicing dentist, but also the aspiring undergraduate dental student and neophyte endodontist. In doing so we have opted to take a slightly different approach to this concept in the second edition, altering the thought process of the problem-solving methodology.

First, by beginning the second edition with a chapter on "success and failure" we have brought to the forefront concepts rarely addressed in undergraduate dental education and which are often buried deep within endodontic texts, so deep that their meaning and applicability are essentially lost or disregarded in the daily struggles of "filing and filling." These concepts form the rationale for treatment and provide a standard of care and evaluation that should never be compromised.

Second, we have tried to emphasize that true problem solving is the key to success in treatment because it demands inspection of the process that produces the finished product and identifies the causes of variations and eliminates them, as opposed to only assessing the final product. The latter approach is not a learning process and invariably leads to a compromise in the treatment rendered—or as it is humorously put, "when all else fails, lower your standards." It is only through an active, cognizant approach to problem solving during the various phases of diagnosis and treatment—with an emphasis on prevention—that success can ultimately be achieved. Likewise, it also creates an introspective, challenging environment in which ego protection can be avoided through an honest appraisal, interpretation, and assessment of past experiences and decisions.

Third, even though many problems encountered in endodontics are primarily technical in nature,

emphasis has been placed on the biological rationale for the problem-solving approach. Ultimate achievement of success within the biological complexities of the oral cavity dictates this consideration throughout the concepts addressed in this edition.

Fourth, we have chosen to expand the realm of problem solving into two timely areas which impact greatly on endodontic diagnosis and treatment—radiology and fractured teeth. Coupled with significant updates in retreatment, access, cleaning, shaping, and obturation, we hope we have provided the reader not only with clear answers and solutions to their questions and problems, but also with a direct challenge to always strive for excellence.

As with any quality endeavor, there exists a number of dedicated people who, through their hard work, make good things happen. Our sincere thanks are extended to Susie Baxter for her professional guidance, support, and patience throughout all phases of this undertaking; to Karen Halm, our production manager, and Fran Perveiler, our copyediting manager, many thanks for your commitment and dedication to achieving a quality, timely publication; and to Sandy Reinhardt for his belief in us that *Problem Solving in Endodontics* could be taken to new plateaus.

Finally, we would like to quote Frederick B. Noyes, who in 1922 expressed the essential philosophy to achieving success in endodontic treatment, a philosophy that should guide all those who choose to provide quality treatment for their patients:

"For our purpose, I shall discuss this subject [Root Canal Treatment] from a biological standpoint. The first theorem that needs to be propounded is perhaps that life is reaction, and whatever you do in the treatment of pulps, in the treatment of peridental membranes, in the treatment of any living tissues is to be measured in biological, not mechanical standards. What you are after is a cellular reaction, a tissue reaction, a biological response. In other words, in everything that involves every one of these subjects, in practice you must think in terms of cell and cell reaction, not in terms of mechanical procedure or drugs. You have a biological problem in the handling of which you must use technical and mechanical skill to control the biological condition.

"The reason we have had to face such a terrible arraignment as a profession [Focal Infection] in the last few years is primarily because we have not been trained to think in terms of biological conceptions, and we have been trained to act in terms of mechanical procedures, and the solution of the pulpless tooth problem will be solved by the profession only when

the majority of all practitioners of dentistry think at the chair, in terms of tissues and tissue reactions."

James L. Gutmann, D.D.S.
Thom C. Dumsha, M.S., D.D.S.
Paul E. Lovdahl, D.D.S., M.S.D.
Eric J. Hovland, D.D.S., M.Ed., M.B.A.

PREFACE

to First Edition

▼

The demand for quality endodontic treatment has significantly increased over the past 25 years. The concomitant explosion in biologic science and technical applications has had a positive impact on our understanding of treatment and its efficient delivery. However, it is very easy to become mired in this plethora of new information and high-tech devices. As the dental professional tries to integrate these changes into the delivery of care, basic concepts of successful treatment may be lost from daily practice. This situation is very real and has become evident to the authors over many years of educating dental professionals in schools and continuing education programs, as well as through the active practice of endodontics. It is this set of circumstances which provided the impetus to develop this text.

The problem-solving approach used in this book is undoubtedly unique to endodontics. It is designed to alert the dental professional to means of avoiding frustrations and failures in treatment, and ways to achieve a consistently high level of quality care in endodontics. We chose to focus on key areas most often identified by the dental professional as causing the most difficulty in diagnosis and treatment. Each of these key areas is addressed in a systematic problem-solving manner designed to *prevent* problems in treatment, to *identify* problems if they are already present or occur during treatment, and to *manage* the problems once they are recognized by the astute practitioner.

Although a multitude of treatment modalities exist in endodontics, and many techniques can be used to manage difficult diagnostic and treatment situations, we have focused on cognitive and psychomotor problem-solving skills which are time tested and proven and can be mastered by the dental professional. We emphasize that the key to problem solving in endodontics is not just another technique or a new device, but rather a cognizant, preventive approach to diagnosis and treatment. This is the essential ingredient of success, the essential ingredient to providing the highest level of patient care.

James L. Gutmann, D.D.S.
Thom C. Dumsha, M.S., D.D.S.
Paul E. Lovdahl, D.D.S., M.S.D.

CONTENTS

▼

PROBLEM SOLVING in
ENDODONTICS

▼

Problems in the Assessment of Success and Failure, Quality Assurance, and Their Integration into Endodontic Treatment Planning

James L. Gutmann
Paul E. Lovdahl

"A few moments' consideration of the original cause of trouble at the apex of roots will enable us to realize what is required to be accomplished in the way of successful treatment. If the original cause is admitted to be irritation from decomposing pulp, its removal will in most cases effect a cure."*

The concepts of success and failure in endodontics are often relegated to positions of secondary importance. This is evident in textbooks, in which chapters on these issues, if present, are situated deep into the written material, whereas those chapters that deal with canal cleaning and shaping, obturation, surgery, and so forth are in the forefront. Dental school lectures are conducted in a similar manner, and those curricula that are limited in time also overlook these issues. Many aspiring professionals are never faced with the concepts of success and failure in didactic courses, and certainly not in clinical training: *in a requirement-driven curriculum, success is erroneously assumed once treatment is completed.* This approach undermines the entire process of treatment planning because the clinician is never able to learn from the ultimate successes or failures of choices made in providing treatment. When faced with future compromised situations,

the clinician is unable to apply and integrate the concepts of success and failure into the treatment plan chosen. Under these circumstances quality assurance is impossible. This frequently leads to the provision of no treatment, poor treatment, or the wrong treatment. In the medical profession the common phrase "Take two aspirin and call me in the morning" is often an indictment of the treatment provided (or lack thereof). Similar phrases characterize the dentist's dilemma, such as, "I don't see anything on the radiograph"; "I'll give you some antibiotics and pain medication and we'll see what happens"; or "I'm not sure what's wrong, but you don't need that tooth and I can make you a bridge." What appears to be in vogue in contemporary dental practice is the automatic identification of an implant as being far better than natural tooth structure.

> The dental professional is faced with a daily continuum of clinical situations requiring an integration of facts, experiences, interpretations, applications, and analyses. The ability to confront these situations in a systematic and successful manner characterizes the problem-solving approach to treatment and evaluation.

*From Whitehouse W: *Br J Sci* 27:238-240, 1884.

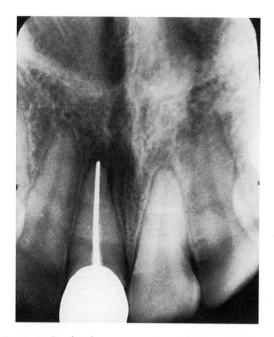

Fig. 1-1 *Single silver-cone root canal fill 4 years after obturation. Radiolucency present and patient symptomatic to pressure on the tooth.*

The purpose of this initial chapter is to emphasize for the dental practitioner the importance of the concepts of success and failure and to encourage the problem-solving approach in the determination of success and avoidance of failure. Once these concepts are grasped, quality assurance is routinely achievable. Integration of these concepts into realistic and thoughtful treatment planning of endodontic problems will be demonstrated with specific case scenarios in this chapter and throughout this text. It is hoped that the information gleaned from this chapter will be integrated into the problem-solving concepts advocated throughout the subsequent chapters. Likewise, a review of this chapter during assimilation of the information in the remainder of this book is highly recommended to ensure the daily performance of all dental treatment at or above the standard of care.

HISTORICAL AND CONTEMPORARY VIEWS ON SUCCESS AND FAILURE

Historically the concept of success or failure of endodontic therapy has centered on the "sterilization" of the root canal system, coupled with the perceived need to achieve a hermetic apical seal. Both research and clinical studies focused on these issues as the priorities in successful treatment. The basis for this focus was Hunter's[14] focal infection theory,

Rosenow's[29] concept of elective localization, and the hollow-tube theory of Rickert and Dixon.[28] These postulates shaped the tenets of success and failure in endodontics into the 1950s, when support for the lack of a complete apical seal as the primary cause for endodontic failure dominated the scene.[5] Even today, these concepts find support despite contemporary views. To put these archaic theories and questionable concepts into contemporary perspective, the following should be considered.

1. "Sterilization" of the root canal system in its purest form is all but impossible because bacteria can remain after root canal cleaning and shaping.[4,18,30,35]
2. The focal infection "theory" is highly speculative and lacks scientific evidence, as does that of elective localization.[19]
3. The hollow-tube theory was convincingly disproved in the 1960s.[8,20,40,41]
4. Dye-leakage studies are nothing more than a static evaluation of a dynamic process and grossly oversimplify the process of long-term coronal and apical leakage into the obturated root canal system.
5. Most early major studies evaluating canal leakage during the 1950s and 1960s dealt with canals that either were not properly cleaned and shaped three-dimensionally or were obturated with single-cone techniques that did not stress three-dimensional obturation (Fig. 1-1) (see Chapter 6). This has led to the emphasis on lack of apical seal as the major cause of failure.
6. Well-designed, contemporary studies evaluating leakage subsequent to root canal treatment have demonstrated that root canal obturations are not thoroughly sealed and that leakage is to be expected.[15] In essence, there are no materials or techniques currently available that can predictably guarantee an impervious seal of the root canal system, whether from the apical or the coronal aspects. *Root canal fillings leak!*
7. Although bacteria are definitely implicated in pulp disease and degeneration and its periradicular (periapical) sequelae,[1,2,36] the process encompasses significant inflammatory and immunologic components.[2,34]

To incorporate the problem-solving approach into these conflicting views, the true factors that influence success must be elucidated and clarified. The historical endodontic triad of "sterilization +

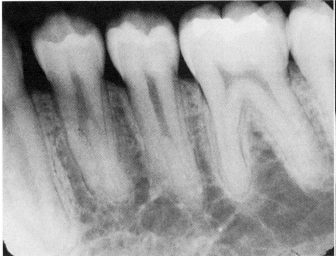
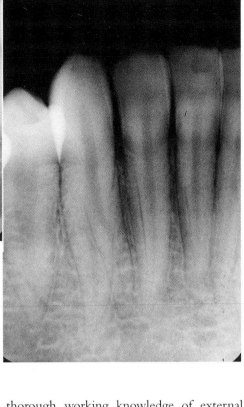

A

B

Fig. 1-2 *A, Wide variation in root and root canal anatomy in mandibular left quadrant. Both premolars exhibit multiple canals and roots. The molar anatomy suggests a four-canaled tooth. B, Even anterior teeth have significant variations. Note the bifurcation of the root structure in the mandibular canine. The practitioner must be aware of these variations and anticipate them before initiating root canal treatment.*

débridement + apical seal = *success*" must be questioned as to the relative importance of its components. A more thorough understanding of pulpal and periradicular disease processes indicates that the key to success in endodontic therapy is the débridement and neutralization of any tissue, bacteria, or inflammatory products within the root canal system. To achieve this end, and to support this leg of the proposed contemporary triad for success (diagnosis + anatomy + débridement = success), there must be a concomitant focus on the need for proper diagnosis and a thorough knowledge of dental anatomy that can be integrated into a repair-predictive, treatment-oriented approach to case management (see Chapter 9).

> A proper diagnosis requires the thorough integration of subjective information about the patient's chief complaint with the objective findings obtained through clinical and radiographic examinations and appropriate pulp tests.

Once integrated, the most probable category of tissue health or disease can be determined and a diagnosis, based on treatment designed to ensure reasonable healing of the periradicular tissues, can be made.

A thorough working knowledge of external coronal and radicular tooth anatomy is also essential, along with a three-dimensional appreciation for the internal anatomy of the pulp space (Fig. 1-2). Ultimately, though, success can be achieved only through proper access to the pulp system and thorough débridement of the inflamed, infected, degenerated, or necrotic pulp tissue (Fig 1-3). Therefore it would seem that *débridement* of the canal system through proper cleaning and shaping would be of paramount importance in successful treatment.[7] This does not necessarily negate the role of obturation because the reasons for obturation are to seal the vestiges of contaminants in the root canal system, which cannot be removed by present techniques, and to minimize the potential role of apical percolation and coronal leakage (Fig. 1-4).[12] Rather, if significant attention is focused on canal débridement, the minimal leakage into the root canal system that will occur over time will encounter little debris with which to interact and potentially cause periradicular inflammation.

FACTORS INFLUENCING THE SUCCESS OR FAILURE OF ENDODONTIC THERAPY

Failure to achieve the desired aims of therapy may require the clinician to reassess the treatment pro-

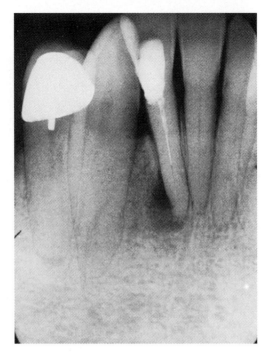

Fig. 1-3 *Failure to clean and shape the canal system in the apical portion of the root, which not only leaves the source of the problem present but also negates the ability to effectively obturate the canal system. Radiographic interpretation suggests the presence of a fractured instrument midroot. Patient presented with a draining sinus tract.*

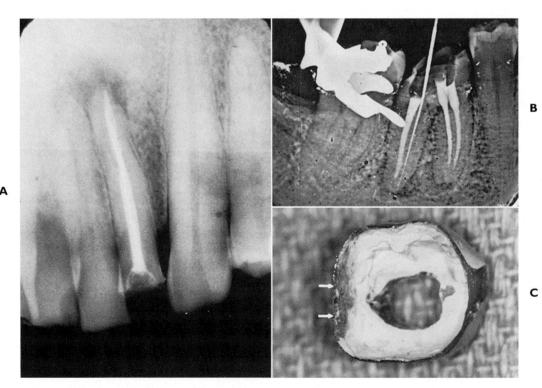

Fig. 1-4 *A,* Poor canal obturation, especially in the apical half, presumably as a result of poor shaping of the canal into a three-dimensional, tapered funnel. Root canal finished 8 months previously; patient fractured crown. Tooth symptomatic to percussion and palpation. *B,* Discovery of a fourth canal in the distal root of the mandibular first molar. *C,* Crown that was on the tooth in *B;* note the leakage evident along the distal margin of the crown (arrows), which provided a straight pathway from the oral cavity down the fourth, uncleaned canal, to the periradicular tissues.

vided in a decision-making, problem-solving manner. As with all dental treatment, multiple integrated factors influence the outcome of endodontic therapy. This requires an astute assessment of the patient's subjective symptoms and objective findings in an attempt to identify the cause of the problem (see Chapter 9). Therefore it is all but impossible to identify any one specific etiologic factor that alone will dictate ultimate success or failure. Likewise, failures of endodontically treated teeth are not always the result of poor root canal treatment. In one study, prosthetic and periodontal reasons were cited as reasons for the failure of root-filled teeth in 91% of teeth treated.[43] Recently an extensive evaluation of the periradicular status of endodontically treated teeth in relation to the technical quality of the root filling and coronal restoration indicated that the technical quality of the coronal restoration was significantly more important than the technical quality of the endodontic treatment for apical periodontal health.[23] For example, a vertical fracture is often identified as the cause for failure after root canal treatment; however, the actual fracture is influenced by occlusion, restoration of the tooth, degree of dentin removal during canal cleaning, shaping and post space preparation, the nature of the post used, previous history of trauma to the tooth, anatomic form of the tooth, and amount of periodontal support.

It is therefore incumbent upon all clinicians who perform endodontic therapy not only to be aware of the factors that affect the success or failure of treatment, but also to comprehend the extensive integration of these factors during the problem-solving thought process that forms the treatment planning of these cases and the assessment of treatment provided.

For rapid identification, the major factors that affect the ultimate achievement of treatment are listed below in categories of importance. The actual nature of these factors are addressed throughout the problem-solving approaches identified in this book. Bear in mind that these relationships are not absolute.

Factors that will Influence Success or Failure in All Cases

1. Radiographic interpretation
2. Anatomy of the root canal system and external root

3. Thoroughness of débridement and apical level of instrumentation
4. Degree of apical seal at the cementum-dentin junction
5. Degree of coronal seal and quality of coronal restoration
6. Asepsis of treatment regimen
7. Health and systemic status of patient
8. Operator skill and expertise

Factors that may Influence the Success or Failure of a Particular Case

1. Pulpal status
2. Procedural accidents (e.g., perforations or broken instruments)
3. Crown or root fractures
4. Periodontal status or disease process
5. Occlusal discrepancies and forces
6. Size of periradicular rarefaction
7. Patient's pain threshold
8. Level of canal obturation—overfill and overextension
9. Time of posttreatment evaluation
10. Degree of canal calcification
11. Accessory communications
12. Presence of root resorption

Factors that have Little Influence on Ultimate Success or Failure

1. Age and sex of patient
2. Cause of pulpal injury or demise
3. Tooth location

CLINICAL ASSESSMENT OF SUCCESS AND FAILURE

Criteria for clinical evaluation are often misunderstood, misapplied, or misinterpreted. This can even happen with the same tooth and the same practitioner on two different occasions. Therefore all clinical evaluation must have reproducible, objective guidelines on which to base the assessment process to make a decision as to the most probable situation.

The criteria for clinical success in the *Quality Assurance Guidelines* published by the American Association of Endodontists (AAE)[22] indicate a clinical outcome in which there are no adverse clinical signs or symptoms. The following subjective and objective criteria can be used clinically to evaluate the outcome of treatment; however, few if any studies base the assessment of success or failure solely on clinical criteria.[11,32,37]

1. Tenderness to palpation
2. Tooth mobility

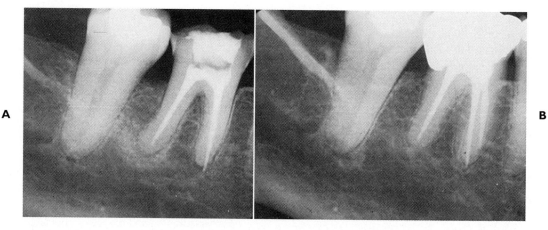

Fig. 1-5 *A, Mandibular first molar with root canal treatment just completed. Note potential straightening of the mesial canals along with overfilling with gutta-percha. B, 3-year recall indicates almost total resolution of the sclerosing osteitis at the apex of the distal root and reformation of a sound lamina dura and periodontal ligament space around all three roots. In spite of the presence of some minor errors in root canal treatment, good cleaning and shaping of the canal along with good obturation and coronal seal promotes a successful response.*

3. Periodontal disease
4. Sinus tracts
5. Sensitivity to percussion
6. Functional tooth
7. Signs of infection or swelling
8. Subjective symptoms

These criteria can be used by the practitioner to classify the treatment into one of three categories.

Clinically Acceptable

1. No tenderness to percussion or palpation
2. Normal mobility
3. No sinus tracts or associated periodontal disease
4. Tooth functional
5. No signs of infection or swelling
6. No evidence of subjective discomfort

Clinically Questionable

1. Sporadic vague symptoms, often not reproducible
2. Pressure sensation or feeling of fullness
3. Low-grade discomfort after percussion, palpation, or chewing
4. Discomfort when pressure is applied by tongue
5. Superimposed sinusitis with focus on treated tooth
6. Occasional need for analgesics to relieve minimal discomfort

Clinically Unacceptable

1. Persistent subjective symptoms
2. Recurrent sinus tract or swelling
3. Predictable discomfort to percussion or palpation
4. Evidence of irreparable tooth fracture
5. Excessive mobility or progressive periodontal breakdown
6. Inability to chew with tooth

Bear in mind, however, that many variables, such as factors related to the patient, case selection, and evaluator bias, can significantly alter perceptions of success and failure. If retention of the tooth in symptom-free clinical function is the aim of endodontic therapy, then many cases can be classified as clinically acceptable using only the above criteria. Likewise, many clinically symptom-free teeth may have pathologic changes at the root apices along with minimal or extensive radiographic changes.[2] Even in the presence of an apparently normal radiographic appearance, a clinically symptom-free tooth may exhibit pathologic changes in the periradicular tissues.

The use of the term *adequate clinical function*[32] may be more realistic and satisfy the needs of the practitioner if retention of the tooth in function is the ultimate aim of treatment. Likewise, this clinical perspective probably satisfies the needs of most patients. Nevertheless, ultimate success or failure must identify a middle ground where the integration of all factors—clinical, radiographic, histologic—and their ultimate effects can be recognized and accepted (Fig. 1-5). However, despite the assessment of all these factors, failure will at times occur, and a realistic perspective must be maintained.

Between the parameters for success and those for failure—which would imply the presence of one or more adverse clinical findings, such as pain to chewing or spontaneous pain—lies a classification of clinically questionable. Often patients in this category exhibit vague, nonspecific symptoms that follow no predictable pattern, an occasional tenderness to biting or percussion in specific directions, or an occasional sensation of "fullness" or pressure. Symptoms are hard to reproduce, or specific areas of discomfort cannot be routinely identified. Radiographic findings are noncontributory. In some situations continued observation is indicated, and the patient should be advised of the possible continuation or termination of symptoms and the potential need for future treatment. In other cases, referral is necessary to address the complex nature of the patient's problem.

All clinicians must resist the temptation to prescribe antibiotics and narcotics automatically for these patients in an attempt to control or alleviate the symptoms or for the convenience of the dentist. This is especially important in those cases in which the patient telephones with symptoms and is not initially seen by the practitioner to determine the cause of the problem.

In all cases, neither the presence nor absence of clinical symptoms alone should determine the success or failure of a case without integrating other factors.

RADIOGRAPHIC EVALUATION OF SUCCESS AND FAILURE

The radiographic evaluation of the periradicular tissues is highly dependent on subjective evaluation and interpretation. Objective criteria for treatment have been published by the American Association of Endodontists (AAE) in *their Quality Assurance Guidelines.*[22] Radiographs should show a dense, three-dimensional filling that extends as close as possible to the cementum-dentin junction (see Fig. 6-21 in the *Quality Assurance Guidelines* as a standard for this guideline). Gross overextensions of the filling material into the periradicular tissues and underfilling or undercompaction in the presence of

patent canal space are undesirable, as are ledges and perforations (Fig. 1-6).

The AAE's quality assurance guidelines specify the absence of breakdown of the supporting periodontium. In addition, if a tooth had a periradicular radiolucency indicative of chronic periradicular periodontitis at the time of filling, the subsequent radiographs should ideally demonstrate a return to an intact lamina dura and a normal periodontal ligament space around the entire root or roots under observation (see Fig. 1-5). Also, if at the time of canal obturation a tooth had a normal periodontal ligament space and an intact lamina dura around the root or roots, the subsequent postoperative radiographic appearance should remain the same.

Unfortunately, radiographic evaluation and interpretation can vary greatly between observers (Fig. 1-7). Agreement between the interpretations of independent observers on the presence or absence of periradicular rarefactions has been found to be less than 50% by several investigators.[6,9,10] This disagreement even occurs with the same observer at subsequent examinations.[24,44] In addition, observer bias is a major factor in interpreting success or failure radiographically.[17,44] These findings make the formalized structuring of all radiographic evaluative studies essential.[13,26,27] Further data indicate that clinical decisions are the result of a cognitive process that includes several concurrent factors, such as facts revealed by the scientific community, the decision maker as a unique individual, and the decision maker as an interactor with other individuals.[13] Therefore studies that do not evaluate large numbers of cases, that do not use multiple observers, and that do not use calibrated agreed criteria or take into account chance agreement may be suspect as to the reliability of findings and observer judgment.[16,24]

The determination of success or failure based solely on radiographic criteria is ill advised, because clinical findings must be included in the decision-making process.

However, specific guidelines that will clarify the evaluative process and provide reasonable radiographic criteria for the postoperative assessment of teeth can be identified for the clinician. These criteria can be classified into three categories.

Radiographically Acceptable (see Figs. 1-5 and 1-6, C)

1. Normal to slightly thickened (<1 mm) periodontal ligament space

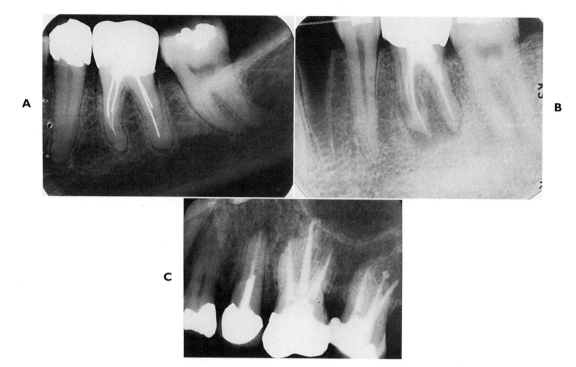

Fig. 1-6 *A, Symptom-free mandibular molar with less than ideal root canal preparation and obturation. The tooth shows radiographic signs of chronic inflammation resulting from failure to fully debride the canal space. **B,** Poorly obturated root canal system in a mandibular molar. The presence of a persistent periradicular lesion and root resorption suggests the source of the failure has not been properly eliminated. **C,** A radiograph of the maxillary left quadrant provides a wide range of radiographic interpretation of root canal treatment. The premolar result would be classified as unacceptable owing to the poor canal obturation and presence of a persistent lesion along with root resorption. The first molar would be classified as acceptable, evidencing well-shaped and obturated canals within the confines of the tooth. The second molar would be classified as questionable because of the extensive filling material beyond the root apex. Ultimate diagnostic classification would require an integration of clinical findings.*

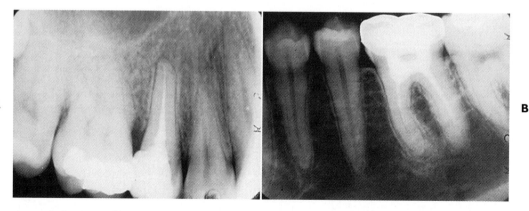

Fig. 1-7 *A, A maxillary second premolar, which was viewed by one practitioner as acceptable and by another as unacceptable. Note the poorly shaped and obturated canal in the apical half of the root. Also, it is possible there are two canals, as indicated by the radiolucent line in the apical half of the root. **B,** Recently performed root canal treatment; radiograph sent to an insurance carrier for payment. Patient symptom-free; however, criteria for radiographic acceptability and achievement of the standard of care in endodontic treatment have not been met.*

2. Elimination of previous radiolucency
3. Normal lamina dura in relation to adjacent teeth
4. No evidence of resorption
5. Dense, three-dimensional obturation of the visible canal space within the confines of the root-canal space, extending to the cementum-dentin junction (approximately 1 mm from the anatomical apex)

Radiographically Questionable (see Figs. 1-6, C and 1-7, A)

1. Increased periodontal ligament space (<2 mm)
2. Radiolucency of similar size or slight evidence of repair
3. Irregularly thickened lamina dura in relation to adjacent teeth
4. Evidence suggestive of slight progressive resorption
5. Voids in density of the canal obturation, especially in the apical third of the canal
6. Extension of filling material beyond the anatomic apex

Radiographically Unacceptable (see Figs. 1-3 and 1-6, C)

1. Increased width of periodontal ligament space (>2 mm)
2. Lack of osseous repair within a periradicular rarefaction, or increase in size of radiolucency
3. Lack of new lamina dura formation
4. Presence of osseous radiolucencies in periradicular areas where previously none existed, including lateral radiolucencies
5. Visible, patent canal space that is unfilled or represents significant voids in canal obturation
6. Excessive overextension of filling material with obvious voids in the apical third of the canal
7. Definitive evidence of progressive resorption

For proper assessment of the radiographic findings at the time of canal obturation and at subsequent evaluations, all radiographs must be of good quality with minimal distortion (see Chapter 2). In addition, angulations, both vertical and horizontal, must be consistent and provide a true representation of the root anatomy and canal configuration. Finally, differences in the observation time for the evaluation of success or failure can greatly change the practitioner's perspective of the role of radiographs in case evaluation. Ideally, recall examination and evaluation should take place annually for a minimum of 4 years, especially in questionable cases[25]; in practice, however, this may be impossible because of the mobility of contemporary society, the unwillingness of patients to make time for treatment evaluation when the tooth feels fine clinically, or patient concerns about radiation exposure. In this respect, patient education and communication are essential to achieve high levels of compliance with long-term treatment evaluation.

HISTOLOGIC ANALYSIS OF SUCCESS AND FAILURE

Histologic assessment of success and failure is relatively meaningless in the clinical practice of endodontics; however, if true healing of the periradicular tissues after root canal treatment embraces the absence of inflammation and complete osseous and periodontal ligament regeneration, success rates for treatment decrease significantly. Brynolf's study[3] in 1967 revealed that complete healing occurred in a very small percentage (7%) of the teeth treated, with chronic inflammation present in the other 93%. Several studies[21,30,31] have supported this concept; apparently patients can exist in this state of chronic inflammation without measurable symptoms. This may be common in cases placed in the clinically or radiographically questionable categories, inasmuch as vague symptoms may occur, coupled with a slightly increased periodontal ligament space or the lack of complete osseous repair as viewed on the radiograph. As an aid to the clinician, histologic criteria of assessment are listed to facilitate an understanding of the nature of the periradicular tissues when treatment evaluation is questionable or unacceptable.

Histologically Acceptable

1. Absence of inflammation
2. Regeneration of periodontal fibers adjacent to or inserting into healthy cementum (Sharpey's fibers)
3. Layering or repair of cementum with new cementum into or across apical foramen (rare)
4. Evident osseous repair along with healthy osteoblasts surrounding the newly formed bone
5. Absence of tooth resorption; previous areas of resorption demonstrate cemental deposition

Histologically Questionable

1. Presence of mild inflammation
2. Areas of cementum undergoing concomitant resorption and repair

3. Lack of periodontal fiber organization
4. Minimal osseous repair along with evidence of osteoclastic activity

Histologically Unacceptable

1. Presence of severe inflammation
2. Lack of osseous repair with concomitant resorption of surrounding bone
3. Active resorption of cementum with no evidence of repair
4. Presence of bacteria and zones of necrotic tissue
5. Presence of granulation tissue and possible epithelial proliferation

INTEGRATION OF EVALUATIVE FACTORS IN THE DETERMINATION OF SUCCESS AND FAILURE: ESTABLISHING A NEW TREATMENT PLAN

A clear consensus of what constitutes success or failure does not necessarily exist among all practitioners,[37] especially when the parameters used are often manipulated to meet the needs of the professional as opposed to those of the patient. Intellectual manipulation of clinical scenarios in specific situations often rationalizes the final case assessment. Therefore the ability of the clinician to assess objectively the treatment rendered (both that rendered personally and that of other professionals) is heavily influenced by personal experience, bias, case information, and cognitive dissonance. The latter concept is defined as "the existence of views, attitudes or beliefs which are inconsistent or incompatible with one another but, nonetheless, are held simultaneously by the same person."[33]

The success or failure of endodontic treatment must be determined on the basis of not only the final outcome but also the additive procedures that yield a final level of attainment. Each subsequent chapter is dedicated to this latter concept; however, there are multiple variables intertwined in the decision-making process. Therefore the best approach to ultimate quality and success is the prevention of problems before they occur; this simplifies the assessment of both the process and the product.

Prevention of problems in endodontics begins with diagnosis and treatment planning.

However, in addition to identifying and managing teeth that exhibit signs and symptoms of pulpal and periradicular pathosis, the clinician is frequently required to assess the success of previously completed endodontic treatment and make judgments about its prognosis in the course of routine examinations and treatment planning. Also, endodontically treated teeth are often found in areas in which the patient is experiencing symptoms. These situations present a significant diagnostic challenge to distinguishing endodontic failure from other possibilities. When faced with clear indications of endodontic failure, however, there are only three treatment alternatives: nonsurgical retreatment, surgical retreatment, or extraction.

CLINICAL PROBLEM 1: *The Evaluation of Previous Endodontic Treatment during Routine Examination*

In the last 50 years, a variety of theories and techniques have been introduced into endodontic care. Research and successful clinical experience indicate that endodontic therapy is most successful when the root canal system has been thoroughly cleaned to the apical constriction and sealed (Fig. 1-8). In the case of root fillings that terminate 2 mm or more from the radiographic apex, it is obvious that there may be uninstrumented and unfilled canal space, which are a potential cause of failure. The lack of a visible canal on the radiograph is no assurance that the space is calcified (Fig. 1-9).

Root canals filled with pastes, silver cones, or other materials have questionable success rates as compared with well-condensed gutta-percha (Fig. 1-10) (see Chapter 6). The presence of these former materials in symptom-free teeth represents a significant potential for failure because their removal in retreatment situations almost invariably shows evidence of a poor seal. Paste materials are most often little more than mushy debris. Silver cones most often show evidence of corrosion and lack of sealer, even in canals that radiographically appeared to be successful (see Chapter 7). Often a symptom-free, grossly carious tooth exhibits apparently successful root canal treatment. (Fig. 1-11) Although it might be assumed that the canal seal is adequate, numerous studies indicate that the seal is as vulnerable (perhaps more) to failure from coronal leakage as from apical leakage (Fig. 1-12).[31,38,39,42] It would be unwise to proceed to the restoration of any tooth in which the endodontic filling has been exposed to saliva or caries for an extended period of time.

Solution: No treatment would be indicated for any symptom-free tooth without evidence of pathosis, regardless of the potential for failure, if no restorative treatment is required. For teeth requiring reconstruction by the use of posts or that may be key abutments, retreatment would be

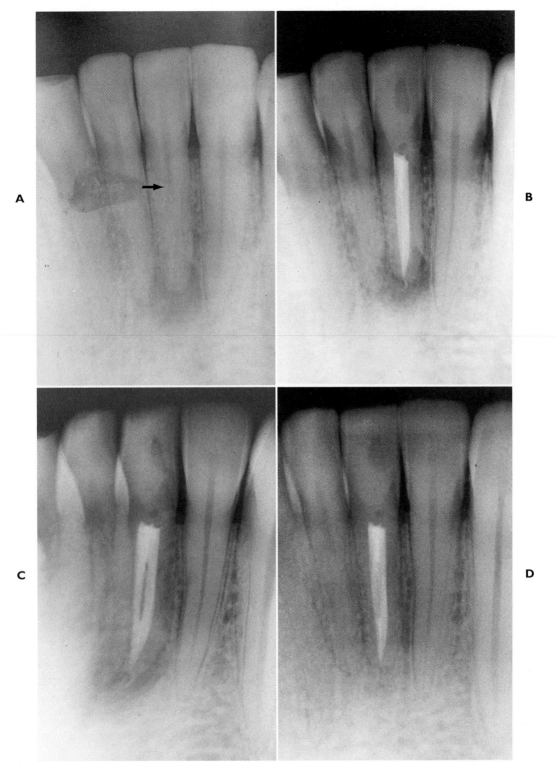

Fig. 1-8 *A, Preoperative radiograph of a nonvital mandibular incisor. Note bifurcation of canal at the midroot level (arrow). B, Immediately following root canal treatment. C, An angled view of the obturation showing the entire canal system. D, A 21-month reevaluation radiograph showing satisfactory healing of the periradicular bone.*

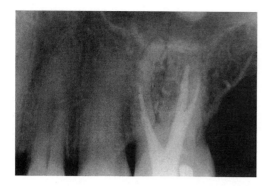

Fig. 1-9 *Mandibular molar with root canal treatment. The tooth was symptom-free. All canals were filled far short of the ideal apical position. Long-term prognosis is questionable.*

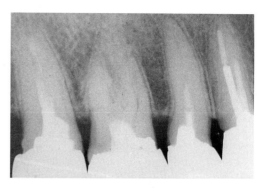

Fig. 1-10 *Multiple maxillary posterior teeth with a history of paste-filled root canals at least 5 years before present examination. All teeth are symptom-free.*

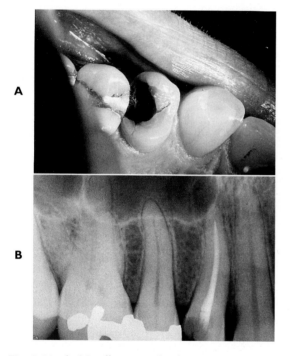

Fig. 1-11 *A, Maxillary premolar demonstrating extensive coronal caries. B, Radiograph of the same tooth shows root canal treatment of acceptable quality; there is a periradicular radiolucency, however.*

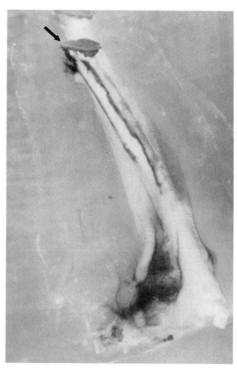

Fig. 1-12 *A demineralized and cleared tooth specimen of an extracted tooth showing leakage staining from the pulp chamber to the root apex. Note also, there is a root-end filling present (arrow) that did not stop the leakage pattern.*

appropriate before restoration. If retreatment is performed on a symptom-free, short-filled tooth with no periradicular pathosis, and it is not possible to get all the way to the apical constriction, restoration should proceed in a normal fashion. Periradicular surgery would be indicated in case of failure, since there would be no advantage in attempting canal reentry (Fig. 1-9).

All cases of previous root canal treatment in which the root fillings have been exposed to caries require retreatment. Any tooth in which the canals have been exposed to saliva for any longer than a few days, as in the case of a coronal fracture, should be retreated (see Fig. 11-7). Teeth with recently completed root canal treatment that exhibit a poorly sealed temporary restoration should be suspect.

CLINICAL PROBLEM 2: *Establishing a Differential Diagnosis of Endodontic Failure: Percussion Tenderness*

It is not unusual to receive a patient referral with a diagnosis of endodontic failure, only to find on examination that the endodontic treatment is satisfactory. Other causes have been overlooked in the initial diagnosis and treatment plan. In these cases it is worthwhile to consider the test results and the history of the complaint to be confident that (1) endodontic failure has truly occurred and (2) the failure is the cause of the symptoms for which the patient has a complaint. The signs and symptoms of endodontic failure usually originate in the periradicular tissues. Swelling, tenderness to palpation or percussion, and development of or increase in a periradicular lesion are common. Occasionally the patient may complain of thermal sensitivity, which must be explained, especially if the tooth identified exhibits a periradicular lesion.

Consider a case in which there are no radiographic signs of endodontic failure or signs of endodontic pathosis on any adjacent tooth (Fig. 1-13). There are several commonly encountered symptomatic problems. First, the patient presents with percussion tenderness only. There are only three potential causes for percussion tenderness: (1) recent trauma; (2) occlusal trauma; or (3) failing root canal treatment.

Solution: Recent trauma is easy to diagnose, and percussion tenderness alone would be expected to resolve gradually without specific treatment, as long as the tooth is not in abnormal occlusal contact. In cases requiring occlusal management, reduction of occlusal contacts in centric and lateral occlusion by grinding is usually sufficient. Occasionally fixation for a few weeks may be necessary to keep the tooth out of occlusion, as in the case of a lingually displaced maxillary incisor. Usually direct bonding to adjacent teeth is sufficient after application of finger pressure to move the tooth out of occlusion. Percussion tenderness associated with trauma is not an indication of endodontic failure and would not require endodontic intervention.

A second commonly encountered situation is that of a tooth in occlusion in which there is tenderness to percussion and there has been no injury. Occlusal abnormalities should be considered, especially when there is evidence of bruxism or wear facets (Fig. 1-14). In these cases the occlusion should be relieved in centric and in lateral excursions. Even though bruxism and clenching are common, evidence of these conditions, such as wear facets or symptoms of temporomandibular disorder (TMD), may not be apparent. It is worthwhile also to inquire whether the patient is expe-

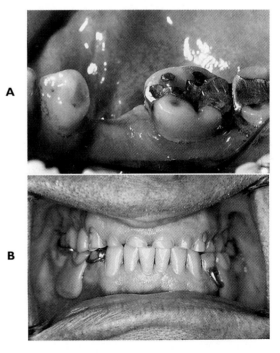

A

B

Fig. 1-14 *A,* Occlusal wear facets on a mandibular molar. *B,* Extreme occlusal wear consistent with bruxism.

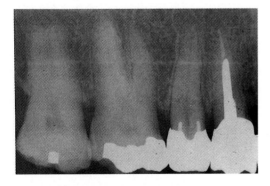

Fig. 1-13 *Radiograph of a maxillary first premolar. Clinically, periodontal probings were normal and there was no palpation tenderness. The tooth was in occlusion. Root canal treatment and post crown restoration was completed 7 years earlier. Adjacent teeth were normal to pulp tests.*

riencing unusual stress. Realization of the connection between a stressful event and bruxing may account for the onset of percussion symptoms in an area without a history of problems. This connection will often aid in treatment because the patient will understand that the bruxing and the symptoms will diminish as the effect of the stressful event passes.

Third, a root canal–treated tooth remains percussion tender 2 weeks after elimination of occlusal contacts or presents initially without an opposing tooth. Assuming that examination with the periodontal probe has ruled out root fracture and the root canal treatment is not recent, the diagnosis of endodontic failure is probably in order. Vertical root fractures often can be present without radiographic changes. A fracture located on the buccal or lingual surface of a mandibular molar may not cause sufficient bone loss to affect the radiographic image of the bone to the mesial or distal side of the image of the root (see Fig. 11-5).

Since it is not unusual to observe percussion tenderness in a recently completed endodontic case, diagnosis of failure would be premature. Likewise, since the periradicular inflammation associated with failure is due to loss or lack of an apical seal, or remnants of tissue debris, symptoms of failure do not usually appear until months after completion of treatment. Inflammation persisting continuously from the time of treatment is problematic but probably not a failure. It is reasonable to monitor such cases, assuming occlusal contacts have been relieved. If symptoms are severe, reentry or periradicular surgery may be necessary, but waiting and watching is usually appropriate. Symptoms of this type generally resolve gradually.

CLINICAL PROBLEM 3: *Establishing a Differential Diagnosis of Endodontic Failure—Discomfort to Thermal Stimulus*

Discomfort to a thermal stimulus without exception requires the presence of dental pulp tissue in the tooth that hurts. It is not possible for a tooth to respond to thermal stimulation if the pulp has been removed. This is true even if the canal is not even filled. In a clinical situation in which the patient complains of thermal sensitivity or discomfort originating from an endodontically treated tooth, only two possibilities exist: either there is an untreated canal in the endodontically treated tooth, or the discomfort originates from another tooth.

Solution: Thermal testing is the only means to identify the source of the symptoms. It is evident

that the object of the testing should be to reproduce the symptoms described by the patient. If cold sensitivity is the complaint, test with ice (Fig. 1-15). If heat is the complaint, hot temporary stopping is effective for testing (Fig. 1-16) (see Chapter 9). It is important to recall at the outset which teeth might have additional canals and where they might be located. It is wise to begin testing on presumably normal teeth in the quadrant to establish a basis for comparison. Choose unrestored, noncarious teeth if possible. It is easy and helpful to test each tooth in the quadrant successively from anterior to posterior, if the complaint seems to be located posteriorly. If it is an anterior tooth, begin testing three or four teeth on one side of the suspected location and continue to three or four teeth on the opposite side. Contralateral teeth are also tested as controls, with previously endodontically treated teeth, if present, also serving as controls. As each tooth is tested, the buccal Class V areas will usually be most responsive. On presumably normal teeth, one normal response will be sufficient. On heavily restored teeth, carious teeth, or suspected teeth, it is wise to test multiple surfaces of the same

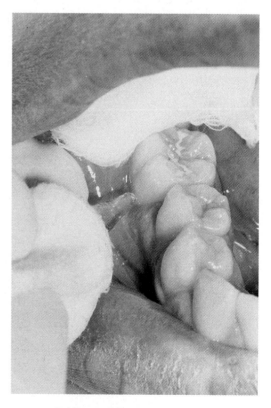

Fig. 1-15 *Cold test performed with an ice stick to the gingival area of the molar.*

tooth before progressing to the next tooth. Test directly on large metallic intracoronal restorations last. Full crowns should also be tested on all exposed surfaces. Since some thermal responses are delayed, it is also wise to test slowly and give each tooth time to respond to each test. No special consideration should be given to the endodontically treated tooth. If isolation is a problem, a rubber dam can be easily placed and moved from tooth to tooth. A response to thermal testing on the endodontically treated tooth should be repeated. If the response is immediate and duplicates the patient's symptoms, it would indicate an untreated canal (see Fig. 7-9). Because of the frequent presence of large restoration contacts, thermal testing on one tooth may elicit a delayed response on an adjacent tooth. Usually when the second tooth is tested directly, the abnormal response will be much more obvious and immediate. Knowledge of canal anatomy should give a clue as to the location of an untreated canal. In maxillary molars, for example, it is usually the second mesial canal in the mesiobuccal root (mesiopalatal), or in mandibular molars it is usually a second canal in the distal root.

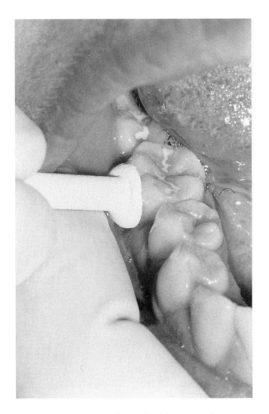

Fig. 1-16 *Heat test performed with warmed temporary stopping.*

In mandibular incisors and premolars it is a second canal located lingually to the other canal. These canals are usually not visible on a radiograph. The action of choice is to find and treat this canal. The second possibility indicated for a painful thermal response is a tooth in the quadrant other than the endodontically treated tooth. The decision to treat in these cases should be based on criteria given in Chapter 9.

CLINICAL PROBLEM 4: *Establishing a Differential Diagnosis of Endodontic Failure—Radiographic Signs of Endodontic Failure*

There is little question that the development of a periradicular radiolucency on an endodontically treated tooth would be diagnostic for endodontic failure. The same would be true for a periradicular lesion that failed to heal or increased in size after the root canal treatment. In the following clinical cases, it should be assumed that there are no symptoms present, treatment is over 2 years old, and periodontal probings are normal.

CLINICAL PROBLEM 4A: *Interpretation of Minimally Widened Apical Periodontal Ligament Space*

Solution 4A: There are three possibilities that may exist. A normal periodontal ligament superimposed over an anatomic void in the bone. The most common example is a normal root tip superimposed over the maxillary sinus (Fig. 1-17). Other common examples are superimposition over the mandibular canal, the incisive canal foramen, or a cystic cavity caused by another tooth. Second, a periradicular lesion may be developing from failing root canal treatment (Fig. 1-18). Third, scar tissue may be present after the healing of a periradicular radiolucency (Fig. 1-19). In all three cases, without a history of symptoms and without clinical signs of pathosis, the best course is to wait and observe the area. A new radiograph would be appropriate after 6 to 12 months. If symptoms or clinical signs of pathosis reappear at any time, reevaluation would be indicated.

CLINICAL PROBLEM 4B: *Interpretation of a Periradicular Lesion on a Tooth with Prior Endodontic Treatment*

Solution 4B: Although the same three possibilities exist as for the previous problem, superimposition over normal structures is found much less frequently, since only a large foramen would have the approximate shape of an apical lesion. Rarely will the incisive canal and foramen or mental foramen be confused for a periradicular lesion. Healing lesions could also be ruled out as a possibility if we are looking at a tooth 2 years after treatment (Fig.

1-20). Teeth treated 1 year previously may be followed radiographically for healing. In the distinct majority of endodontically treated teeth, the presence of periradicular lesions represents failure for which nonsurgical retreatment would be the treatment of choice.

CLINICAL PROBLEM 4C: *Interpretation of Very Large Periradicular Lesions Associated with the Apex of an Endodontically Treated Tooth*

Solution 4C: Occasionally a normal sinus might be misinterpreted as a large periradicular lesion. Extremely large narrow spaces in the mandible might also appear to be lesions of pulpal origin. In most cases, a normal periodontal ligament space and lamina dura are visible and would rule out pathosis. If such a large lesion has no symptoms and no evidence of drainage, a biopsy might be indicated if normal anatomy cannot account for the radiographic presentation. It is uncommon but not impossible for a large periradicular lesion to develop from an endodontic failure (Fig. 1-21). It is more likely that the original lesion for which the endodontic treatment was presumably done failed to heal. This is true in cases where the endodontic treatment is obviously inadequate and in those that appear to be well filled. Lesions of nonpulpal origin must always be suspected, and a biopsy to provide a differential diagnosis may be indicated.

CLINICAL PROBLEM 4D: *Interpretation of Radiographic Lesions Enveloping an Entire Root*

Solution 4D: Lesions that appear to involve significant bone loss limited to a single root and extending to the crest of bone should be suspected of having a severe periodontal defect, a vertical root fracture, or a failing root canal treatment that would be capable of healing (Fig. 1-22). The periodontal probe will be of greatest value in arriving at the correct diagnosis. Severe periodontal defects will probe deeply over a broad circumferential area of the root (see Chapter 12). When such a probing pattern is found with obvious periodontal bone loss affecting other teeth, the diagnosis is straightforward. Treatment options are either tooth extraction or root resection.

It is more difficult to reach a diagnosis of advanced periodontitis where such a lesion seems to be solitary. One might logically conclude the bone loss is of endodontic origin. In terms of prognosis, however, if the probing pattern confirms deep pocketing and loss of attachment over a wide area of the root circumferentially, the prognosis is nearly hopeless regardless of the cause. An appropriate treatment plan to consider, if endodontic etiology is suspected, would be to remove the root filling materials, reclean the canals, and close the tooth for 2 to 3 months. If reattachment should occur, retreatment can be completed. Patients should be advised, however, of the limited potential for healing in such cases.

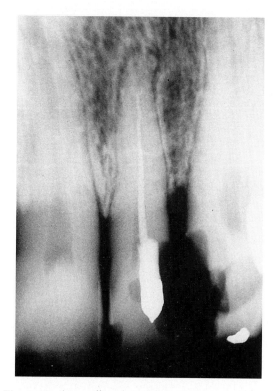

Fig. 1-18 *A maxillary lateral incisor with very poor quality root canal treatment. The widened apical periodontal ligament space is evidence of pathosis.*

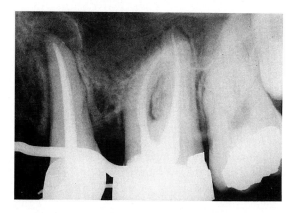

Fig. 1-17 *Two endodontically treated maxillary posterior teeth with apices near or above the sinus floor. The molar appears to have a widened apical periodontal ligament space. This is normal. The premolar has a periradicular lesion.*

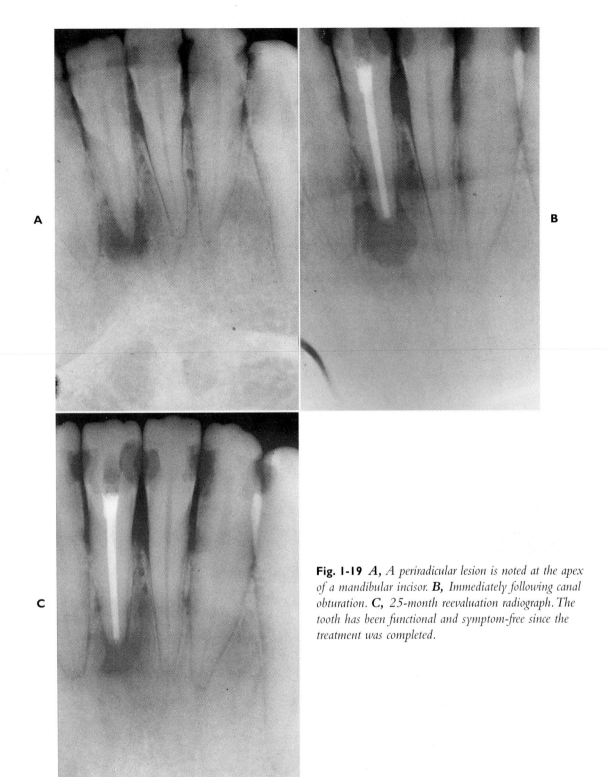

Fig. 1-19 *A, A periradicular lesion is noted at the apex of a mandibular incisor.* ***B,*** *Immediately following canal obturation.* ***C,*** *25-month reevaluation radiograph. The tooth has been functional and symptom-free since the treatment was completed.*

Clinical Problem 5: Establishing a Differential Diagnosis of Endodontic Failure: Clinical Signs of Pathosis

CLINICAL PROBLEM 5A: *Clinical Signs of Pathosis Associated with Endodontic Problems Generally Result from Infection*

When a patient presents with palpation tenderness, swelling, or drainage in an area with an endodontically treated tooth, the problem is not whether pathosis is present but rather whether it is the result of endodontic failure. Other possible causes are a periodontal lesion, a vertical root fracture, and a lesion arising from an adjacent tooth.

Solution 5A: In Fig. 1-23 two key pieces of information are on the radiograph: root canal treatment has been performed, and there is no periradicular lesion. In view of the gingival inflammation associated with the distal root, a vertical root fracture should be suspected. To confirm this, a fine periodontal probe is used to probe in 0.5 to 1 mm increments circumferentially around the entire tooth. The presence of a narrow deep probing defect over the distobuccal aspect of the tooth is diagnostic for a vertical fracture. Occasionally the same pattern of probing will be found on the lingual aspect of the root as well. This would indicate a complete fracture of the root.

Most vertical root fractures occur on the buccal or lingual of the root; consequently, radiographic changes are often absent. When bone destruction associated with a vertical root fracture is sufficient to cause radiographic changes, the periodontal ligament will usually appear distinctly and uniformly widened around the entire root to the crest of bone (Fig. 1-24) (see Chapter 11).

It is well recognized that any apical lesion may establish drainage through a sinus tract on the mucosa or a sinus tract exiting through the gingival sulcus (see Chapter 12). A sulcus drainage tract may probe like a vertical fracture. Clinically, sulcus drainage tracts associated with failing root canals are extremely uncommon relative to the incidence of vertical fractures. The only way to distinguish between these two possibilities is to reflect a mucoperiosteal flap over the probing defect and

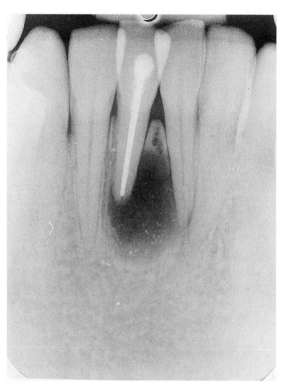

Fig. 1-20 *A large periradicular lesion on a mandibular central incisor. Root canal treatment was completed with a silver cone approximately 18 years earlier.*

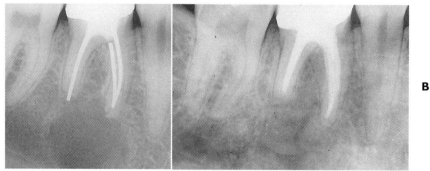

A   B

Fig. 1-21 *A, Large periradicular lesion associated with failing root canal treatment on a mandibular molar. B, Reevaluation 7 months after nonsurgical retreatment.*

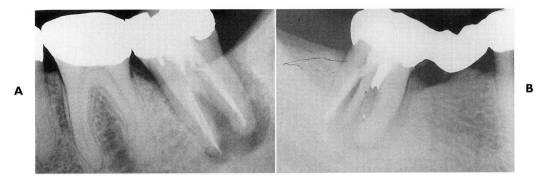

Fig. 1-22 *A, Periradicular radiolucency enveloping the entire distal root of a mandibular second molar. Periodontal probings were consistent with advanced periodontal disease. B, Periradicular radiolucency around the entire mesial root of a mandibular molar. Clinical examination and probings confirmed a vertical fracture of the distal root. Note the untreated mesial root and the repaired furcation perforation.*

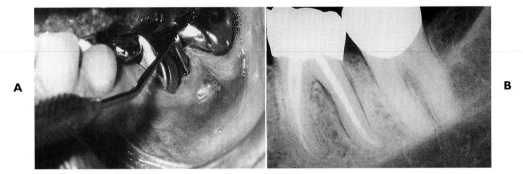

Fig. 1-23 *A, Deep, narrow probing defect over the buccal aspect of the distal root. Note the sinus tract opening on the mucosa. B, Radiograph of the same tooth. There is no apical lesion evident. When this occurs, the clinician must determine the source of the drainage.*

observe the root surface (see Fig. 11-6). It is critical to make an accurate diagnosis since retreatment of a failing root canal treatment would likely result in healing of any sinus tract. On the other hand, retreatment of any kind on a vertical root fracture would be futile. A final point is that if on the same endodontically treated root the clinician finds both a mucosal sinus tract and a narrow vertical probing pattern the diagnosis will always be vertical root fracture (Fig. 1-23, *A*).

CLINICAL PROBLEM 5B: *A Patient Presents with Draining Mucosal Sinus Tract Associated with an Endodontically Treated Tooth*

Solution 5B: Assuming the probings are normal, there are two radiographic possibilities: a radiographic lesion or the absence of a radiographic lesion. The lack of a radiographic lesion would indicate a cause somewhere on the surface of the root adjacent to the sinus tract opening. Only exploratory surgical tissue reflection will reveal the exact cause

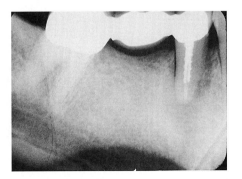

Fig. 1-24 *Bone loss around a mandibular premolar consistent with a vertical root fracture. This was confirmed with probings.*

(see Chapter 12). These occur most often at the midroot level (Fig. 1-25). Other possibilities are a post perforation, retentive pin perforation, and localized root fractures or craze lines. Typical treatment will be direct repair if the cause is small. Extraction may be indicated if there are unmanageable periodontal defects. If there is radiographic evidence of bone loss, the location of the radiolucency will give a clue to the cause. Apical lesions will most likely be the result of endodontic failure. Knowledge of canal anatomy is important, however. Frequently the cause of pathosis is an untreated second canal in the same root (see Chapter 7). If a second canal is likely and radiographs exposed from different angles are not helpful, the tooth should be reopened for retreatment. It is sometimes possible to treat only an untreated canal without retreating the filled canals.

A midroot radiolucency presents various possibilities. If the root is straight and the canal appearance does not suggest perforation, a lateral canal could be the cause (Fig. 1-26). Retreatment may be effective. The obvious success of retreatment would be the resolution of the draining sinus tract within 2 to 3 weeks.

A radiolucency at the point of a midroot curvature most likely signifies a stripping perforation that occurred during instrumentation (see Fig. 5-25). Even though the radiograph may not show filling material extruding through the perforation, it must be remembered that roots frequently have external invaginations on their proximal surfaces (see Chapter 5). As a result, the distance between the canal and the periodontal ligament is smaller than it appears on the radiograph. Even where a perforation has not occurred, condensation pressures on very thin canal walls will result in cracking, which will also produce a lesion.

Finally, a midroot radiolucency at the level of the termination of a post most often signifies a post perforation (see Chapter 13). Once again excessive thinning of the canal wall can also result in a lesion. There is no effective treatment for a

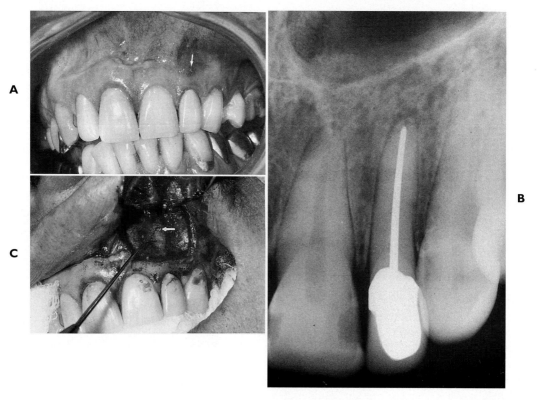

Fig. 1-25 *A, Draining sinus tract over the lateral incisor* (white arrow). *B, Radiograph of the same tooth. The apical periodontal ligament space is minimally widened. C, Surgical exposure of the root surface reveals a lateral lesion* (white arrow).

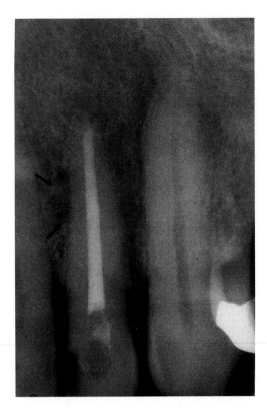

Fig. 1-26 *A lateral periradicular lesion* (arrows) *consistent with failing root canal treatment at the site of a lateral canal.*

midroot perforation. Sometimes it can be repaired (see Fig. 10-26), and root resection or tooth extraction is often indicated.

A draining sinus tract may appear in the attached gingiva over the furcation of a molar or near the gingival crest of a premolar with two roots. Assuming probings are normal, the radiograph may show some furcal bone loss at the crest in the case of the molars. In the case of premolars, there may be crestal disruption of the bone on the mesial or distal of the root, seldom both. This pattern represents a furcal perforation. Surgical exploration is usually necessary to confirm the cause. If the surgery is planned correctly and the furcation is not too deep relative to the crestal bone, the problem may be treated by a crown-lengthening approach. Otherwise, root resection or tooth extraction is necessary.

The determination of endodontic failure in the absence of symptoms is difficult. In most cases where accurate diagnosis is not possible, a wait and watch approach is best. Fortunately, most cases of endodontic failure can be diagnosed accurately

because of the presence of more diagnostic information. Percussion tenderness may be accompanied by a periradicular radiographic lesion. Palpation tenderness may be present to confirm pathosis where the radiographic image is uncertain. Numerous other combinations are common. The prudent diagnostician must collect as much information as possible and construct a rationale for the diagnosis made.

The clinician who performs endodontic therapy must understand the level of diagnosis, treatment planning, and treatment necessary to achieve success and to attain that level on a consistent basis. The wise and prudent clinician will be able to assess both the process and the completed treatment, with the proper integration of clinical and radiographic factors, in an environment that minimizes the shackles of bias and the dictates of cognitive dissonance. This is the essence of problem solving.

References

1. Baumgartner JC, Falkler WA: Bacteria in the apical 5 mm of infected root canals, *J Endod* 17:380-383, 1991.
2. Bergenholtz G: Pathogenic mechanisms in pulpal disease, *J Endod* 16:98-101, 1990.
3. Brynolf I: A histologic and roentgenological study of the periapical region of human upper incisors, *Odontol Rev* 18:1-176, 1967.
4. Bystrom A, Sundqvist G: Bacteriologic evaluation of the efficacy of mechanical root canal instrumentation in endodontic therapy, *Scand J Dent Res* 89:321-328, 1981.
5. Dow PR, Ingle JI: Isotope determination of root canal failures, *Oral Surg Oral Med Oral Pathol* 8:1100-1104, 1955.
6. Duinkerke ASH, Van de Poel ACM, DeBoo T et al: Variations in the interpretation of periapical radiolucencies, *Oral Surg Oral Med Oral Pathol* 1975; 40:414-422, 1975.
7. Fuchs C, Friedlander C, Rosenberg E et al: Statistical models for evaluating the penetrating ability of endodontic instruments, *J Dent Res* 1990; 69:1617-1621, 1990.
8. Goldman M, Pearson A: A preliminary investigation of the "hollow tube" theory in endodontics: studies with neotetrazolium, *J Oral Therap Pharmacol* 1:616-626, 1965.
9. Goldman M, Pearson AH, Darzenta N: Endodontic success—who's reading the radiograph? *Oral Surg Oral Med Oral Pathol* 33:432- 437, 1972.
10. Goldman M, Pearson AH, Darzenta N: Reliability of radiographic interpretations, *Oral Surg Oral Med Oral Pathol* 38:287-293, 1974.
11. Grossman LI, Shephard LI, Pearson LA: Roentgenologic and clinical evaluation of endodontically treated teeth, *Oral Surg Oral Med Oral Pathol* 1964; 17:368-374, 1964.
12. Gutmann JL, Dumsha T: Cleaning and shaping the root canal system. In Cohen S, Burns RC, editors: *Pathways of the pulp,* ed 4, St Louis, 1987, Mosby.

13. Halse A, Molven O: A strategy for the diagnosis of periapical pathosis, *J Endod* 12:534-538, 1986.

14. Hunter W: The role of sepsis and of antisepsis in medicine, *Lancet* 1:79-86, 1911.

15. Kersten HW: *Leakage of root fillings—an in vitro evaluation,* Amsterdam, 1988, Krips Repro Meppel.

16. Koran LM: The reliability of clinical methods, data and judgments, *N Engl J Med* 293:642-646, 695-701, 1975.

17. Lambrianidis T: Observer variation in radiographic evaluation, *Endod Dent Traumatol* 1:235-241, 1985.

18. Martin H: Bacteriology and endodontics, *J Dist Col Dent Soc* Summer:13-15, 1978.

19. Morse DR: Microbiology and pharmacology. In Cohen S, Burns RC, editors: *Pathways of the Pulp,* ed 4, St Louis, 1987.

20. Phillips JM: Rat connective tissue response to hollow polyethylene tube implants, *Can Dent J* 33:59-64, 1967.

21. Pitt Ford TR: Vital pulpectomy—an unpredictable procedure, *Int Endod J* 1982; 15:121-126, 1982.

22. *Quality Assurance Guidelines,* Chicago, 1994, American Association of Endodontists.

23. Ray HA, Trope M: Periapical status of endodontically treated teeth in relation to the technical quality of the root filling and the coronal restoration, *Int Endod J* 28:12-18, 1995.

24. Reit C: The influence of observer calibration on radiographic periapical diagnosis, *Int Endod J* 20:75-81, 1987.

25. Reit C: Decision strategies in endodontics: on the design of a recall program, *Endod Dent Traumatol* 3:233-239, 1987.

26. Reit C, Grondahl H-C: Endodontic decision-making under uncertainty: a decision analytic approach to management of periapical lesions in endodontically treated teeth, *Endod Dent Traumatol* 3:15-20, 1987.

27. Reit C, Hollender L: Radiographic evaluation of endodontic therapy and the influence of observer variation, *Scand J Dent Res* 91:205-212, 1983.

28. Rickert UG, Dixon CM: The controlling of root surgery, in *Proceedings of the 8th International Dental Congress,* Section IIIa, 1931, pp 15-22.

29. Rosenow EC: Studies on elective localization. Focal infection with special reference to oral sepsis, *J Dent Res* 1:205-268, 1919.

30. Rowe AHR, Binnie WH: The incidence and location of microorganisms following endodontic treatment, *Br Dent J* 142:91-95, 1977.

31. Saunders WP, Saunders EM: Coronal leakage as a cause of failure in root-canal therapy: a review, *Endod Dent Traumatol* 10:105-108, 1994.

32. Seltzer S: Root canal failures. In *Endodontology,* ed 2, Philadelphia, 1988, Lea & Febiger.

33. Seltzer S, Bender IB: Cognitive dissonance in endodontics, *Oral Surg Oral Med Oral Pathol* 20:505-516, 1965.

34. Seltzer S, Naidorf IJ: Flare-ups in endodontics. I. Etiological factors, *J Endod* 11:472-478, 1985.

35. Shovelton DS: The presence and distribution of micro-organisms within non-vital teeth, *Br Dent J* 117:101-107, 1964.

36. Simon JHS: Pathology. In Cohen S, Burns RC, editors: *Pathways of the Pulp,* ed 5, St Louis, 1991, Mosby.

37. Stabholz A, Friedman S, Tamse A: Endodontic failures and retreatment. In Cohen S, Burns RC, editors: *Pathways of the Pulp,* ed 5, St Louis, 1991, Mosby.

38. Swanson K, Madison, S: An evaluation of coronal microleakage in endodontically treated teeth. I. Time periods, *J Endod* 13:56-59, 1987.

39. Torabinejad M, Ung B, Kettering JD: *In vitro* bacterial penetration of coronally unsealed endodontically treated teeth, *J Endod* 16:566-569, 1990.

40. Torneck CD: Reaction of rat connective tissue to polyethylene tube implants, part 1, *Oral Surg Oral Med Oral Pathol* 21:379- 387, 1966.

41. Torneck CD: Reaction of rat connective tissue to polyethylene tube implants, part 2, *Oral Surg Oral Med Oral Pathol* 24:674-683, 1967.

42. Trope E, Chow E, Nissan R: In vitro endotoxin penetration of coronally unsealed endodontically treated teeth, *Endod Dent Traumatol* 11:90-94, 1991.

43. Vire DE: Failure of endodontically treated teeth, *J Endod* 17:338-342, 1991.

44. Zakariasen KL, Scott DA, Jensen JR: Endodontic recall radiographs: how reliable is our interpretation of endodontic success or failure and what factors affect our reliability? *Oral Surg Oral Med Oral Pathol* 57:343-347, 1984.

Chapter 2

Problems in Radiographic Technique and Interpretation

Thom C. Dumsha
Eric J. Hovland

"The greatest difficulty lies primarily in a lack of understanding of normal roentgenographic anatomy, and the variations in normal bony structure, and in the assumption that every dark space is indicative of infection. Far too often, the roentgenographic equipment is used to impress the patient rather than as an aid in finding conditions not visible clinically. Almost without exception, dentists who bring or mail in roentgenograms for interpretation invariably accompany their request with profuse apologies for the poor quality of the film sent."[*]

Although the patient's dental history and the clinical findings are of major importance to the clinician, radiographs are as fundamental to diagnosis as gutta-percha is to obturation.

Radiographs are a necessary adjunct in endodontics, and accurate radiographic techniques and proper interpretation are essential for sound diagnosis and treatment.

Radiographic findings also are used for determining tooth and pulpal anatomy prior to endodontic access openings, for establishing working lengths, confirming master-cone placement, and for evaluating the success of treatment. In addition, the clinician can obtain significant information regarding case difficulty and long-term prognosis from a radiograph, before treatment is initiated.

Furthermore, in the present litigious society in which clinicians must practice their skills, it is imprudent and unjustified to practice poor radiographic technique and interpretation when the

---

[*]From Sommer RF: *J Am Dent Assoc* 25:595-600, 1938.

cost of such behavior can be so devastating. Even under controlled conditions, it has been demonstrated clearly that radiographic interpretation is difficult at best. Goldman et al in a classic work that compared several clinicians' radiographic interpretation of successful and failing root canal therapy provided a stunning demonstration of how radiographic evaluation can and does change with time and perhaps other factors.[4] The clinicians reviewed immediate postoperative films and recall radiographs of patients and then these same radiographs were reviewed 6 to 8 months later. The clinicians agreed with their own interpretation of success and failure only between 72% and 88% of the time. This work merely demonstrates that even under controlled conditions radiographic interpretation is at best difficult and consistency and reproducibility present even a greater challenge.

Radiographic techniques and interpretation during root canal treatment, particularly during the working-length and master-cone procedures, are perhaps two of the most critical aspects of endodontics and are, at times, some of the most difficult procedures encountered by the clinician. Likewise, a major concern is to minimize the amount of radiation exposure to the patient while ensuring that quality of care is not compromised. Therefore, the major purposes of this chapter are to discuss various techniques for exposing radiographs during root canal treatment, common problems in radiographic technique, and methods to correct problems encountered during radiographic exposure and interpretation.

DIAGNOSIS AND RADIOGRAPHIC INTERPRETATION
Initial Endodontic Radiograph (Start Film)

The purpose of the initial radiograph is to assist in making a diagnosis and to demonstrate tooth, pulp chamber, and root canal anatomy before access.

In most situations a single periapical radiograph will provide the necessary information. It is rarely necessary to expose multiple radiographs at different angulations to determine the number and location of canals and roots. This information is obtained by a properly angled working-length film. To produce the most accurate initial radiograph and to provide a reproducible angle and cone placement for subsequent recall films, a paralleling device such as the Rinn XCP (Rinn Corp, Elgin, Illinois) should be used (Fig. 2-1). Occasionally, an initial supplemental bite-wing radiograph will be useful to detect recurrent decay, to determine the depth of a calcified pulp chamber, or to reveal a pulp chamber obscured by a large amalgam (see Chapter 3).

CLINICAL PROBLEM: A 52-year-old female patient presents with a complaint of previous severe pain in the maxillary right molar and premolar area. Sometimes there was extreme sensitivity to cold with the pain lasting for several hours. At other times cold did not cause pain. In the last 24 hours the pain has abated. All teeth in this quadrant responded normally to the electric pulp test, cold tests, and the percussion test. A periapical radiograph demonstrates large amalgam restorations in the two maxillary premolars and the first molar (Fig. 2-2, *A*). The radiograph did not reveal periapical pathosis. With a previous history of severe and spontaneous pain lasting for several hours, along with severe pain to cold liquids and cold foods, the most likely diagnosis is a tooth with irreversible pulpitis. However, today the patient is symptom free and the practitioner cannot determine which tooth has been causing the problem.

Solution: Expose an additional radiograph at a different angle, in this case a bite-wing. This additional bite-wing radiograph may provide supplementary information not seen on the periapical film. In this case, the bite-wing radiograph demonstrated recurrent decay under the restoration in the maxillary second premolar (Fig. 2-2, *B, arrows*). The restoration was removed, and upon excavation of the decay a carious pulp exposure resulted. Root canal treatment was indicated.

If a sinus tract or fistula is present, it should be traced to the area of pathosis. This is accomplished by threading a fresh gutta-percha cone (size 30 to 40) through the tract and exposing a radiograph (Fig. 2-3). If the sinus tract cannot be penetrated with the gutta-percha cone, it may be necessary to reopen the tract with an explorer tip or periodontal probe by gentle probing. After penetration, the gutta-percha cone can be inserted with special care to ensure that the cone is inserted to its maximum depth.

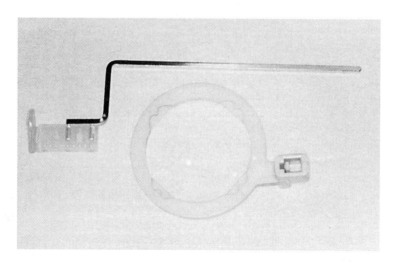

Fig. 2-1 *Rinn XCP film holder showing bite block, tubehead ring positioner, and positioning bar.*

Radiographic Support in Diagnosis

The following concepts are essential for proper interpretation of radiographic findings when diagnosing pulpal and periradicular disease.

1. Teeth with irreversibly inflamed pulps often fail to demonstrate periradicular changes radiographically. However, changes ranging from a slightly thickened lamina dura to a significantly widened periodontal ligament and loss of lamina dura are possible (Fig. 2-4). It should be noted, however, that radiographic angulation can and often does play a significant role in confusing the diagnosis for a particular tooth when the symptoms are not clear.

> The clinician must remember the tenet that radiographic angulation can sometimes make normal anatomy appear as pathologic and, by the same notion, periapical pathosis can be hidden by angulation and appear as normal anatomy.

For example, Fig. 2-5, *A*, demonstrates what appears to be both the loss of lamina dura and periodontal ligament space widening. The clinician might be inclined to diagnose this tooth in need of root canal therapy because of the

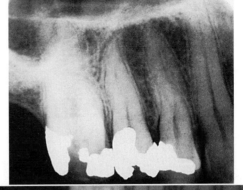

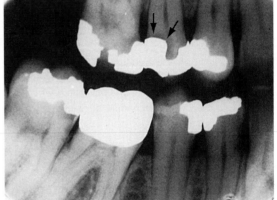

Fig. 2-2

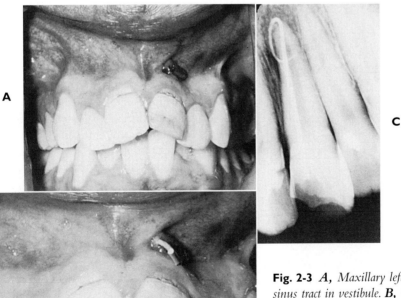

Fig. 2-3 *A, Maxillary left central incisor with draining sinus tract in vestibule. B, Gutta-percha point (No. 30) threaded into sinus tract. C, Periapical radiograph demonstrating how the gutta-percha point traces to the periapical pathosis.*

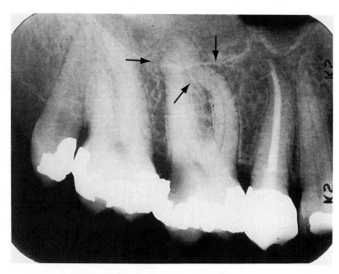

Fig. 2-4 *Periapical radiograph of an irreversibly inflamed maxillary first molar with a widened periodontal ligament and some loss of lamina dura around the buccal roots* (arrows).

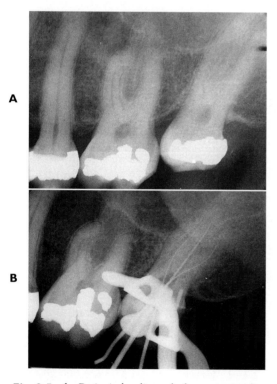

Fig. 2-5 *A, Periapical radiograph demonstrating loss of lamina dura and widening of the periodontal ligament space around mesiobuccal root of maxillary first molar. B, Same tooth from a different angle denotes normal periapical anatomic features demonstrating normal lamina dura and periodontal ligament space.*

radiographic appearance of the mesiobuccal root. However, as can be clearly demonstrated in Fig. 2-5, *B,* from a slightly different angulation, the lamina dura and the periodontal ligament space are completely normal and undisturbed by any form of pathosis.

2. Teeth with necrotic pulps do not necessarily have associated periradicular lesions that are radiographically discernible. However, more often than not, some radiographic change will be noted, which may range from a widened periodontal ligament to an obvious radiolucency (Fig. 2-6).

3. Periradicular radiolucent lesions of pulpal origin will routinely demonstrate the loss of the apical lamina dura in association with the radiolucency (Fig. 2-6).

4. Vertical angulation can also be used as a diagnostic aid in determining tooth-related pathosis. Fig. 2-7, *A,* demonstrates what appears to be a lesion associated with the maxillary second premolar. The tooth had been treated endodontically with a silver point, and therefore thermal tests were inappropriate as a diagnostic tool. A slightly different vertical angle caused the radiolucent lesion to move toward the sinus, and such movement confirmed that the lesion was not associated with the tooth. In addition, a normal lamina dura and periodontal ligament space was evident (Fig. 2-7, *B*).

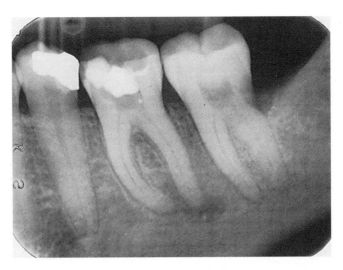

Fig. 2-6 *Large radiolucent lesion demonstrating significant bone loss around the distal root of a mandibular first molar.*

Radiographic Support in Assessing Tooth Anatomy

The initial radiograph will often reveal the presence of multiple canals or aberrant canal or tooth anatomy. When evaluating the radiograph for these possibilities, application of the following principles will assist the clinician in a more thorough assessment.

1. When a radiograph reveals root canal space is not in the center of the root, an extra canal should be suspected.[5,10] If there is only one canal in a root, it will always appear radiographically in the center of the root regardless of radiographic angulation, whereas, if the canal is asymmetrically located within the root, toward the mesial or distal periodontal ligament (PDL) space, there is a high probability of an additional canal (Fig. 2-8).

2. In single-rooted teeth, a sharp or rapid change (fast break) in the visible density of the root canal space usually indicates one of the following situations: (a) a broad pulp chamber has split into two canals; (b) one large canal has split into two canals; or (c) two canals that were superimposed upon each other have now diverged in separate directions[10], often seen in radiographs of premolars and mandibular incisors (Fig. 2-9). If the rapid change in density occurs in the apical third of the root, it is possible that the canal exits on the buccal or lingual surface of the root.

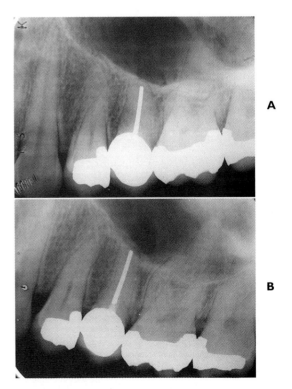

Fig. 2-7 *A, Radiolucent lesion seemingly associated with the second premolar. B, Another angle from a less severe vertical angulation demonstrates that lesion moves superiorly and is not associated with tooth.*

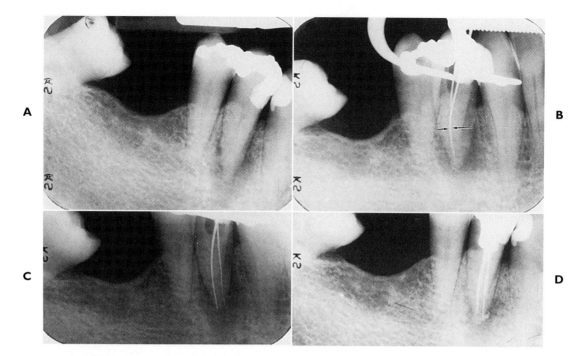

Fig. 2-8 *A, Start film of a mandibular first premolar showing a large radiolucent lesion. B, Working length with two files in the same canal. Notice that the files are skewed significantly to the distal area of the root, indicating the presence of a second canal toward the lingual side, since the radiograph was exposed from a mesial angulation. Length of each arrow indicates relative width of underlying root. C, Working-length with files in lingual and buccal canals. D, Six-month recall film demonstrating partial healing of bone.*

CLINICAL PROBLEM: A 30-year-old male patient presents with pain on biting in the mandibular incisor area. Percussion demonstrated sensitivity with the right lateral mandibular incisor. A radiograph shows a periapical radiolucency associated with the tooth (Fig. 2-10, *A*). The diagnosis was failing root canal treatment. The radiograph demonstrated the gutta-percha fill was not in the center of the root but was closer to the mesial periodontal ligament (PDL) than to the distal PDL (Fig. 2-10, *A, arrows*). This indicates the presence of a second canal (see Chapters 3 and 4). Although the cause of the root canal failure could have been a leaking temporary restoration, or short and poorly obturated canal, the most likely cause was an uninstrumented and unfilled second canal.

Solution: Access was made, gutta-percha was removed from the previously treated canal, and the second canal was located. Correct working length was established for both canals (Fig. 2-10, *B*). Both canals were obturated, and post space was prepared for the buccal canal and a proper temporary was placed (Fig. 2-10, *C*) A post, core, and crown were subsequently placed (Fig. 2-10, *D*).

RADIOGRAPHIC FILM HOLDERS

Numerous types of film holders or positioners are available. One of the most popular types of film holders is the Rinn XCP (Rinn Corp, Elgin, Illinois). This device allows an accurate reproduction of the intraoral structures with the least amount of distortion because of its positioning ring and bite block (see Fig. 2-1). Although the XCP is ideal for endodontic start and final films, it is not effective for either master-cone or working-length films, or any additional films that must be exposed during treatment when a rubber dam is in place.

Because recall radiographs are an essential aspect of case assessment, it is imperative to reproduce the same angulation for the recall film as was achieved for the start or final film.

This same angulation is necessary to determine actual changes in the periradicular area versus artifacts that arise from different horizontal or vertical angulations. The XCP is the film holder of choice for endodontic recall radiographs because of its ability to provide the same radiographic angle, a

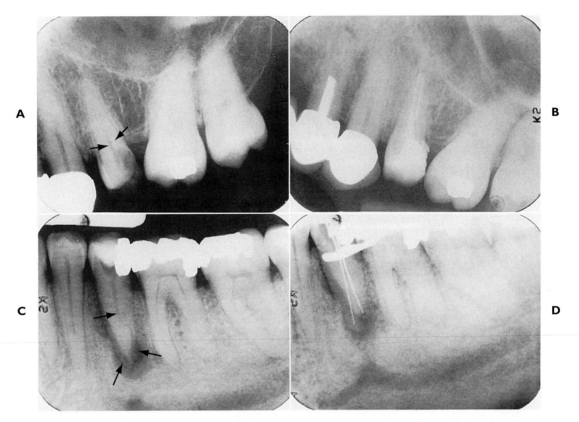

Fig. 2-9 *A, Radiograph of maxillary second premolar showing radiolucent canal that stops abruptly in the coronal third (arrows) of the root indicating a "fast break." B, Premolar after obturation of both canals. C, Mandibular second premolar with a "fast break" at midroot (arrow), indicating a high probability of a two-rooted, two-canal system. Periradicular area also indicates the likelihood of two roots (arrows). D, Working-length film exposed at a 20-degree angle confirms the presence of two canals and two roots.*

characteristic that ensures a valid method for comparing radiographs to determine treatment outcome and prognosis.

The Snap-A-Ray (Rinn Corp, Elgin, Illinois) is also a widely used film holder, though it requires more expertise and experience for its proper use (Fig. 2-11). The main difference between the XCP and the Snap-A-Ray is the lack of a positioning ring. The Snap-A-Ray relies on the ability of the clinician to position the x-ray beam based on an educated estimate of the location of the intraoral film and its angle with respect to the tooth. With practice, however, extremely accurate radiographic reproductions of intraoral structures can be obtained. The advantage with this device is that it can be used during all aspects of treatment, including working-length and master-cone film exposures.

The Snapex (Dunvale Corp, Gilberts, Illinois) system is similar in shape to the Snap-A-Ray except that it is made to house a ring-positioning bar and therefore has the advantages of both the XCP and the Snap-A-Ray (Fig. 2-12). Its size, however, has caused some clinicians to choose other, simpler devices.

The Crawford Film Holder (CFH Co, Indian Wells, California) has all the advantages of the above-mentioned film placement devices with few if any disadvantages. This device is a hybrid of an XCP and a hemostat. Therefore it has the benefit of a positioning ring with which to align the x-ray head and a hemostat, which can hold and position the film without discomfort to the patient (Fig. 2-13).

Although there are additional commercial film holders and positioning devices available, most are

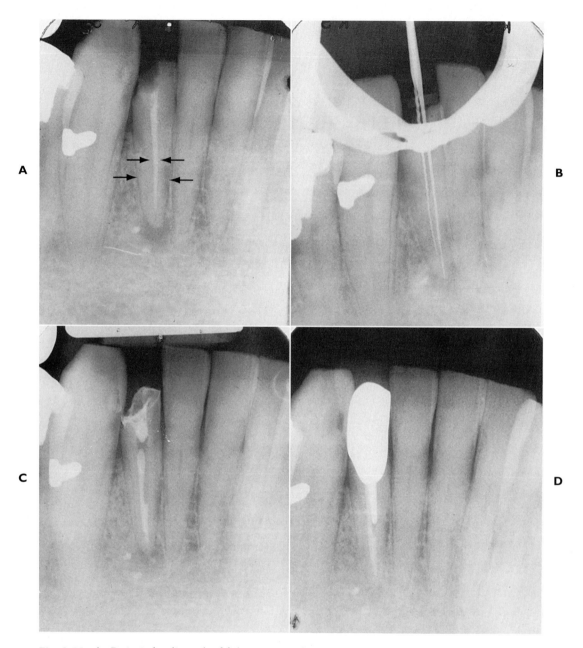

Fig. 2-10 *A, Periapical radiograph of failing root canal treatment in a mandibular lateral incisor. Notice the asymmetry of the gutta-percha and its closer approximation to the mesial periodontal ligament (PDL) than to the distal PDL of the root (arrows). **B,** Working length after removal of gutta-percha demonstrates the presence of two canals. **C,** Immediately after obturation of both canals. **D,** Twelve-month recall radiograph showing healing of periradicular tissues.*

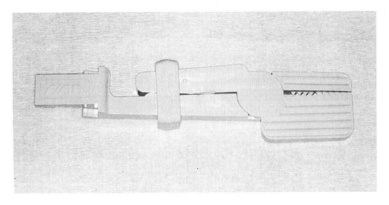

Fig. 2-11 *Snap-A-Ray film holder.*

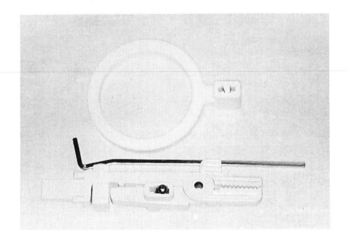

Fig. 2-12 *Snapex film holder and x-ray tubehead positioning ring.*

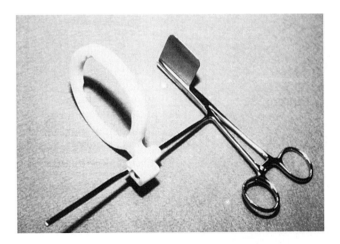

Fig. 2-13 *Crawford film holder. The film holder has a positioning ring similar to that of the XCP and Snapex. (Courtesy Dr. Frank Crawford, Indian Wells, California.)*

variations of those discussed. The last film-holding device that is mentioned is the hemostat. This, the most elementary and perhaps the most common among endodontists, is routinely used for exposing films when a rubber dam is in place. Although it takes more time and experience to develop a reliable technique with the hemostat, once mastered it is the method of choice because of its availability and modest price, and it should be routinely included as part of all basic endodontic tray setups.

Commercially available film-positioning devices used for endodontic films have one very important consideration in common if an undistorted and diagnostic radiograph is desired. This common factor is the necessity for the film and the x-ray cone to be placed intraorally such that the x-ray beam is perpendicular to the film. Lack of this proper alignment is one of the most common problems encountered when exposing radiographs with the rubber dam in place during root canal treatment. Effective use of the hemostat can virtually eliminate all radiographic distortion. Fig. 2-14 illustrates this concept using a hemostat handle as a guide. Because it is difficult and at times impossible to visualize the angle of the film after it has been placed intraorally, an extraoral reference point (the finger and thumb hole of the hemostat) must be utilized for accurate alignment of the x-ray beam.

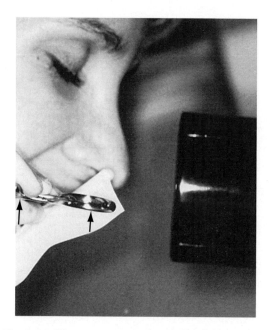

Fig. 2-14 *Hemostat positioned with film in place. The thumb and finger holes* (arrows) *are the external reference point with which to align the x-ray tubehead.*

The following guidelines for the use of the hemostat will prevent most problems encountered with obtaining quality endodontic radiographs.

Film Placement in the Hemostat. Before the hemostat is placed intraorally, the film must be properly positioned within the beaks of the hemostat.

1. The film should neither be bent nor "cornered" to facilitate placement or patient comfort. By repositioning the film intraorally, the same objective will be accomplished, but, more importantly, accidental distortion because of a warped film will be prevented.

2. The film should be aligned in the hemostat so that the beaks clamp on the dimple (an embossing of the negative that frequently makes any superimposed object unreadable, e.g., the tip of a file or a radiographic apex) (Fig. 2-15, *A*). This procedure prevents critical intraoral images from being distorted by the dimple.

3. The film must be completely positioned within the beaks so that a majority of the film is supported by the hemostat, thereby eliminating accidental bending when the film is positioned. Placing only the corner or a portion of the edge of the film in the hemostat (Fig. 2-15, *B* and *C*) ensures a high probability of film rotation within the beaks of the hemostat when the film is placed. This error will result in an invalid external reference point and distortion of the film, producing a nondiagnostic image. Also, long-beaked hemostats, as opposed to needle holders or shorter-beaked instruments, provide a more secure grip on the film and less possibility of intraoral film movement (Fig. 2-15, *D*).

Intraoral Film Placement. Once the film is properly secured by the beaks of the hemostat, it can be positioned intraorally. One very basic rule applies to the placement of the film with respect to intraoral radiographs. This rule states that the top edge of the film should always be placed as close as possible to the occlusal surface or incisal edge (Fig. 2-16). Such placement will ensure that the entire tooth and root will be imaged on the radiograph.

The rubber dam frame need never be removed during a radiographic exposure when using this technique.

Preventing Foreshortening or Elongation. By design, the beaks with respect to the hemostat handle are at a 90-degree angle to each other,

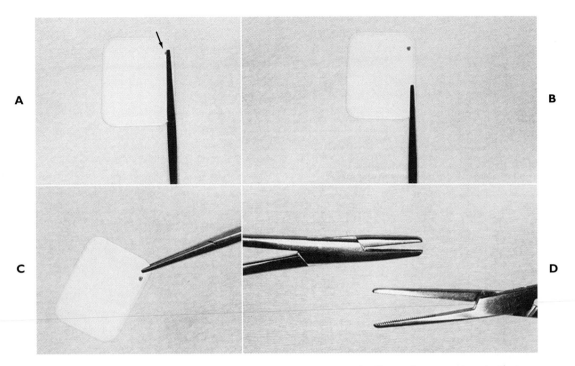

Fig. 2-15 *A, Proper positioning of the beaks of the hemostat on the film pack. Notice that the beaks are placed over the dimple (arrow). B, Improper grasping of the film pack with the hemostat. An inadequate amount of the film pack is positioned in the beaks. C, Example of another common error when grasping the film pack. This error allows the film to rotate on the tip of the hemostat beak when placed intraorally, and a cone cut or lack of desired tooth structure is the result. D, Needle holders (top) are sometimes mistakenly used for film positioning. The beak is significantly shorter than the hemostat (bottom) and cannot grasp the film pack as securely.*

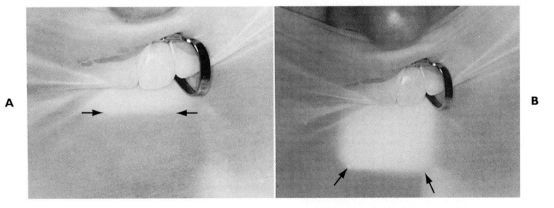

Fig. 2-16 *A, Proper positioning of the film pack for anterior teeth. Notice that the edge of the film pack (arrows) is positioned approximately along the incisal edge of the anterior teeth. B, Improper positioning of the film pack (arrows) for an anterior radiograph. This usually occurs because the patient unconsciously lowers the hemostat when the dentist or assistant is positioning the x-ray tubehead.*

which positions the intraoral film perpendicularly to the handle. Therefore the hemostat handle can be used as an external reference point. By aligning the x-ray cone perpendicularly to the plane of the hemostat handle, as is demonstrated in Fig. 2-17, the central beam of the x-ray head will strike the intraoral film at a 90-degree angle. This will virtually eliminate all distortion, provided that the film has been properly positioned.

This same principle with one slight modification is used with multirooted teeth. Fig. 2-18, *A* demonstrates how the x-ray beam has been moved 20 to 30 degrees mesial of perpendicular to the buccal surface of the mandibular first molar (Fig. 2-18, *B*). This minor amount of angulation change will not result in a distorted image of the root, but will provide an adequate "separation" of the files within a given root. Note in Fig. 2-19 that this change in angulation results in both the mesial and the distal roots being separated so that a diagnostic working-length film is obtained for each of the four canals. Some clinicians place a Hedström file in both lingual or both buccal canals to differentiate canal position (Fig. 2-19). However, by proper application of the standard guidelines of the buccal object rule

(see Locating Working Length later in this chapter) this procedure becomes unnecessary.

Always assume, perhaps except for maxillary incisors, that every tooth undergoing root canal treatment has more than one canal, until proved otherwise.

For this reason, all working-length films, except for maxillary molars, whose roots are naturally separated when viewed from perpendicular to the buccal, should be exposed at a slight angle, mesial to perpendicular (20 to 30 degrees), as previously described. These basic principles of radiographic technique will provide both the clinician and the dental assistant with a reliable and accurate method for exposing radiographs during treatment.

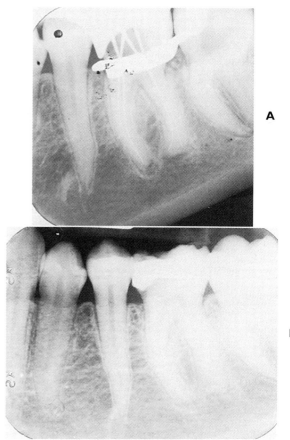

A

B

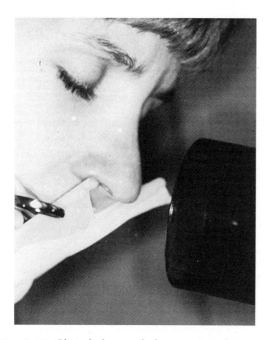

Fig. 2-17 *Clinical photograph demonstrating the correct positioning of the tubehead using the hemostat handle as an external reference. The x-ray beam will strike the film at a 90-degree angle, thereby preventing most types of distortion.*

Fig. 2-18 *A, Radiograph of a mandibular first molar with four canals exposed at a 20-degree angle. Notice the absence of distortion and the clarity of the apical anatomy. B, Start film of same tooth exposed with an XCP.*

PROBLEMS ASSOCIATED WITH RADIOGRAPHIC TECHNIQUE AND INTERPRETATION

Distortion: Errors in Vertical Angulation

Several types of distortion can occur when radiographs are improperly exposed. One of the most common errors is elongation, which is easily resolved by knowing the cause of the problem. There are two major causes that result in an elongated film: (1) the film is not perpendicular to the x-ray beam, or (2) the film is not parallel to the object being radiographed.

The problem of elongation occurs typically in the maxillary canine and molar regions (Fig. 2-20) because of the difficulty of film placement in this area (shallow palate, small mouth, and so forth) and difficulty associated with aligning the x-ray tubehead perpendicular to the object and to the film. The first problem is prevented by placement of the film adjacent to the opposing arch, while maintaining a parallel alignment of the film to the tooth being radiographed. The second problem is prevented by following the principles highlighted with the use of the hemostat. That is, by using the fact that the hemostat handle is perpendicular to the film within its beaks, if the tubehead is positioned at an angle that is perpendicular to the handle, the central x-ray beam will be perpendicular to the film. Fig. 2-21 clearly demonstrates how the clini-

cian can determine if the tubehead is properly aligned by examining the path of the x-ray beam and comparing it with a plane perpendicular to the handle of the hemostat. If the x-ray beam does not strike this plane at a 90-degree angle, an elongated film will result (see Fig. 2-20).

Another form of distortion, foreshortening, occurs when the central x-ray beam is at too steep an angle (excess vertical angulation) compared with the film or object being radiographed (Fig. 2-22). Although the film may be parallel to the object (tooth), if the beam is too steep, the object will be foreshortened and in many cases a nondiagnostic film will result. Foreshortening is not necessarily detrimental and can sometimes be used to delineate the apical anatomy of buccal and palatal roots. However, if working-length files are incorrect and adjustments are necessary, a foreshortened radiograph is of little value. The clinician cannot accurately judge how much change (even in small increments) is necessary because the film no longer represents a one-to-one reproduction of the tooth. Therefore, changing the file length 2 mm to increase the length toward the apex because the original working length was 2 mm short will not, in all likelihood, result in the correct length. The rationale behind this statement is that the file is foreshortened the same degree as the root, and, since the amount of foreshortening cannot be

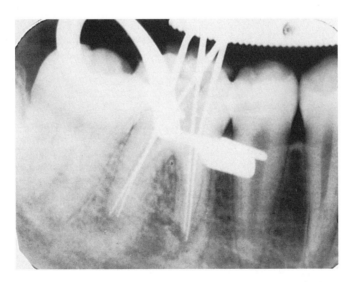

Fig. 2-19 *Working-length film of a mandibular first molar with four canals. The two buccal canals each have a Hedström file in place verifying that the film was exposed at a 20-degree angle from the mesial.*

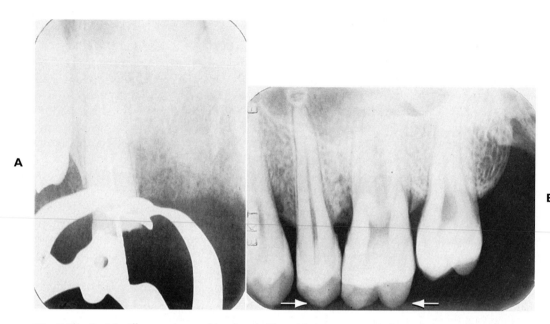

Fig. 2-20 *A, Maxillary canine working-length film with improper vertical angulation resulting in an elongated image and loss of periapical detail. **B,** Maxillary posterior radiograph with correct intraoral film positioning* (arrows demonstrate film positioned at occlusal plane), *but improper vertical angle of x-ray beam results in elongated buccal roots and loss of detail of the palatal root. Notice also the improper positioning of the film in the hemostat, with the dimple being located in the apical region, superimposed on the apex of the second premolar.*

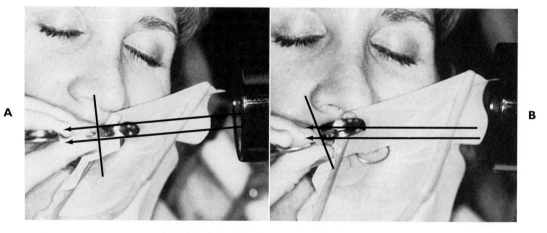

Fig. 2-21 *A, Clinical example of the correct method for aligning the x-ray beam with respect to a plane perpendicular to the hemostat handle. **B,** Incorrect alignment of the tubehead resulting in a greater than 90-degree angle between x-ray beam* (lines with arrows) *and film pack* (line without arrow), *producing an elongated image of the tooth.*

accurately ascertained, the clinician can only guess at how much to add or subtract when correcting an error in working length based on a foreshortened or elongated radiograph. However, a parallel radiograph will give a very close one-to-one approximation of root length. Therefore, if the file is short or long of the desired length, adding or subtracting the estimated distance based on the actual parallel radiographic image will result in a valid and corrected working length.

Lack of Clarity or Definition: Horizontal Position of the X-ray Tube

Lack of clarity or image definition results when the tube head is at too severe a horizontal angle with respect to the radiographed object (Fig. 2-23). This is prevented by use of a small horizontal angulation (20 degrees from perpendicular) to produce a separation of images (such as files, roots) on the film. Too severe an angulation usually results in an undiagnostic film, additional exposure for the patient, and increased chair time for the procedure.

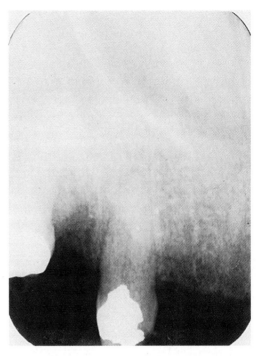

Fig. 2-22 *Radiograph of a maxillary canine exposed at too severe a vertical angle, causing the image to be foreshortened. Notice that film placement was correct. Compare with Fig. 2-18, A.*

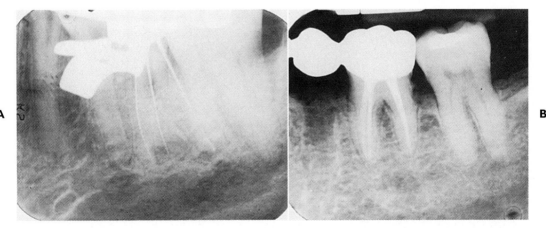

A **B**

Fig. 2-23 *A, Working-length radiograph of a mandibular first molar exposed from too great a mesial angle. Although the mesial roots are separated, the severe angle results in loss of definition of the periodontal ligament, lamina dura, and radicular structures. Superimposition of the mesial roots from the second molar on the distal root of the first molar also occurs with this exaggerated angulation. B, Final film of a mandibular molar exposed at the proper angle. Notice that the contacts do not significantly overlap, an indication that only a slight amount of mesial angulation is necessary to adequately separate canals within the same root.*

It should be noted, however, that it is incumbent upon the clinician to take properly angled radiographs to obtain the true clinical picture rather than an artificial radiographic presentation created by improper film placement or inappropriate angulation of the x-ray beam.

CLINICAL PROBLEM: A 25-year-old female patient returning for completion of root canal therapy in her left maxillary second molar complains of a periodic discomfort to chewing in her upper left canine and premolar area. The pain was never severe but she states that over the last 2 weeks she noticed an occasional bad taste in her mouth. The patient's entire maxillary dentition is restored with 3- and 4-unit porcelain-fused-to-metal bridges as a result of trauma several years ago. Clinical exam reveals a sinus tract exiting in the attached gingiva between the first and second premolars. A size 35 gutta-percha cone was slowly threaded into the sinus tract and a radiograph exposed (Fig. 2-24, *A*). As can be noted from the radiograph, the gutta-percha appears to indicate that the first premolar is the cause of the patient's discomfort. Since all teeth are restored with crowns and porcelain, electric pulp tests are inappropriate. Cold tests are inconsistent and therefore inconclusive.

Solution: The clinician decided to save the patient from additional radiation and obturated the molar. When the final film was exposed for the molar, gutta-percha was again threaded into the sinus tract and a radiograph was exposed (Fig. 2-24, *B*). The gutta-percha traced to the midroot level of the premolar region where a midroot radiolucency was observed. In addition, this film also demonstrated a radiolucent lesion at the apex of the second premolar. This tooth was opened without anesthesia, and a necrotic pulp was verified. The second premolar was obturated with gutta-percha and sealer, and a lateral canal was noted adjacent to where the gutta-percha had traced (Fig. 2-24, *C, arrow*). The sinus tract resolved within several days, and the patient's symptoms and bad taste were alleviated.

In using the radiograph as an aid in endodontic diagnosis, the clinician must realize that periradicular pathosis or bone destruction may be present but not radiographically apparent.

Radiographic bone loss is not evident until there is significant erosion of the cortical plate.[1,8] There-

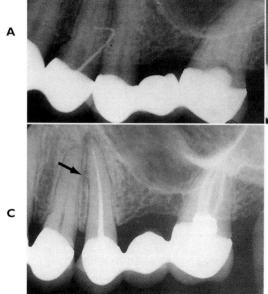

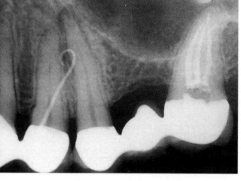

Fig. 2-24 *A, Periapical radiograph of premolar with gutta percha threaded into sinus tract. B, Final film of molar root canal and gutta percha is again threaded into sinus tract, revealing quite a different picture from the previous radiograph. C, Completed root canal therapy on premolar. Notice cement-filled lateral canal adjacent to lesion.*

fore periradicular radiolucencies will not appear on the radiograph even though there may be considerable bone destruction if the bone loss is confined to the cancellous bone. In addition, roots situated close to the cortical plate or where the cortical bone is thin are more likely to demonstrate a radiographic change than those more distant from the cortex or with thick overlying cortical bone.[8,9] For example, mandibular first molars demonstrate areas of rarefaction more often around the mesial root in contrast to the distal root because of its closer position to the buccal cortical plate.[8,9] Maxillary anterior teeth and buccal roots of maxillary molars are close to the labial or buccal cortical bone, and therefore radiolucencies are more often visible around these roots.

Film Placement

Although proper film placement is essential for diagnostic films, it is often perceived as a difficult procedure in the presence of a rubber dam. Many clinicians remove the rubber dam frame when placing working-length or master-cone films. In fact, there are no valid reasons to remove the frame to obtain excellent quality, diagnostic films. At the same time, however, multiple reasons can be cited for leaving the frame in place such as maintaining an aseptic field, ensuring patient comfort, and, most importantly, preventing the aspiration or the swallowing of endodontic files.

Proper film placement requires application of the following principles.

1. Place as much film in the beaks of the hemostat as possible, closing the beak on the dimple (Fig. 2-15, *A*).
2. The film must be intraorally positioned so that it is parallel to an imaginary mesiodistal line running through the object tooth and one tooth mesial and distal to it.
3. The top edge of the film, held by the hemostats, must be no higher than the occlusal surface of the tooth being radiographed (see Fig. 2-16, *A*).
4. The x-ray tubehead must be perpendicular to an imaginary plane created by the hemostat handle (see Fig. 2-21, *A*).
5. The tubehead must be positioned so the central beam is perpendicular to the facial or buccal surface of the tooth being radiographed, or if an angled radiograph is desired, the central beam must be only 20 to 30 degrees mesial or distal to perpendicular.

Adherence to these guidelines will prevent most types of distortion and will consistently result in

excellent diagnostic radiographs. Although applicable to most teeth when working-length or master-cone films are desired, slight modifications are required for anterior and posterior teeth. In Fig. 2-15, *A,* the film is positioned within the beaks of the hemostat in the same manner for both anterior and posterior teeth; however, the hemostat is inserted differently. If the shorter edge of the film is grasped with a hemostat (Fig. 2-25, *A*) and inserted intraorally so that it exits the mouth at a 90-degree angle to the long axis of the anterior teeth (Fig. 2-25, *B*), it often results in the bending of the film. This is due to a shallow palate or misalignment of the film because of the inability to visualize the actual film position. The film will be

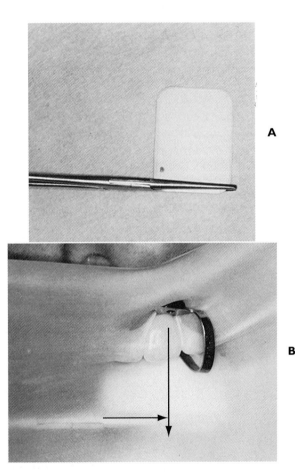

Fig. 2-25 *A, Improper film placement in the hemostat for anterior teeth. B, Incorrect method of exposing anterior working-length films. Hemostat is at a 90-degree angle to the long axis of the tooth, which can result in a distorted film. The lack of rigidity resulting from the hemostat beak grasping the film pack along the incorrect edge allows warping of the film when placed intraorally.*

subject to less flexing (less distortion) if the longer edge of the film is firmly positioned within the beaks of the hemostat (see Fig. 2-15, *A*). When inserted parallel to the long axis of anterior teeth, it allows better manipulation of the film and easier handling by the patient.

Locating Working Length

Before exposing working-length film, a file should be placed into each canal that has been identified. This is preferable to placing only one or two files at a time into a tooth and to exposing a radiograph two or three times to obtain a working length for each canal. This minimizes patient exposure to radiation, reduces chair time for obtaining proper working length, and provides a comparative relationship of the working length of each canal to the other(s). It is an extremely rare clinical situation in which three or four files, with stops, cannot be properly placed in an access opening to obtain a working-length film.

Upon review of the working-length film, if the distance between the root apex and file tip is greater than 1 mm, another film is strongly recommended to obtain the proper working length.[5] It has been demonstrated that it is unlikely for a clinician to estimate accurately the added or subtracted length needed to correct a provisional file length to proper working length (based on a radiograph) if the amount of correction is greater than 1 mm.[3]

When treating teeth with buccal and lingual canals, application of the buccal object rule is essential to proper working-length determination. This rule is also termed the *SLOB rule* (same lingual opposite buccal). Although this concept is thoroughly addressed in dental school curriculums, many clinicians fail to apply it routinely in their daily practice. As the x-ray tube head is moved from posterior to anterior (that is, to the mesial), objects imaged on the film that are on the lingual aspect (palatal roots, mesiolingual roots, distolingual roots) will be positioned mesially (the position of the x-ray tube). Objects located on the buccal will be shifted distally (Fig. 2-26). This is most obvious if one examines a radiograph of a maxillary molar that has been exposed from a mesial angulation (Fig. 2-27). The palatal root will always shift in the direction of the tubehead, while the buccal roots shift away from the tubehead. The clinician can therefore determine whether the exposure was at a mesial or distal angulation (Fig. 2-28).

CLINICAL PROBLEM: A 42-year-old female patient presents with pain to chewing in the upper right quadrant. A porcelain-fused-to-metal crown is present on the two premolars. A periapical radiograph reveals a radiolucent lesion associated with the right maxillary second premolar, and the tooth gives an abnormal response to percussion (Fig. 2-29, *A*). The patient states that she had root canal treatment on this tooth several years ago.

SOLUTION: The astute clinician suspects a second canal, which was neither instrumented nor obturated. However, with the presence of a porcelain crown and amalgam core present, the difficulty

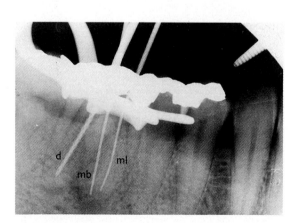

Fig. 2-26 *Mandibular molar working length radiograph exposed with the cone head on the mesial pointing in a distal direction. The distal most file (d) is in the distal canal, the middle file is in the mesiobuccal canal (mb), and the mesial most file is in the mesiolingual canal (ml). The buccal object, "the mesiobuccal canal and file" has moved to the distal.*

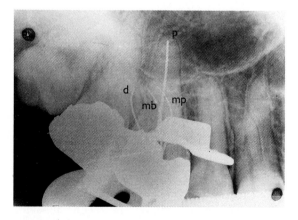

Fig. 2-27 *Maxillary molar with four files in the root canals. A mesially angulated radiograph (cone head angled from mesial to distal) shows four distinct files (canals): d, distal; p, palatal; mb, mesiobuccal; mp, mesiopalatal.*

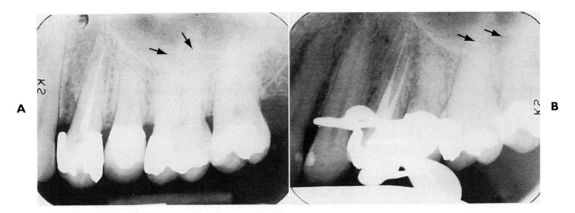

Fig. 2-28 *A, Final treatment film of a maxillary first premolar. The XCP radiograph superimposes the two canals on each other. Notice that the buccal roots of the maxillary first molar are anatomically separated (arrows). B, Radiograph of the maxillary first premolar during obturation. Without knowing at what angle the radiograph was exposed, the clinician can still determine that the longer canal is in the palatal root because the palatal root of the maxillary first molar is positioned mesially and the buccal roots have been shifted (arrows).*

arises with respect to where to look for the second canal. Was the obturated canal the buccal or the lingual? After finding the canal that was obturated with gutta-percha, take an angled working-length film from the mesial. In this case the palatal canal was obturated, and the buccal canal must now be identified and cleaned, shaped, and obturated (Fig. 2-29, *B*). The master-cone film is exposed (Fig. 2-29, *C*) and the canals obturated (Fig. 2-29, *D*). A 1-year recall film demonstrates nearly complete resolution of the lesion (Fig. 2-29, *E*).

Finally, the working-length file should be placed to the full length of the canal to determine the morphology of the canal system. Because the apical foramen may exit coronally to the radiographic apex, a file must be inserted to the complete length of the root to ascertain where the foramen is located with respect to the radiographic apex (see Fig. 2-18, *A*). This is particularly true for mandibular molars in which the distal canal often exits coronal to the radiographic apex.

Calcified Canals

It is often necessary to penetrate with a bur deep into the canal system because of severe calcification (see Chapter 4). At times this can be a risky decision because of the high probability of perforation. However, by applying the previously discussed fundamentals about radiographic interpretation and

the SLOB rule, this task can be performed with an added degree of confidence.

If a file or bur is placed within the access opening, an angled film will reveal if the instrument is penetrating in a buccal or a lingual direction. However, this describes only the buccal or lingual relationship of the canal to the instrument, and no information is available regarding its mesiodistal position in the root. By exposing a second film that is parallel and identical to the angle of a bite-wing and that encompasses the radicular structure, the mesiodistal position can be determined. These two films will then provide all information necessary to determine the exact location of the instrument with respect to the center of the root and will allow for opportunity to correct its orientation in the pursuit of the actual canal.

Film Processing: Quick Developing Units
Underdeveloped and Overdeveloped Radiographs

There are numerous problems associated with quick-developing units that are easily prevented. The most common problem that occurs with quick-developing units are films that appear too light and undiagnostic. This problem is primarily due to the time of development. When the film is too light, the working-length file is often difficult to see and the clinician often guesses where it is with respect to the apex (Fig. 2-30). This only compromises the quality of care by reading errors into the

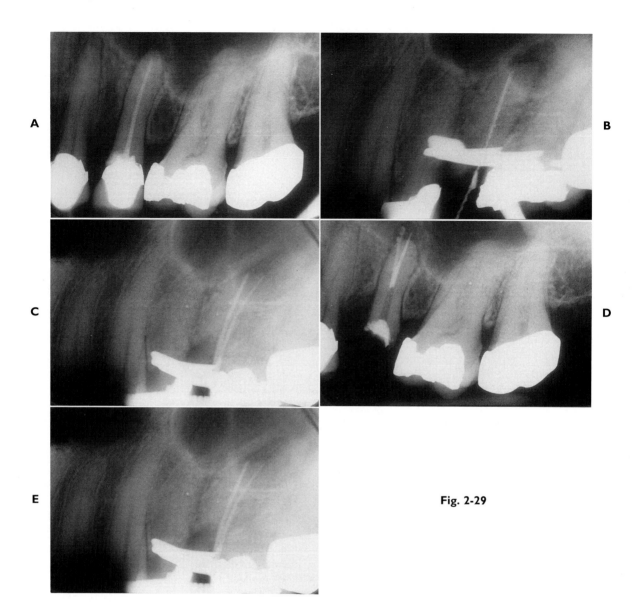

Fig. 2-29

film or by creating anatomy (periradicular structures), which may or may not be present.

Radiographs that are too light (underdeveloped film) cannot be made diagnostic (darkened) after being placed into the fixative. Therefore, with most quick-developing methods, it is prudent to err on the side of overdeveloping. Most overdeveloped films (too dark) can be corrected by being placed in the quick fixative solution an additional amount of time to lighten the radiograph to diagnostic quality. Unfortunately, this may take 10 to 20 minutes (unless the solution is changed daily), and although this amount of time makes the corrective procedure clinically unfeasible for working-length or master-cone films, it can be a useful technique for correcting start or final films.

Radiographs that Turn Brown or Darken

Another common problem with developing units is that radiographs may turn dark brown within hours to days after fixing. This problem is the result of improper washing. All films should be washed in water for at least 15 to 20 minutes after removal from the fixative solution. After the film has been rinsed under tap water for approximately 10 seconds, the film should be placed into a cup of water for at least 15 minutes.

Dark Films: Proper Exposure and Development Time

Although the radiograph may have been properly developed, if it is not placed into the fixative solution for an adequate period of time, it may not be of diagnostic quality. Fig. 2-31 illustrates a film that has been adequately developed but improperly fixed for a short period of time. It is scarcely readable with respect to the working length. No light can be transmitted through the film, which is the tell-tale sign of improper fixation. Light transmission through the negative will indicate proper fixation. If the film has a generalized dark brown color immediately upon removal from the fixative, improper fixation time is the likely cause, and periradicular structures will not be sufficiently distinct for proper interpretation of the image. The solution to this problem is to replace the film in fixative for an additional 1 to 3 minutes.

Superimposition of Anatomic Structures

Root Structure

The superimposition of roots is readily prevented by moving the cone only 20 to 30 degrees from perpendicular. A common problem occurs, however, with excessive angulation, which results in the superimposition of other structures over the desired area of interest. This can occur in mesiodistal and superoinferior dimensions. The basic rule to follow is that a very small change in horizontal tubehead angulation will result in a significant and diagnostically valuable separation of superimposed roots. This is particularly true for the mesiobuccal root of the maxillary first molar. The two canals that are often present in this root, mesiobuccal and mesiopalatal, are extremely difficult to separate without the resulting superimposition of other anatomic structures obscuring the periradicular area. If the horizontal angulation is moved only a slight amount (20 to 30 degrees), the desired separation will result without distortion or superimposition (Fig. 2-32).

Osseous Structures

The zygoma, or zygomatic arch, is an anatomic landmark that routinely interferes with the interpretation of maxillary periapical films.

Tamse and coworkers[11] have shown that the bisecting-angle technique is inferior and unreliable for diagnostic radiographs in the maxillary molar region. Preventing the zygoma from interfering with the interpretation of tooth structure in this area can be accomplished by positioning the tubehead with less vertical angulation than that presented in Fig. 2-33. If the vertical angulation is too great, the zygoma will be superimposed on the buccal and palatal roots making interpretation of periradicular structures impossible (Fig. 2-34). However, a less severe angle will demonstrate all periradicular structures without loss of critical information regarding the morphology of the tooth.

APEX LOCATORS

Electronic apex locators, though a relatively new addition to the armamentarium of clinicians, are rapidly gaining more acceptance. McDonald[6] recently reviewed the numerous studies on electronic apex locator accuracy and reported that they tend to be accurate (within ±0.5 mm) between 83% and 93.4% of the time.[6] Although few are advocating the use of apex locators as a replacement for radiographs, many recommend apex locators as an adjunct to assist in endodontic treatment. Presently there are two major types of electronic apex locators available to the clinician. These are the older but continually improving resistance type of apex locators and the more newly introduced frequency-dependent type.[2]

Resistance Type of Apex Locators

The resistance type of locators are based on the principle that the electric resistance between the periodontal ligament and the oral mucosa is a constant value. This value is built into the circuitry of the apex locators. Therefore, when one lead of the apex locator is placed on the oral mucosa (lip clip) and the other lead on the root canal file, the clinician is able to determine the working length when the file reaches the PDL (apical foramen). There are additional electronic physical principles that also effect the performance so that the operation of these apex locators can at times be inconsistent.

For the greatest accuracy, resistance type apex locators require a reasonably dry environment. In addition, they require that the file fit snugly in the canal. These requirements can cause some difficulty when initially attempting to determine working length in a fluid- or blood-filled canal. The operator must also be aware that the file cannot touch any metal, such as amalgam or pins when operating the unit. Despite these potential problems manufacturers continue to improve the resistance type of apex locators with improved circuitry, easy-to-use

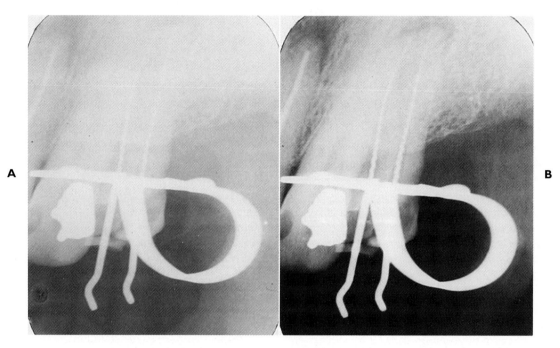

Fig. 2-30 *A, Improperly developed working-length film. The lack of periapical definition is a result of too short a developing time. B, Working-length film of same tooth with appropriate developing time. Periradicular anatomy is well defined.*

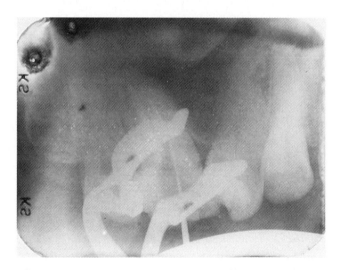

Fig. 2-31 *Improperly fixed working-length film. Generalized darkened color in film indicates that a longer fixing time is needed.*

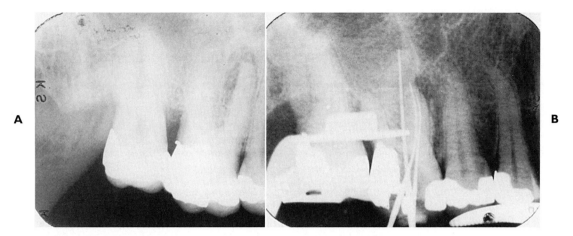

Fig. 2-32 *A,* *Maxillary first-molar start film.* **B,** *Working-length verification film exposed with a very slight mesial angulation. The two mesiobuccal root canals are separated with this technique without superimposition of other structures.*

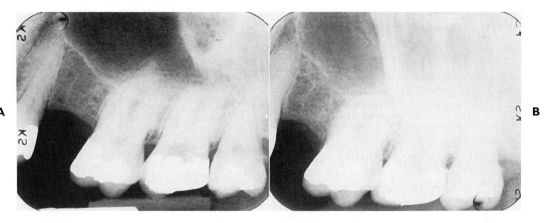

Fig. 2-33 *A,* *Start film of a maxillary second molar demonstrating periradicular anatomy.* **B,** *Final film exposed at approximately the same horizontal angulation but with a significant change in vertical inclination of the tubehead, which results in the superimposition of the zygoma and complete loss of detail in the periradicular region.*

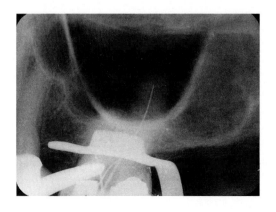

Fig. 2-34 *Superimposition of the zygomatic process and the flange from the rubber dam clamp make interpretation of the working length of this maxillary molar impossible.*

digital readouts and decreasing size and weight. Examples of these type of apex locators are NeoSono (Amadent, Cherry Hill, New Jersey) and Foramatron (Parkell, Farmingdale, New York).

Frequency-Dependent Apex Locators

Recently frequency-dependent apex locators have become available. These apex locators operate by comparing the rates of difference between a high- and low-frequency signal. As the file advances to the apex, this ratio changes and is maximally different at the apical constriction.

Those units operate in a wet environment so that sodium hypochlorite, pus, or blood appear to have little effect on the measurements. Like the other type of apex locators, these require that the file fit the size of the canal snugly. These apex locators use an electrical output of very low voltage in comparison with the resistance type. This eliminates the occasional patient complaint of a tingling sensation when the unit is being used. Examples of frequency-dependent apex locators are the Endex (Osada Electric Co., Tokyo, Japan) and the Root ZX (J. Morita Corp., Tustin, California).

Apex locators can be used as an adjunct in determining working lengths where problems with anatomic variations obscure visualization of the periradicular area. In addition, they may be used to determine perforations or in patients where radiation exposure needs to be reduced. What must be recognized, however, is that the apex locators are no substitute for high-quality radiographs that yield invaluable information regarding root morphology and curvature, calcification, number of canals and roots, and anatomic anomalies, a concept succinctly stated by Provan in 1916:

"It seems to me that, on account of the very uncertain number and complex conditions of roots and canals, it ought to be taken as an axiom that the radiograph should be employed in all cases where treatment of these roots or canals is to be carried on."[7]

References

1. Bender IB, Seltzer S: Roentgenographic and direct observation of experimental lesions in bone. I & II. *J Am Dent Assoc* 62:152-160, 708-716, 1961.
2. Christie, WH, Peikoff, MD, Hawrish, CE: Clinical observations on a newly designed electronic apex locator, *Can Dent J* 59:765-772, 1993.
3. Cox VS, Brown CE, Bricker SL, et al: Radiographic interpretation of endodontic file length, *Oral Surg Oral Med Oral Pathol* 72:340-344, 1991.
4. Goldman M, Pearson A, Darzenta N: Reliability of radiographic interpretations, *Oral Surg Oral Med Oral Path* 38:287-293, 1974.
5. Gutmann JL, Leonard JE: Problem solving in endodontic working length determination, *Comp Contin Educ Dent* 16:288-304, 1995.
6. McDonald NJ: The electronic determination of working length, *Dent Clin North Am* 36:273-307, 1992.
7. Provan WF: Roots and their treatment, *Dent Summary* 36:675-680, 1916.
8. Schwartz SF, Foster JK: Roentgenographic interpretation of experimentally produced bone lesions. I. *Oral Surg Oral Med Oral Pathol* 32:606-612, 1971.
9. Seltzer S: *Endodontology: biologic considerations in endodontic procedures*, ed 2, Philadelphia, 1988 Lea & Febiger, pp 155-156.
10. Slowey R: Radiographic aids in detection of extra root canals, *Oral Surg Oral Med Oral Pathol*, 37:762-772, 1974.
11. Tamse A, Kaffe I, Fishel D: Zygomatic arch interference with correct radiographic diagnosis in maxillary molar endodontics, *Oral Surg Oral Med Oral Pathol* 50:563-565, 1980.

▼

Chapter 3

Problems Encountered in Tooth Isolation and Access to the Pulp Chamber Space

James L. Gutmann
Paul E. Lovdahl

"The first step in the treatment of a tooth . . . is the adjustment of the rubber dam over the diseased tooth to preclude the possibility of the entrance of any germs in the oral secretions into the pulp chamber. This should be the invariable rule."*

"The first essential in getting at any root-canal is to gain direct access, and not to try to work around corners, whatever tooth-structure may have to be sacrificed."†

The main purpose of a lingual or occlusal endodontic access opening is to create an unimpeded passageway to the pulpal space and the apical foramen of the tooth. This unrestricted opening should be specifically designed for each tooth to facilitate proper canal cleaning, shaping, and obturation. In some cases, a problem-solving approach may dictate the need to initiate the access opening in a surface other than the lingual or occlusal surface (Fig. 3-1). Although rare, these creative approaches should be used only when standard entries to the canal system are impossible or the loss of tooth structure permits.

A properly prepared endodontic access opening can eliminate many of the technical difficulties encountered in root canal treatment.[28,29] In fact, many of the problems that are discussed in this book in regard to locating and negotiating fine and calcified canals, cleaning and shaping, obturation, and retreatment may often be avoided or eliminated with a proper endodontic access opening.

The major consideration in all access openings is that coronal conservation of tooth structure should never preclude the proper design and execution of the access opening.

This admonition does not imply that radical removal of the coronal tooth structure is necessary simply to obtain unimpeded access to the pulpal space. Rather, it implies that the practitioner must be thoroughly knowledgeable about pulpal anatomy and external root anatomy and must be capable of proper radiographic assessment of the three-dimensional relationship of the pulpal space within the confines of the tooth.[23] When these factors are all considered, a properly placed and shaped access opening can be prepared. Failure to approach this initial technical step in root canal treatment in this manner not only invites problems during access opening preparation, but also unleashes a plethora of technical problems in all phases of treatment. Subsequently, treatment may be compromised or teeth unnecessarily lost.

This chapter identifies and discusses common problems in access preparation. Potential sequelae of the problems are noted in an effort to assist the practitioner in determining the true cause of prob-

---

*From Eidt: *Dominion Dent J* 12:231-233, 1900.
†From Hofheinz RH: *Dent Cosmos* 34:182-186, 1892.

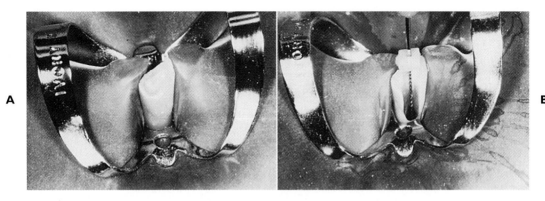

Fig. 3-1 *A, Isolation of a facially tipped mandibular incisor. The adjacent teeth have shifted in behind this tooth, blocking entry for a lingual access opening. B, Facial-incisal access opening.*

lems encountered in other phases of treatment. For example, failure or inability to locate a canal orifice or to properly shape a curved canal may be attributed to problems in canal preparation when in fact it may result from errors in access opening.

CLINICAL PROBLEM: A 37-year-old female presents with irreversible pulpitis in the mandibular left first molar (Fig. 3-2, *A*). Root canal treatment was initiated on the tooth, and the final radiograph shows poorly condensed canals with significant canal space apical to the gutta-percha filling in all canals (Fig. 3-2, *B*). The practitioner indicated that the mesial canals had been prepared to a size #30 and the distal canal to a size 35 K-file. The working length had been established 1 mm from the radiographic apex, and the final file sizes went to the full length in the root.

Solution: An assessment of the tooth in Fig. 3-2, *B* indicates that the roof of the pulp chamber has not been removed *(arrow)*. Failure to remove this anatomic obstruction would force the practitioner to prepare and obturate the canals through the pulp horns. A major constriction of this nature, because of an improper access opening, would significantly influence the quality of the canal cleaning and shaping and obturation. Yet the practitioner's problem focused on errors in obturation.

CONSIDERATIONS IN TOOTH ISOLATION

All access openings should be performed with a well-fitted and disinfected rubber dam in place.[25] Once placed, disinfection is performed with the use of 2.5% sodium hypochlorite.[16]

> The use of the rubber dam serves multiple purposes, which focus on patient protection and comfort, practitioner protection, and facilitation of treatment.

Adherence to this approach is especially important to ensure compliance with infection control guidelines. Studies have shown that microorganisms can be reduced to levels approaching 100% when the rubber dam is properly used.[7] Combined with gloves, mask, and protective eyewear, the rubber dam provides an excellent barrier to the potential spread of infection in the root canal system and within the environment of the dental office. Certain cases, however, may dictate subtle modifications of this injunction; the pertinent situations will be reviewed. Whenever possible, however, the entire access opening preparation should be performed with a rubber dam in place.[2,15,33] Specific tips in isolation are available in multiple publications[19,20] and can also be found later in this chapter and in Chapter 8.

MAJOR PROBLEMS (ERRORS) IN ACCESS OPENINGS

Errors in endodontic access openings generally occur in one of the following key problem areas:

1. Failure to identify and excavate all caries and to remove unsupported, weak tooth structure or faulty restorations.
2. Failure to establish proper access to the pulp chamber space and root canal system.

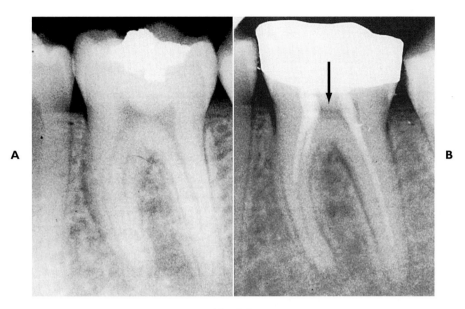

Fig. 3-2

3. Failure to identify the angle of the crown to the root and the angle of the tooth in the dental arch.
4. Failure to recognize potential problems in access openings through crowned teeth or teeth with excessively large restorations.

Failure to Identify and Excavate All Caries and Remove Unsupported, Weak Tooth Structure or Faulty Restorations

Removal of all compromised tooth structure is necessary for sound restorative dentistry. Removal of compromised tooth structure before the actual pulpal access is created not only ensures that sound, restorable tooth structure remains and that an uncontaminated environment can be established for aseptic root canal treatment, but also prevents the development of various problems during access preparation and subsequent treatment phases, such as:

1. Salivary and bacterial contamination of the canal system and periradicular tissues during and between treatment[21]
2. Inadequate assessment of the restorative needs of the tooth[21]
3. Loosening and packing of alloy or composite particles in the canals[17,32]
4. Fracture of tooth structure between treatments with loss of measurement reference points or loss of tooth[30]

CLINICAL PROBLEM: A 54-year-old man presents with episodic pain in the mandibular left quadrant. All teeth in this quadrant are extensively restored (Fig. 3-3, *A*). He thinks the pain is coming from the first molar, but he is not sure. There is pain to percussion on the first molar, with all others responding normally. Cold also elicits prolonged pain on the first molar, with normal responses on the adjacent and contralateral teeth. Periodontal probings are normal, as is palpation. An explorer can be placed under the mesiobuccal margin of the crown on the first molar. A radiograph shows an invasive carious lesion on the mesial of the first molar along with radiolucencies at the apices of both roots. The diagnosis is irreversible pulpitis with acute periradicular periodontitis (see Chapter 9). The dilemma with this case focuses on the access opening. Preparation of an access through the crown creates a situation where all the above problems (listed 1 to 4) can occur.

Solution: All potential problems with gaining access to the pulpal space can be prevented with crown removal. The tooth is isolated, and in this case the crown is cut off using a bur to cut a groove from buccal to lingual (Fig. 3-3, *B*). Attempting to retain the crown for future use is futile because the margins are seriously compromised. Figs. 3-3, *C* to *E* show the extent of the decay under the crown and the core. Ultimate removal of the core and the

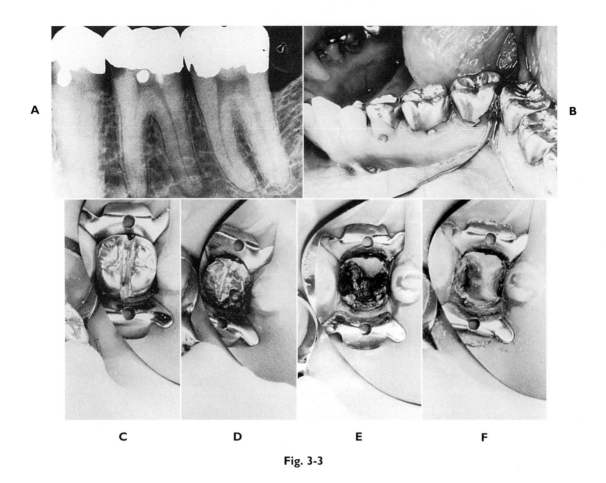

Fig. 3-3

decay (Fig. 3-3, *F*) provides excavated tooth margins, sound tooth structure, and the ability to assess the restorative needs (see Chapter 13), and direct and unimpeded access into the pulp chamber.

During excavation of the tooth that is being considered for root canal treatment, the peripheral carious tooth structure is removed first, and then caries is removed inward toward the pulp chamber (Fig. 3-4). Penetrating a pulp chamber where pulp is hyperemic or purulence has accumulated creates the difficulties of working in a confined space in a pool of blood or pus (Fig. 3- 5). Attempts to unroof a chamber or to enlarge the access at this point can lead to crown or furcation perforation. Careful excavation around the pulp chamber before penetration will generally avert this problem.

Along with caries excavation, removal of unsupported tooth structure and weakened or faulty restorations will enhance access to the canal system and visibility of tooth fractures (Fig. 3-6; see also Chapter 11) and help prevent fracture of fragile enamel walls and possibly the entire tooth during treatment. It will also remove restorations from the borders of the access opening, thereby preventing the loosening of alloy or composite particles that may enter and block the root canal system (Fig. 3-7), a common occurrence when large pin restorations or crowns are present. If the restoration is intact, total removal is not necessary. In these cases the operator should (1) use water during the access opening preparation to eliminate the debris and (2) flare the walls occlusally in an accentuated manner to enhance straight-line access (Fig. 3-8). This also prevents scraping of the metallic margins with the intracanal instruments and the carrying of metallic particles into the canal. However, removal of foreign debris inadvertently carried into the canal has been demonstrated with gentle ultrasonic canal instrumentation.[36] In cases where a temporary restorative material such as zinc oxide–eugenol, or Cavit (Premier Dental Products Co, Norristown, Penn.) is present, removal of the entire restoration is recommended except in those areas where avenues of leakage may be opened. However, crown lengthening may be the preferred alternative to leaving deep temporary restorations in place

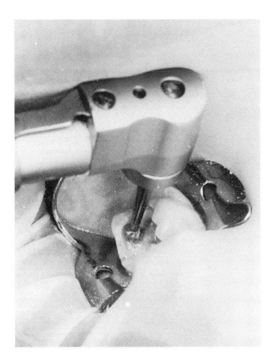

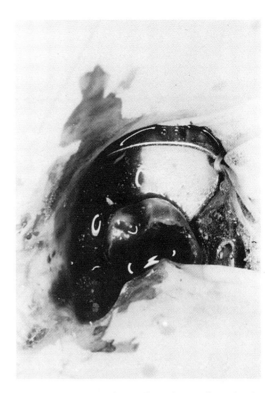

Fig. 3-4 *Caries around margins and under cusps must be excavated before the endodontic access opening is made.*

Fig. 3-5 *Excessive hemorrhage from inflamed pulp tissue can impair visualization of the pulp chamber.*

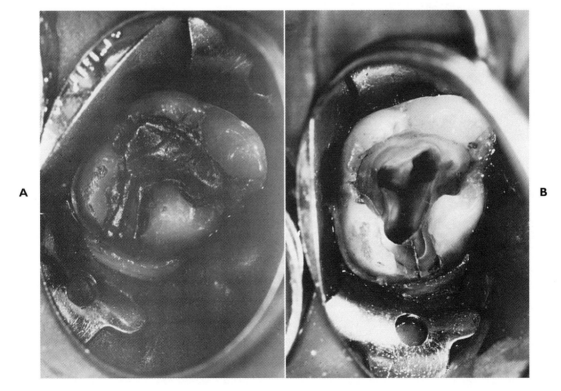

Fig. 3-6 *A, Maxillary molar requiring root canal treatment. Amalgam restoration has recurrent decay at its broken margins. B, Removal of the amalgam reveals a vertical fracture on the palatal margin.*

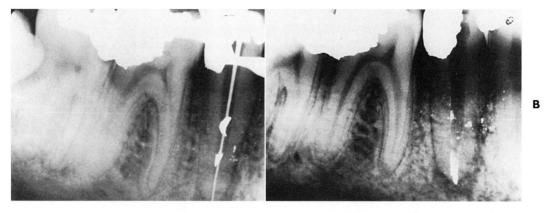

Fig. 3-7 *A,* *Alloy particles loosened around the margins of the access opening have entered the canal space.* ***B,*** *Aggressive attempts to remove alloy particles caused packing of the foreign material in the apical third of the canal.*

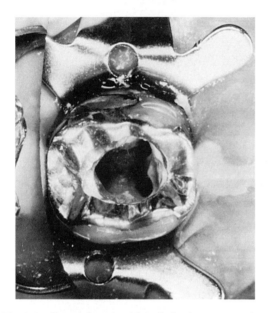

Fig. 3-8 *Crowned tooth with endodontic access opening. There is visibility of all canals when viewed from the occlusal.*

▼ **Table 3-1** Specific indications for restoration removal

COMPELLING REASONS TO REMOVE RESTORATIONS

- Evidence of continued leakage during treatment
- Unexpected carious invasion beneath restorations, especially full crowns
- Fractures uncovered during access preparation
- Loose, defective, or undermined restorations
- Treatment-planned restoration replacement

REASONS OF CONVENIENCE TO REMOVE RESTORATIONS

- Malpositioned teeth or restorations, which may impede direct access to the canals
- Need to search for calcified orifices
- Need to establish tooth restorability, especially with possible chamber perforations
- Need to enhance clinician orientation

(see Chapter 8). Indications for restoration removal can be found in Table 3-1.

Failure to Establish Proper Access to the Pulp Chamber Space and Root Canal System

Pulp chamber spaces are generally located in the center of the crown (Fig. 3-9, *A* and *B*).[41,42] However, age changes or pulpal response to irritation (such as caries, restorative procedures) will change the dimensions of the space visible on a good-quality two-dimensional radiograph (Fig. 3-9, *C* to *F*). In many cases, especially when large restorations are present, bite-wing radiographs are necessary for proper visualization of the chamber space (Fig. 3-9, *G* and *H*). Often, angled radiographs (from the mesial and distal aspects) will also be necessary when teeth are rotated or have abnormal root configurations.

Access opening preparation is a dynamic, three-dimensional process.[23] The old adage in access opening preparation, "Go for the pulp horns," is

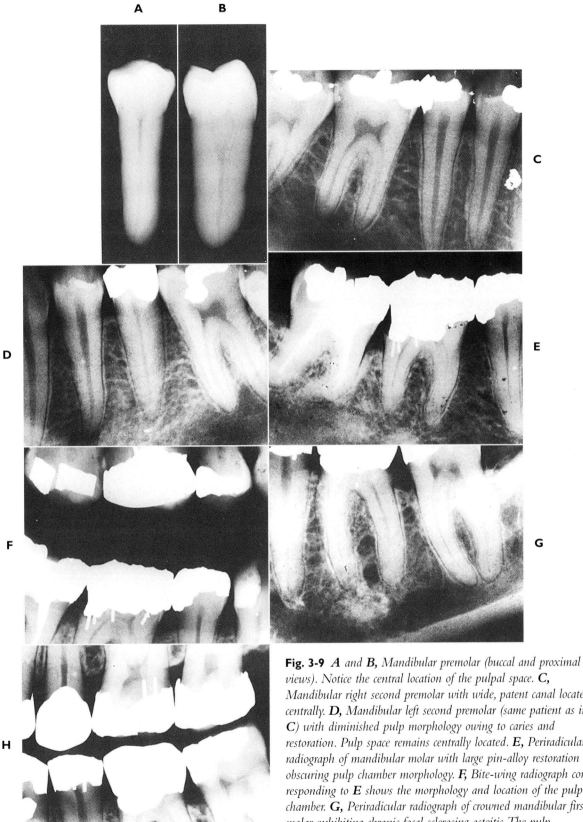

Fig. 3-9 *A and B, Mandibular premolar (buccal and proximal views). Notice the central location of the pulpal space. C, Mandibular right second premolar with wide, patent canal located centrally. D, Mandibular left second premolar (same patient as in C) with diminished pulp morphology owing to caries and restoration. Pulp space remains centrally located. E, Periradicular radiograph of mandibular molar with large pin-alloy restoration obscuring pulp chamber morphology. F, Bite-wing radiograph corresponding to E shows the morphology and location of the pulp chamber. G, Periradicular radiograph of crowned mandibular first molar exhibiting chronic focal sclerosing osteitis. The pulp chamber is not visible. The canals are very fine, with linear calcification. H, Bite-wing radiograph corresponding to G reveals now-visible pulp chamber on the mesial aspect as a result of the presence of an alloy under the crown. The presence of the alloy further complicates access to the mesial aspects of the chamber.*

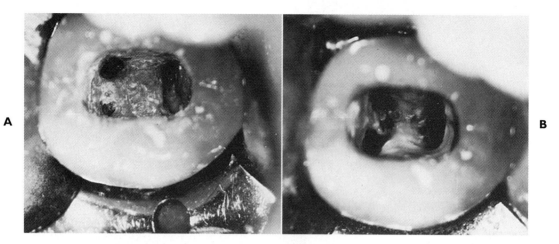

Fig. 3-10 *A, Mandibular molar with access opening, referred for treatment because of constant pain during attempts to enter the canal orifices. Notice that only pulp horns are exposed and pulp chamber roof is intact. **B,** Ideal access with roof removed.*

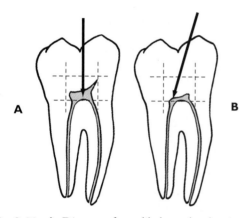

Fig. 3-11 *A, Diagram of mandibular molar showing anticipated parameters of the pulp chamber. Access entry must proceed into the center of these parameters (arrow). **B,** Access entry may be directed to the largest canal (arrow) in cases of tooth misalignment, calcification, or lack of visible pulp chamber.*

reasonable in cases of severely diminished pulp-chamber spaces only to the extent that the practitioner understands the pulp horns represent only a very small area of the pulp chamber at its borders. The dentin between the horns must also be removed (Fig. 3-10).

Entry into the chamber within the coronal-apical and mesiodistal parameters is more efficient and effective and less conducive to errors in misdirection and misalignment of the bur.

It also minimizes the failure to distinguish the pulpal horns from the canal orifices. In some cases this may mean directing the bur toward the largest or the only visible chamber and canal space,[37] such as the distal canal of mandibular molars or the palatal canal of maxillary molars (Fig. 3-11). Therefore time must be spent by the practitioner to (1) assess accurately the pulp chamber morphology, (2) note the coronal-apical and mesiodistal dimensions of the space, and (3) identify the positions of the orifices as they leave the pulp chamber (Fig. 3-12). Failure to operate within these parameters commonly leads to the following problems[12]:

1. Failure to completely unroof the pulp chamber
2. Failure to locate all canals
3. Excessive gouging in the chamber walls and floor
4. Perforation of the chamber wall or floor

Anterior Teeth‡

In anterior teeth, removal of the lingual ledge and incisal edge is essential to obtain straight-line access to the canal system. Ideally these anatomic obstructions should be removed by cutting using an outstroke to prevent gouging or perforation (Fig. 3-13). Once they have been removed, complete access to the canal space is achieved, and such access allows penetration to the apical constriction and enhances thorough canal cleaning and shaping (Fig. 3-14, *A*). In addition, proper removal of

---

‡Burs recommended for penetration: Nos. 2 and 4 round. Burs recommended for refinement: No. 4 round with tapered diamond shank; No. 557R or 701R; Gates-Glidden burs.

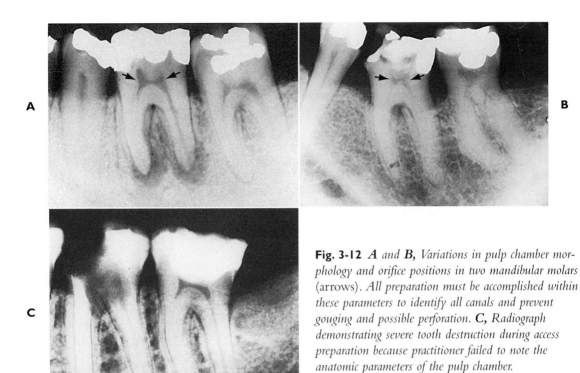

A

B

C

Fig. 3-12 *A and B, Variations in pulp chamber morphology and orifice positions in two mandibular molars (arrows). All preparation must be accomplished within these parameters to identify all canals and prevent gouging and possible perforation. C, Radiograph demonstrating severe tooth destruction during access preparation because practitioner failed to note the anatomic parameters of the pulp chamber.*

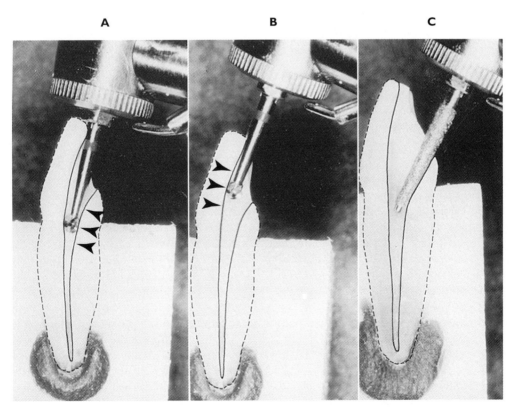

A   **B**   **C**

Fig. 3-13 *Cross-sectional diagrams illustrating removal of the lingual ledge, **A,** and incisal edge, **B.** All cutting is done on the outstroke. A safe-ended diamond bur, **C,** can also be used to flare the walls of the access opening.*

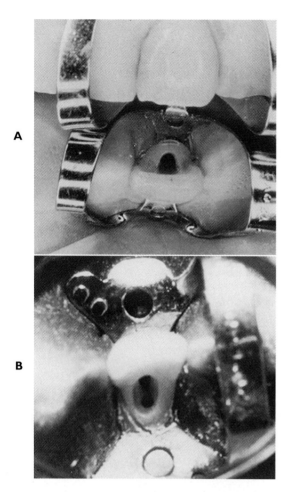

Fig. 3-14 *A, Access opening in maxillary central incisor, demonstrating straight-line access to the pulp space. B, Access opening in mandibular incisor extended lingually. Note second canal located under the cingulum.*

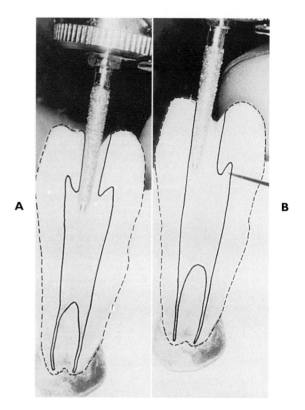

Fig. 3-15 *A, Safe-ended diamond bur is placed adjacent to the overhanging ledges of the pulp chamber roof. B, Lateral cutting will safely remove the roof of the pulp chamber and flare the access preparation occlusally.*

the lingual ledge will often uncover extra canals in mandibular incisors, canines, and premolars (Fig. 3-14, *B*). Failure to locate these canals often leads to severe postoperative pain or ultimate treatment failure (see Chapter 1). Often the blame for failure of this nature is transferred to the patient or the tooth, when in fact the practitioner should have full knowledge and control in these situations.

Posterior Teeth§

Failure to remove the entire roof of the pulp chamber is a common problem that precludes locating the canal systems in posterior teeth. To ensure complete removal of the roof, the practitioner should adhere to the following guidelines:

1. Measure the size and depth of the pulp chamber space on the radiograph by holding the mounted bur in the handpiece next to the image of the crown on the radiograph.
2. Place a safe-ended bur adjacent to the overhanging roof and cut laterally to unroof the overlying dentin and to flare the walls of the access opening occlusally (Fig. 3-15).
3. Use a No. 17 or No. 23 explorer to evaluate the removal of the roof or dentin overhangs.
4. Visually inspect the chamber to ensure an unobstructed entry into the canal systems.

Once the pulp chamber of the posterior tooth is opened to good visualization, recognition of the commonly observed anatomic relationships seen on the floor of the chamber is essential to determine the location of the orifices and to prevent perforations. Fig. 3-16 depicts commonly seen

§Burs recommended for penetration: Nos. 4 and 6 round or 701. Burs recommended for refinement: safe-ended tapered diamond burs.

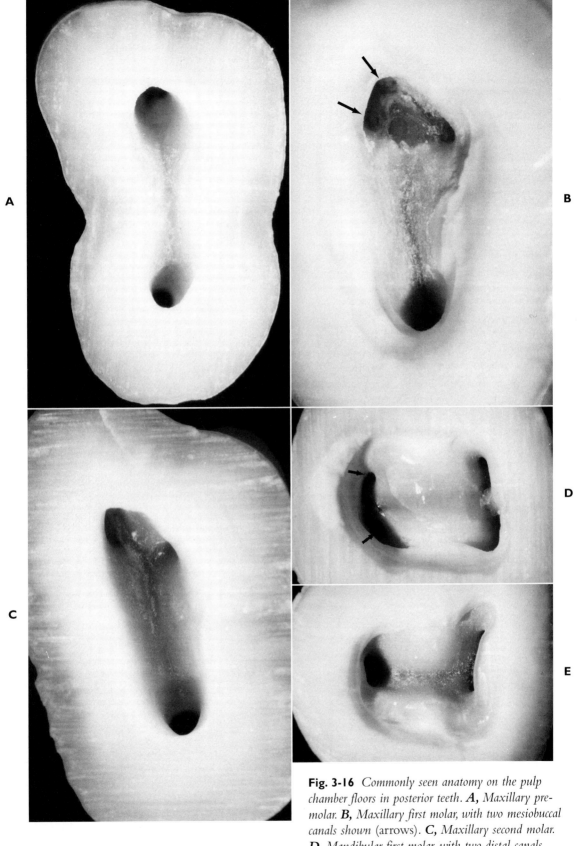

Fig. 3-16 *Commonly seen anatomy on the pulp chamber floors in posterior teeth. **A,** Maxillary premolar. **B,** Maxillary first molar, with two mesiobuccal canals shown (arrows). **C,** Maxillary second molar. **D,** Mandibular first molar, with two distal canals shown (arrows). **E,** Mandibular second molar.*

chamber floors in a maxillary two-rooted premolar, maxillary first and second molars, and mandibular first and second molars. Recognition of these anatomic designs and integration of this information with the radiographic findings will prevent problems during both the access preparation and the canal orifice location.

In the refinement of posterior access openings, removal of cervical ledges is important because these often impede a straight-line entry into the canal or cover up additional canals.[18,37] It is recommended that ledges be carefully removed using lateral cutting while tapering the internal wall occlusally and avoiding any apical penetration.

CLINICAL PROBLEM: Both mandibular and maxillary molars present with cervical ledges or bulges that cover over main and secondary canal orifices. Notice the maxillary molar in Fig. 3-17, *A*. The arrows indicate the location of the ledges. Also these ledges severely constrict the opening in the chamber. Fig. 3-17, *B*, is a cross section of a molar that exhibits the anatomic relationship of these ledges to the pulp horns and chamber. The arrows indicate the ledge location. When accessing the pulp chamber of the molar in Fig. 3-17, *A,* the floor of the chamber with ledges appears in Fig. 3-17, *C*. The challenge to the practitioner is to unroof the ledges and identify the canal orifices without gouging or perforating the tooth structure. Here again, all cutting must be done within the confines of the pulp chamber.

Solution: Using a No. 2 or 4 round bur in a dry chamber, the bur is placed in the position of the mesiobuccal orifice. Carefully it is brought toward the palatal orifice while it cuts into the cervical ledge in a buccopalatal direction. Depth perception is especially crucial to prevent excessive gouging of the chamber floor. The ledge is usually not thicker or deeper than the size of the bur head on a No. 4 round bur. Once the ledge is removed, not only is the main mesiobuccal canal clearly accessible, but also the fourth, or mesiopalatal, canal is unroofed (Fig. 3-17, *D* and *E*).

In addition to identifying extra canal orifices (Fig. 3-17, *D* and *E*), removal of the cervical ledges is especially important to facilitate initial entry into extremely curved canals. This is common in maxillary molars, where the curved mesiobuccal root often contains two canals (Fig. 3-18).[31,40] Failure to locate and clean this canal is a common cause of posttreatment problems such as pain, swelling, sensitivity to heat or cold on an endodontically treated tooth, pain to percussion localized in

the mesiobuccal root, or the development of a sinus tract in the mucobuccal fold adjacent to this root. In addition, failure to remove the cervical ledge that overlies the orifice of extremely curved canals restricts entry into the first 1 or 2 mm of canal space, and ledges often occur in the canal. Additional treatment parameters to correct or eliminate this problem are discussed in Chapters 4 and 5.

Although many errors can occur during access preparations, the most deleterious is perforation of the pulp-chamber space into the oral cavity or periodontal tissues. Attention to the radiographic position of the pulp-chamber space before access opening preparation will most often prevent this problem. Likewise, knowledge of the anatomy of the floor of the pulp chamber and of the location of the canal orifices will also enhance the practitioner's orientation and prevention of perforations. However, if it occurs, it should be recognized as soon as possible. Early recognition will prevent needless irritation and further insult to the periodontal tissues.[35] If the perforation occurs above the osseous crest in the gingival sulcus or above the free gingival margin (Fig. 3-19), consider the following measures:

1. Control the hemorrhage with a dry cotton pellet or the large end of a paper point, or consider epinephrine 1:50,000 on the pellet or other hemostatic agent, such as Cut-Trol (Ichthys Enterprises, Mobile, Ala.), which contains ferric sulfate (Fig. 3-20). *Do not use intracanal medicaments such as formocresol.*
2. Seal with a temporary cement, such as Cavit (zinc oxide–eugenol mixture).
3. Proceed with root canal treatment.
4. Plan to restore the perforated area separately or make such restoration part of the total tooth restoration. Adjunctive periodontal treatment may be necessary (see Chapter 8).[38]

If the perforation is at or below the osseous crest (Fig. 3-21, *A*) or into the furcation region (Fig. 3-21, *B* and *C*), the following steps can be considered; however, the prognosis for these cases is very poor.[17,25,35]

1. The perforation must be sealed immediately.
2. If the perforation is close to a canal orifice, place a file, gutta-percha cone, or silver cone into the canal to prevent the placement of any material in the canal during the repair.
3. Hemorrhage must be controlled and a hemostatic agent is recommended. If it cannot be controlled because of the size of the perforation, calcium hydroxide powder[3,22,25] or a

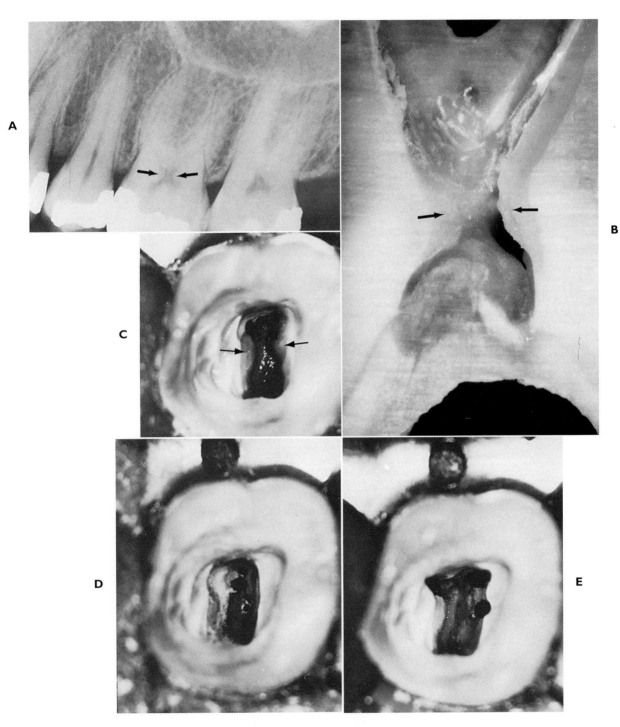

Fig. 3-17

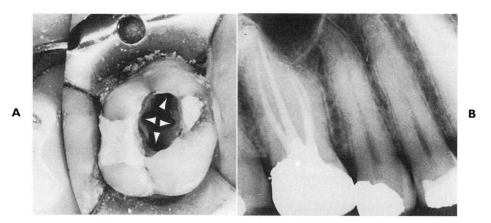

Fig. 3-18 *A, Different maxillary molar with access opening depicting four separate canals after ledge removal (arrowheads). B, Radiograph demonstrating two canals in the mesiobuccal root.*

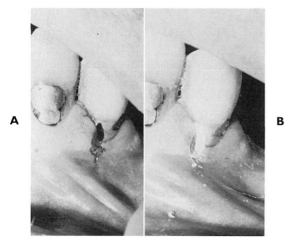

Fig. 3-19 *A, Buccal surface of a mandibular first premolar was perforated at the level of the gingival sulcus during access preparation. B, Temporary sealing of the perforation with Cavit before root canal cleaning and shaping.*

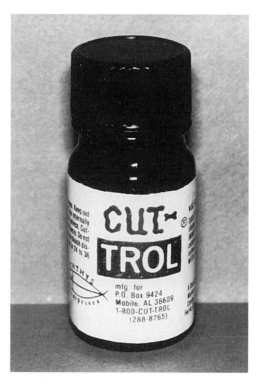

Fig. 3-20 *Liquid hemostatic agent, Cut-Trol, a solution of ferric sulfate.*

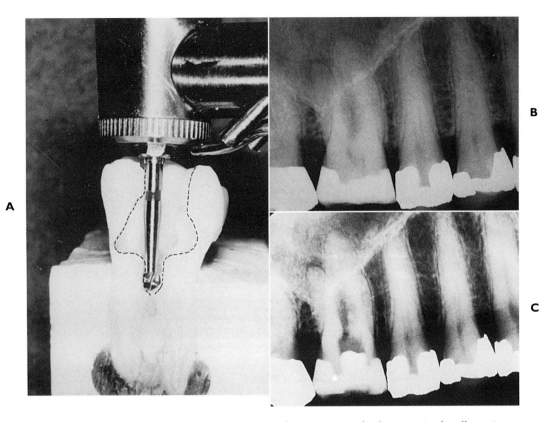

Fig. 3-21 *A, Tooth model illustrating how excessive bur penetration leads to proximal wall gouging and furcation perforation. B, Radiograph showing a reduced pulp chamber space in the maxillary molar. C, Perforation of the furcation during access preparation. Also notice excessive gouging in the mesiodistal parameters based on the morphology of the chamber shown in B.*

fast-setting, pulp-capping agent such as Dycal (LD Caulk Co., Milford, Del.) may be considered. Also effective as a hemostatic agent is the placement of Gelfoam (Upjohn Co, Kalamazoo, Mich.) into the perforation site.[38] In addition to hemorrhage control, the initial placement of Gelfoam into the site provides a scaffold on which to pack Cavit,[14,17] zinc oxide–eugenol,[24] alloy,[1,4,8] or Super EBA (H.J. Bosworth Co., Skokie, Ill.) cement to seal the perforation.[26] All patent orifices must be protected to prevent entry of any filling material. Presently new healing-inductive materials are being evaluated for their use in perforation repair, and the future successful management of these defects looks promising.

4. Try to avoid pushing any sealing material into the periradicular tissues.[4,35]

Although the prognosis for furcation perforations is questionable, some clinical success with

nonsurgical treatment has been reported.[10,14,22] Surgical repair of furcation perforations is futile at best, and often the tooth must be extracted or root or tooth resection (hemisection) must be considered (see Chapters 8 and 12).[9,13,25,38]

In single-rooted teeth, perforations in the cervical third during access preparation also have a highly guarded prognosis. However, with adjunctive periodontal or orthodontic treatment, the cases may be managed with simple surgical repair[9] or root extrusion[34] (Fig. 3-22) (see also Chapter 8).

Failure to Identify the Angle of the Crown to the Root and the Angle of the Tooth in the Dental Arch

Good-quality periradicular radiographs, though only two dimensional, are essential for determining the anatomic relationship of the crown to the root and the angle of the root in the arch.[23] When aberrations are suspected, the practitioner should antic-

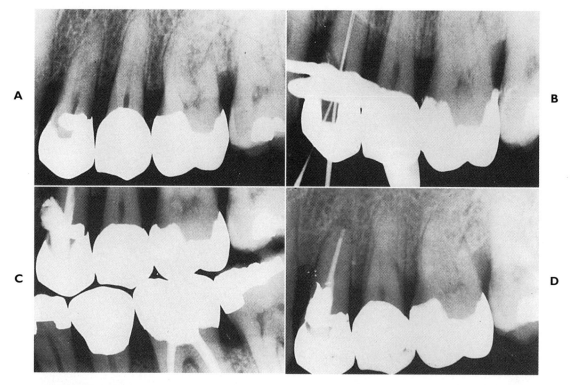

Fig. 3-22 *A, Radiograph of an intact maxillary first premolar exhibiting irreversible pulpitis. **B,** Working-length radiograph. Notice perforation under mesial crown margin at osseous crest in the coronal third. **C,** Zinc oxide–eugenol temporary filling placed at time of obturation. **D,** Alloy seal of root perforation along with slight osseous recontouring.*

ipate possible deviations in the third dimension. Teeth that normally exhibit significant crown-root angulations are maxillary lateral incisors and mandibular first premolars. The crowns of these teeth are often perforated during access preparation as a result of misalignment of the bur with the long axis of the root.

Additional problems that can occur when angulations are not considered include the following:

1. Misidentification of canals (thinking that the mesiolingual canal is the mesiobuccal canal)
2. Inability to locate the canal
3. Missing extra canals
4. Undermining and weakening coronal or radicular tooth structure, even if a perforation does not occur

The best way to manage these problems is to prevent them. As previously mentioned, recognition of deviations and thorough radiographic review are essential (see Chapter 2). As an aid to orientation, the initial outline form and bur penetration during access preparation can sometimes be accomplished without a rubber dam. This facilitates proper bur alignment with the long axis of

the tooth. Second, alignment of bur penetration for both depth and angulation can be confirmed with radiographs (Fig. 3-23). Third, if the tooth is severely misaligned in the arch, removal of specific portions of the crown may be warranted to facilitate an unconventional yet satisfactory access into the pulpal space (see Fig. 3-1).[6]

Failure to Recognize Potential Problems in Access Openings through Crowned Teeth

A significant portion of root canal treatment is performed through existing crowns. The presence of these metallic and porcelain-to-metal restorations can add additional problems to those previously discussed. The following guidelines deserve special attention during access preparations in crowns.

1. All potential avenues of carious leakage under crown margins must be determined and eliminated (see Fig. 3-3). If crowns must be remade or if the periodontal status dictates better marginal relationships of crown to soft tissue and osseous crest, crown removal is indicated to facilitate total tooth treatment (Fig. 3-24).

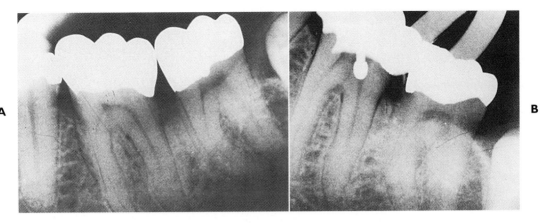

Fig. 3-23 *A,* Mandibular first molar with crown and decreased pulp chamber space visible on the radiograph. *B,* Confirmation of bur position during access preparation. Notice bur angle directed at the largest canal (see Fig 3-11, B).

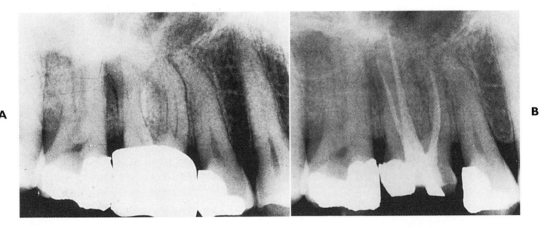

Fig. 3-24 *A,* Maxillary first molar with poorly contoured crown margins. The pulp chamber is not visible. Remake of the crown is indicated, along with assessment of the local periodontium. *B,* Crown removal facilitated restorative and periodontal assessment and enhanced access to the pulp chamber and root canal treatment.

2. Bite-wing radiographs may assist in pulp chamber location in some cases; however, most crowns obscure the pulp chamber space on periradicular radiographs.

3. Root structure or natural crown structure under full-coverage restorations may be rotated or misaligned with normal tooth position and arch configuration.

4. Most crowns have extensive alloy or composite buildups that often impede direct access and chamber or orifice location.

5. Visibility into the dark access openings in crowns is limited.

6. Porcelain-to-metal crowns are subject to fracture or craze lines during access preparation. This is especially true for old porcelain jacket crowns.

7. Newer, nonprecious alloys are very hard and impede access preparation.

8. Failure to use water during access opening preparation in crowns may leave large metallic deposits in the pulp chamber or canal orifices.

9. The artificial occlusal or lingual anatomy of a crown restoration does not serve as a guide to the access opening entry.

10. The presence of crowns may obscure fractures in the tooth structure, especially the proximal walls or floor of the chamber (see Chapter 11).

Most of these concerns can be addressed (or problems prevented) when preparing an access opening through a crown.

As with naturally occurring crown-root angulations, a thorough radiographic evaluation is necessary to identify angled roots. Subsequently, the following recommendations can be considered.

1. Use a fiberoptic system for increased visibility.
2. Prepare the initial access through the crown without a rubber dam.
3. Evaluate the shape of the alveolar process over the root surface in the cervical area below the margin of the crown.
4. Before cutting the access opening, measure the bur against the radiograph to estimate the depth of penetration relative to the position of the furcation.
5. Use water spray and proceed slowly with high-speed diamond burs to protect any porcelain present. Advise the patient ahead of time of a possible fracture.
6. Using a diamond bur under water spray, cut the porcelain in a light, shaving manner (as opposed to using heavy pressure and long cutting times). Once the porcelain has been penetrated, switch to a sharp carbide bur to complete the access preparation.
7. After entry into the pulp space, restrict all cutting to a lateral or outstroke movement; irrigate often.
8. Flare the walls of the access opening to the occlusal side for posterior teeth or the lingual side for anterior teeth to prevent contact with the intracanal instruments.
9. Probe for possible avenues of carious leakage or fractures.
10. If necessary, do not hesitate to open the coronal outline of the access beyond a standard size access to facilitate canal location and exploration. The integrity of the crown resides in the gingival margins, not the occlusal surface. As previously mentioned, conservation of tooth (crown) anatomy does not preclude using the necessary avenue of access (Fig. 3-25), especially if restorations are to be remade.
11. Irrigate the prepared coronal access well before entering any of the canals. This will help prevent carrying metallic or composite fragments into the canal space.

Adherence to these preventive problem-solving approaches will help the practitioner avoid problems in canal identification, creation of artificial canals, missing aberrant canals, weakening of tooth structure, and two very common problems—postoperative discomfort and tooth perforation.

It is important to remember that access preparations are not complete until all the orifices have been properly exposed and convenient, unobstructed access to these orifices has been established.

TIPS IN TOOTH ISOLATION AND ACCESS-OPENING PREPARATIONS

The following tips may be of assistance in unique clinical situations to facilitate tooth isolation and access preparation.

1. If the rubber dam clamp cannot be positioned on the tooth to be treated, consider clamping adjacent teeth (Fig. 3-26). Further control of moisture can be achieved with Cavit, Oraseal (Ultradent Products, Inc., Salt Lake City, Utah), medical adhesives (Stomahesive, Squibb, Novo Inc., Princeton, New Jersey),[5,11] a rubber base, or floss.
2. If isolation can only be achieved by clamping the tissue, then crown lengthening is necessary and should precede definitive root canal treatment (see Chapter 8).
3. Remove temporary crowns before isolation and access whenever possible. This prevents dislodgment during canal preparation, potential contamination during or after treatment, unstable reference points, and leakage of irrigant into the mouth.

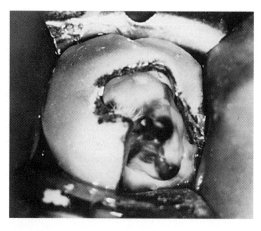

Fig. 3-25 *Buccal and occlusal access opening to facilitate entry through a crown to retreat root canals. Crown was to be remade.*

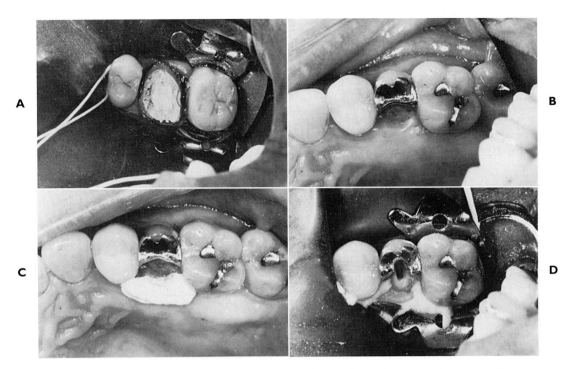

Fig. 3-26 *A, Clamping of adjacent teeth to facilitate isolation of a tooth prepared for a crown. B, Maxillary premolar with subgingivally fractured palatal cusp. C, Placement of Oraseal along the palatal margin. D, Rubber dam sealed in place. Access opening and canal prepared in an isolated field.*

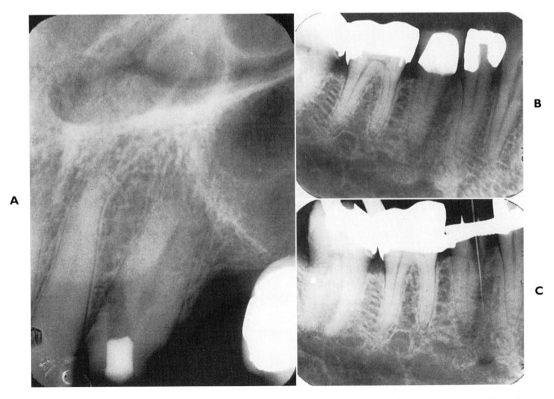

Fig. 3-27 *Incorrect angle of handpiece and bur led to serious subosseous perforation in canine, A, and premolar (B and C).*

4. Draw a line on the crown indicating the angle of the root when creating an access opening under a rubber dam. Failure to determine excessive root angulation often leads to a perforation (Fig. 3-27).

5. Exercise care in crown penetration when using long-shank or surgical-length burs.

6. In severely calcified pulp chambers, consider using only slow-speed burs for penetration through the roof of the chamber.

7. If a perforation should occur and a white material such as calcium hydroxide or zinc oxide–eugenol is used to repair the aberrant opening, place a small amount of dye (such as methylene blue, or red food coloring) in the filling material for easy identification inside the access opening.

References

1. Aguirre R, ElDeeb ME, ElDeeb M: Evaluation of the repair of mechanical furcation perforations using amalgam, gutta-percha, or indium foil, *J Endod* 12:249-256, 1986.

2. Barkmeier WW, Cooley RL, Abrams H: Prevention of swallowing or aspiration of foreign objects, *J Am Dent Assoc* 97:473-476, 1978.

3. Beavers RA, Bergenholtz G, Cox CF: Periodontal wound healing following intentional root perforations in permanent teeth of *Macaca mulatta, Int Endod J* 19:36-44, 1986.

4. Benenati FW, Roane JR, Biggs JT et al: Recall evaluation of iatrogenic root perforations repaired with amalgam and gutta-percha, *J Endod* 12:161-166, 1986.

5. Bramwell JD, Hicks ML: Solving isolation problems with rubber base adhesive, *J Endod* 12:363-367, 1986.

6. Cathey GM: Molar endodontics, *Dent Clin North Am* 18:345-366, 1974.

7. Cochran MA, Miller CH, Sheldrake MA: The efficacy of the rubber dam as a barrier to the spread of microorganisms during dental treatment, *J Am Dent Assoc* 119:141-144, 1989.

8. ElDeeb ME, ElDeeb M, Tabibi A et al: An evaluation of the use of amalgam, Cavit, and calcium hydroxide in the repair of furcation perforations, *J Endod* 8:459-466, 1982.

9. Frank AL: Resorption, perforation, and fractures, *Dent Clin North Am* 18:465-487, 1974.

10. Frank AL, Simon JHS, Abou-Rass M et al: *Clinical and surgical endodontics: concepts in practice*–Philadelphia, 1983, JB Lippincott Co, pp 51-60.

11. Fors UGH, Berg J-O, Sandberg H: Microbiological investigation of saliva leakage between the rubber dam and tooth during endodontic treatment, *J Endod* 12:396-399, 1986.

12. Gutmann JL: Prevention and management of endodontic procedural errors, *NZ Soc Endod Newslett* 23:15-36, 1983.

13. Gutmann JL, Harrison JW: *Surgical endodontics,* St. Louis, 1994, IEA Publishers Inc, pp 409-448.

14. Harris WE: A simplified method of treatment for endodontic perforations, *J Endod* 2:126-134, 1976.

15. Heling B, Heling I: Endodontic procedures must never be performed without the rubber dam, *Oral Surg Oral Med Oral Pathol* 43:464-466, 1977.

16. Hermsen KP, Ludlow MO: Disinfection of rubber dam and tooth surfaces before endodontic therapy, *Gen Dent* 35:355-356, 1987.

17. Jew RCK, Weine FS, Keene JJ et al: A histologic evaluation of periodontal tissues adjacent to root perforations filled with Cavit, *Oral Surg Oral Med Oral Pathol* 54:124-n-135, 1982;.

18. Leeb IJ: Canal orifice enlargement as related to biomechanical preparation, *J Endod* 9:463-470, 1983.

19. Liebenberg WH: Access and isolation problem solving in endodontics: anterior teeth, *Can Dent J* 59:663-671, 1993.

20. Liebenberg WH: Access and isolation problem solving in endodontics: posterior teeth, *Can Dent J* 59:817-822, 1993.

21. Lovdahl PE, Gutmann JL: Periodontal and restorative considerations prior to endodontic therapy, *J Acad Gen Dent* 23:38-45, 1980.

22. Martin LR, Gilbert B, Dickerson AW: Management of endodontic perforations, *Oral Surg Oral Med Oral Pathol* 54:668-677, 1982.

23. Moreinis SA: Avoiding perforation during endodontic access, *J Am Dent Assoc* 98:707-712, 1979.

24. Nicholls E: Treatment of traumatic perforations of the pulp cavity, *Oral Surg Oral Med Oral Pathol* 15:603-612, 1962.

25. Oswald RJ: Procedural accidents and their repair, *Dent Clin North Am* 23:593-616, 1979.

26. Oynick J, Oynick T: Treatment of endodontic perforations, *J Endod* 11:191-192, 1985.

27. Reid JS, Callis PD, Patterson CJW: *Rubber dam in clinical practice,* Chicago, 1991, Quintessence Publishing Co Ltd.

28. Robinson D, Goerig AC, Neaverth EJ: Endodontic access: an update, part I, *Compend Contin Educ Dent* 10:290-298, 1989.

29. Robinson D, Goerig AC, Neaverth EJ: Endodontic access: an update, part II, *Compend Contin Educ Dent* 10:328-333, 1989.

30. Schultz HH, Goerig AC: Helpful hints in endodontics: part I, *Dent Surv* 56:32-38, 1980.

31. Seidberg BH, Altman M, Guttuso J et al: Frequency of two mesiobuccal root canals in maxillary permanent molars, *J Am Dent Assoc* 87:852-856, 1973.

32. Shankle RJ: Extension for convenience in root canal therapy, *J Acad Gen Dent* 29:62-n-64, 1981.

33. Sherard JH Jr: Diffusion update. In Gerstein H, editor: *Techniques in clinical endodontics,* Philadelphia, 1983, WB Saunders Co, p 102.

34. Simon JHS, Kelly WH, Gordon DG et al: Extrusion of endodontically treated teeth, *J Am Dent Assoc* 97:17-23, 1978.

35. Sinai IH: Endodontic perforations: their prognosis and treatment, *J Am Dent Assoc* 95:90-95, 1977.

36. Stamos DG, Haasch GC, Chenail B et al: Endosonics: clinical impressions, *J Endod* 11:181-187, 1985.

37. Strieff JT, Gerstein H: Access cavity preparation. In Gerstein H, editors: *Techniques in Clinical Endodontics,* Philadelphia, 1983, WB Saunders Co, pp 1-41.

38. Tidmarsh BG: Accidental perforation of the roots of teeth, *J Oral Rehabil* 6:235-240, 1979.

39. Walia H, Strieff J, Gerstein H: Use of a hemostatic agent in the repair of procedural errors, *J Endod* 14:465-468, 1988.

40. Weine FS, Healey HJ, Gerstein H et al: Canal configuration in the mesiobuccal root of the maxillary first molar and its endodontic significance, *Oral Surg Oral Med Oral Pathol*–28:419-425, 1969.

41. Wolcox LR, Walton RE: The shape and location of mandibular premolar access openings, *Int Endod J* 20:223-227, 1987.

42. Wilcox LR, Walton RE, Case WB: Molar access: shape and outline according to orifice locations, *J Endod* 15:315-318, 1989.

Chapter 4

Problems in Locating and Negotiating Fine and Calcified Canals

Paul E. Lovdahl

James L. Gutmann

"It is seldom that we see canals in buccal roots of superior molars, or in roots of lower molars, in which a drill can be used; . . . There are canals that are constricted just at the chamber, sometimes so much so that they can scarcely be found . . . There are canals in curved roots and canals obstructed by osseous growths that, if not properly opened, would most likely cause trouble. It is with this difficult class of root-canals that I wish to deal at this time."*

Dystrophic and excessive linear calcification in the root canal system is a frequently encountered problem in root canal treatment.[4] To assess properly the possible nature of this calcific response, thereby facilitating clinical problem-solving techniques, it is necessary to review the types of calcification that can occur in the pulp. The clinician must understand that pulpal calcifications are signs of the pathosis, not the cause.[14,18]

PULPAL RESPONSES TO IRRITATION
Rapid Death with Canal Patency

When the pulp is subjected to a rapid and overwhelming bacterial invasion or traumatic insult, little time exists for reparative dentin formation. The pulp chamber and canal system remain patent and easily accessible (Fig. 4-1). Radiographically the canal space is patent and root canal treatment is straightforward.

---

*From Callahan Jr: *Dent Cosmos* 36:329-331, 1894.

Irritational Response with Pulpal Demise

Often an irritated pulp can mount a reparative response for a variable time before demise. These cases will present with a variety of appearances, such as extensive diffuse calcification (Fig. 4-2), isolated pulp stones (Fig. 4-3), or extensive irregular linear calcification characterized by gnarled, atubular dentin (Fig. 4-4). Radiographically these cases give a hint of a canal space in varying positions in the root. More often than not, these canals can be negotiated and treated nonsurgically.

Extensive Irritational Response and Pulp System Closure

This histologic appearance generally reflects a long-term response to a continuous low-grade irritation. Radiographically this will appear as complete calcification with histologic support confirming complete canal closure, except for a few small areas containing minimal tissue remnants (Fig. 4-5). Successful negotiation of this type of canal to its apical extent is extremely difficult.

Fortunately, only a small percentage of cases that radiographically exhibit fine or unidentifiable canals or calcified blockages prove to be untreatable by nonsurgical root canal techniques. Of the numerous techniques available to the practitioner to locate and negotiate these canals, only those

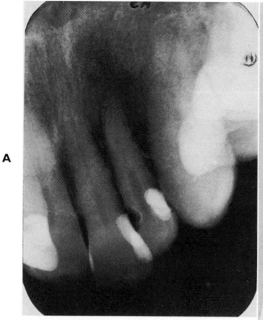

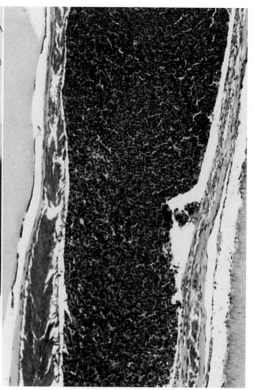

Fig. 4-1 *A,* *Maxillary lateral incisor with evidence of previous caries on distal surface. Pulp chamber and coronal third of the canal are normal in size with canal size reduced in the apical third; however, canal is patent.* ***B,*** *Abscess present in pulp canal; no reparative dentin is noted on walls; patency is ensured. (Hematoxylin and eosin, 100×.)*

procedures known to be most effective in clinical practice are considered here.

Success in negotiating small or calcified canals is predicated on a proper access opening and identification of the canal orifice or orifices.

To locate the calcified orifice, the practitioner first mentally visualizes and projects the normal spatial relationship of the pulp space onto a radiograph of the calcified tooth. Then the two-dimensional radiographic image is correlated with the three-dimensional morphology of the tooth. Thereafter access preparation is initiated, with the rotary instrument directed toward the presumed location of the pulpal space. This approach requires knowledge of the normal pulp chamber location, root canal anatomy, and the long axis of the roots, especially in posterior teeth.[10] Accurate radiographs are essential for preoperative visualization and periodic assessment of bur penetration and orientation (see Chapter 2). Finally, the practitioner must be able to recognize the calcified orifice when it has been reached.

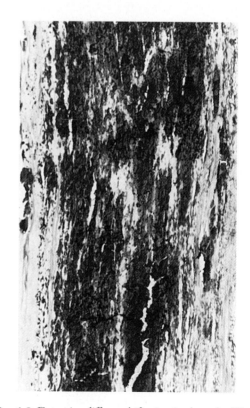

Fig. 4-2 *Extensive diffuse calcification in the pulp. (Hematoxylin and eosin, 100×.)*

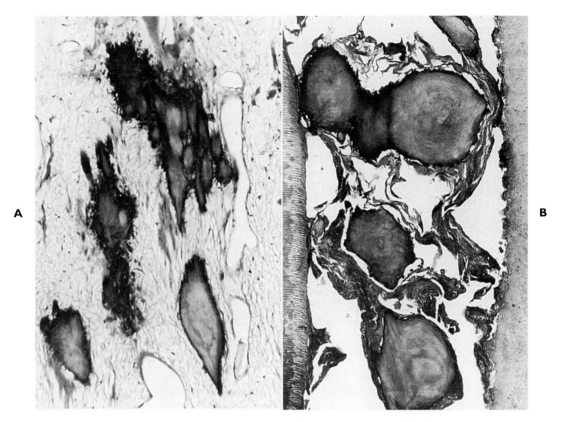

Fig. 4-3 *A and B, Examples of the variability in pulp stone formation or isolated areas of calcification. (Hematoxylin and eosin, 100×.)*

NORMAL ROOT CANAL ANATOMY

In the past textbooks on root canal morphology have often overlooked an important anatomic fact: the canal space is always located in the cross-sectional center of the root (Fig. 4-6). Similarly the pulp-chamber is (or was, before calcification) located in the cross-sectional center of the crown (Fig. 4-7).[24]

In a tooth with a calcified pulp chamber, the distance from the occlusal surface to the projected pulp chamber floor is measured from the preoperative periradicular film, or preferably from a bite-wing film, which maximizes accuracy (see Chapter 3). An access cavity of normal size and shape is created in the crown to a depth equal to that of the pulp-chamber floor in a noncalcified tooth (Fig. 4-8).

A second important aspect of normal root canal anatomy is the geometric pattern of canal orifices found in the pulp chambers of teeth with multiple canals.[26] These geometric patterns and their potential variations must be mentally projected on the calcified pulp-chamber floor, with consideration for the direction of the canals as they leave the pulp chamber. This requires an astute integration of two-dimensional radiographic findings with three-

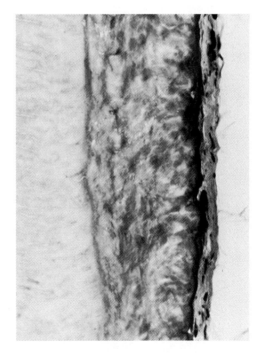

Fig. 4-4 *Irregular linear calcification. Notice the lack of tubules and the gnarled appearance of the reparative dentin. (Hematoxylin and eosin, 100×.)*

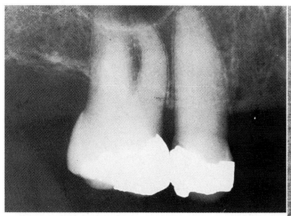

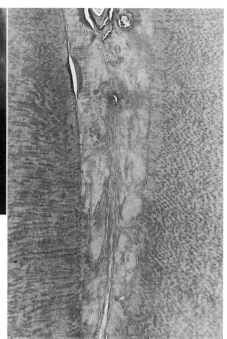

Fig. 4-5 *A,* Maxillary premolar and molar with radiographic evidence of complete calcification. *B,* Complete calcific closure of the pulp canal. Notice the pattern of dentin formation. (Hematoxylin and eosin, 100×.)

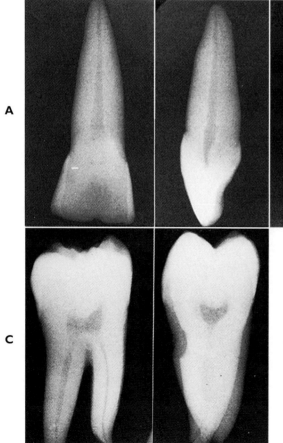

Fig. 4-6 *Facial and proximal views of an anterior tooth, A, a premolar, B, and a molar, C, showing pulp chambers in the cross-sectional centers of the crowns and root canals in the cross-sectional centers of the roots.*

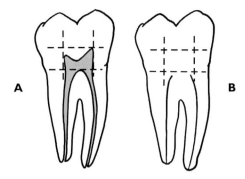

Fig. 4-7 *A, Normal mandibular molar without evidence of dystrophic calcification. Broken lines delineate central location of pulp chamber. **B,** Same tooth as in **A,** with dystrophic calcification. Notice the complete obliteration of the pulp chamber and recession of canal orifices. Broken lines delineate anatomic position of former pulp chamber.*

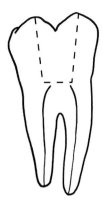

Fig. 4-8 *Same tooth as in Fig. 4-7, B, with access preparation to precise depth and lateral extension as a normal pulp chamber. Notice the coronal flare of cavity walls.*

dimensional tooth anatomy, coupled with a safe and dextrous movement of the rotary instrument on the pulpal floor. To facilitate this approach to the location and negotiation of fine or calcified canals, the following discussion is a consideration of access preparation of the calcified pulp chamber by each tooth type, with canal variations.

Maxillary Central and Lateral Incisor and Canine

A maxillary incisor with dystrophic calcification is diagramed in Fig. 4-9, *A*. The root canal is located in the cross-sectional center of the root.[24] If aesthetics and structural integrity were disregarded, the ideal location of the access preparation would be through the incisal edge; however, the standard access preparation for this tooth is in the exact center of the palatal surface of the crown buccolingually and incisogingivally (see Fig. 4-9, *A*). At an angle of roughly 45 degrees to the long axis, bur penetration of 3 to 4 mm will generally intersect with the pulp chamber in average-sized teeth (Fig. 4-9, *B*). In a calcified chamber, however, continued penetration at 45 degrees to the long axis will eventually pass over the canal entirely and result in perforation of the labial root surface below the gingival attachment (Fig. 4-9, *C* and *D*) (see Chapter 3).

Therefore, when the chamber is calcified and the canal has not been located after 3 to 4 mm of penetration, the bur must be rotated to be as parallel to the long axis of the tooth as possible to prevent perforation (Fig. 4-9, *E* and *F*). Penetration proceeds down the lingual aspect of the access preparation with frequent exploration with the

DG-16 endodontic explorer for the orifice. In deep excavations, the bur may be changed to a long-shank No. 2 round bur. Frequent visual and radiographic reassessment of direction is necessary.

Maxillary Premolars

The point of coronal penetration for access begins in the center of the occlusal surface and follows the long axis of the tooth. Since the pulp chamber is wide buccolingually in both one- and two-canaled premolars, the chamber must be cut wide buccolingually but should remain narrow mesiodistally (Fig. 4-10).[24]

Maxillary Molars

The most common design for access preparation is a triangle formed by the orifices of the two buccal canals and the palatal canal.[24,26] In many molars with calcified chambers or canals, it is common to find one or two orifices without much difficulty but to visualize no additional orifices. In these situations a mental image of the geometric pattern of the canals is invaluable. Initially, it is extremely helpful to establish firmly a visual location of the identified orifices and canals. These canals are negotiated with a small file, typically a No. 8 K-file, to within 2 or 3 mm of the estimated root length (Fig. 4-11, *A*). Once negotiated, the orifice is flared in a circumferential pattern using anticurvature filing in the coronal one third of the canal. A No. 10 K-file is then used in a manner similar to that of the No. 8 file, followed by a No. 20 Hedström file (Fig. 4-11, *B* and *C*). All instrumentation of this type requires copious irrigation with a 2.5% to

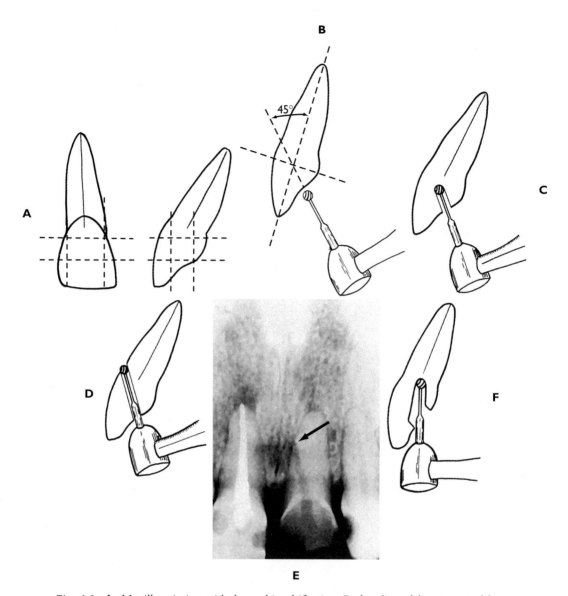

Fig. 4-9 *A, Maxillary incisor with dystrophic calcification. Broken lines delineate central location of former pulp chamber. **B,** Angle of access penetration is approximately 45 degrees to the long axis of the root. The access opening should extend incisogingivally to include the full middle third of the crown. **C,** No pulp chamber will be found in the calcified canal. Continued bur penetration may result in a facial perforation. **D,** Mesiofacial perforation resulting from excessive bur penetration without adequate radiographic control for bur angulation and pulp canal depth. **E,** Perforation of mesial wall of central incisor (arrow) resulting from improper bur angulation. **F,** Angle of bur is changed from 45 degrees to an angle as close to parallel as possible with the long axis of the root.*

5.25% solution of sodium hypochlorite (NaOCl). After filing, the orifices are further enlarged with a succession of Nos. 2, 3, and 4 Gates-Glidden (GG) drills or Hedström files in a stepwise manner. The No. 2 GG drill penetrates roughly to the midroot level; the penetration of the No. 3 GG drill is 2 mm shorter. The No. 4 GG drill is used *only* to flare the orifice itself (Fig. 4-11, *D* to *F*). This approach to initial penetration has been termed *preflaring,* and various alternatives have been described that employ both instruments[5-7,12,13] and ultrasonics.[21]

Once the pulp chamber has been irrigated and dried, the clear position of the located and instrumented canals will indicate the likely location of the calcified orifices (Fig. 4-12). It should be assumed that all maxillary molars have four canals until each potential site has been excavated with a long-shank No. 2 round bur to a depth of 1 mm. For a second canal in the mesiobuccal root, a slot or trench is usually excavated in a straight line toward the palatal orifice from the primary mesiobuccal canal orifice. Generally, if a second mesiobuccal orifice is present it will be anywhere from 0.5 to 5 mm toward the palatal orifice and often located under a cervical ledge (see Chapter 3, Fig. 3-17). Occasionally the orifice to the fourth

canal will actually be located 1 to 2 mm into the mesiobuccal orifice or even the palatal orifice (Fig. 4-13). The management of these cases is discussed in the next two sections of this chapter.

Mandibular Incisors, Canines, and Premolars

The most common canal morphology for each of these teeth is a single canal; however, a second canal, if present, will almost invariably be found lingual to the first canal (see Chapter 3, Fig. 3-14, *B*).[2,24] In the incisors and canines, second canals are particularly

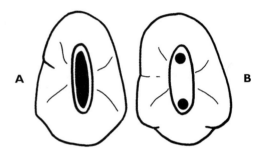

Fig. 4-10 *Typical access shape and canal morphology of a single-canal premolar,* **A,** *and a two-canal premolar,* **B.** *The access is wide buccolingually and narrow mesiodistally.*

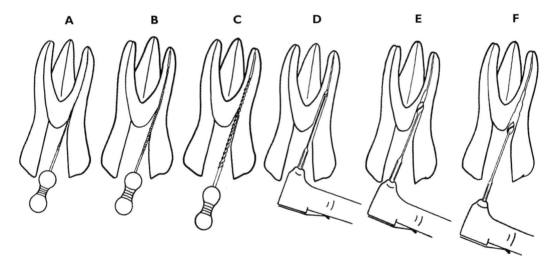

Fig. 4-11 *A, Orifice widening or preflaring begins with a No. 8 K-file to the estimated working length. It is important to reach this length before advancing to a larger file. B, No. 10 K-file is used to continue the canal flaring. Irrigate frequently and recapitulate often with the No. 8 K-file. C, Use a No. 20 Hedström file to flare and straighten the coronal half of the canal; use anticurvature filing. D, Continue preflaring with a No. 2 GG drill to midroot. Do not force the GG drill apically. Flush often. E, Use a No. 3 GG drill to a depth 2 mm shorter than the No. 2 GG drill. F, Final orifice widening may be completed with a No. 4 GG drill introduced only to the length of the bur head. Use copious irrigation, and recapitulate with a No. 8 K-file.*

difficult to locate (even where minimal calcification is present) because of angulation of the anatomic crown or the location of the standard access cavity on the lingual aspect (Fig. 4-14). After the main canal is located and debrided, it is important to widen the orifice lingually and probe for the second orifice using a No. 8 or No. 10 K-file with an abrupt curve placed 1 or 2 mm from the tip of the file. If the canal is not located with this technique, the use of a No. 2, 3, and 4 Gates-Glidden drill on the lingual surface may be very helpful in uncovering the orifice of a lingual canal. The drill is used in the manner of the round bur and is drawn up the lingual surface in a sweeping motion.

Breakage of these instruments may occur during this motion, however, the fracture occurs high on the shank, and such a position allows easy removal of the segment. If the canal is found with either technique, even a normal-sized second canal is usually as fine as any calcified canal and should be penetrated in the manner described in last section of this chapter.

Mandibular Molars

The most common morphology for access preparation in mandibular molars is a trapezoid formed by the two canals in the mesial root and the oval canal in the distal root.[24,26] It is common to find the distal

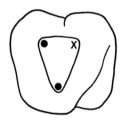

Fig. 4-12 *Occlusal view of a maxillary molar with a standard access preparation. By locating and preflaring the orifices of two canals, the practitioner can determine the location of the third canal (X) consistently and accurately.*

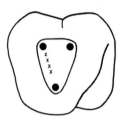

Fig. 4-13 *After the three primary canals have been located, the orifice of the second mesiobuccal canal can be located by troughing 0.5 to 5 mm toward the palatal canal orifice. Most second canals will be found 1 to 3 mm from the primary mesiobuccal canal orifice, X's.*

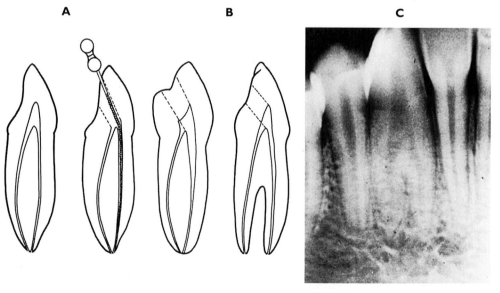

A   B   C

Fig. 4-14 *A, In a two-canal mandibular incisor, the standard access preparation will invariably place the initial instrument in the facial canal, passing over the orifice of the second canal. B, Second canals in mandibular canines and premolars are almost always found on the lingual aspect. Most diverge at significant angles from the facial canals and require negotiation with very fine instruments. C, Radiograph demonstrating a rotated two-rooted mandibular canine.*

canal to be wide buccolingually, with a morphology that requires separate preparation of the buccal and lingual aspects of the canal. In roughly 30% of cases the distal canals will be separate, making it necessary to make a wide buccolingual excavation in the distal root in calcified canals (Fig. 4-15) (see Chapter 3, Fig 3-16, *D*). A small percentage of second molars will have only one canal in each root. If one canal is located in the mesial root, it is wise to enlarge its orifice as described above and assess the symmetry of the orifice geometry. In a two-canal morphology both canals will be in the mesiodistal midline (Fig. 4-16, *A*). If after orifice widening the mesial canal is asymmetrically located to the buccal or lingual side relative to the distal canal, the mesial root probably has two canals, and the second canal can be envisioned as completing

the trapezoid described initially (Fig. 4-16, *B*). Again, it is wise to make a groove in excavating for the calcified orifice because it may be either quite close to the located canal or as far as 3 to 4 mm away. As with the fourth canal in the maxillary molar, the orifice of either the mesiobuccal or mesiolingual canal may be located 1 to 2 mm into the singly identified mesial orifice.

RECOGNITION OF THE ORIFICE
Location and Penetration

The most important instrument for orifice location is the DG-16 explorer. In firm probing during excavation of the pulp chamber floor, the explorer will not penetrate and "stick" in solid dentin; however, if an orifice is present, firm pressure will force

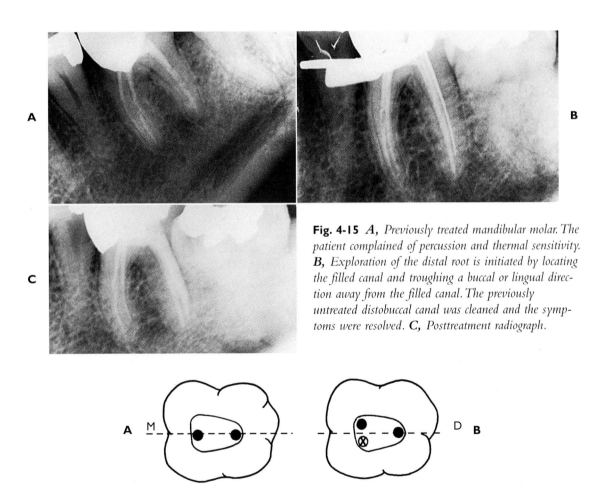

Fig. 4-15 *A, Previously treated mandibular molar. The patient complained of percussion and thermal sensitivity. B, Exploration of the distal root is initiated by locating the filled canal and troughing a buccal or lingual direction away from the filled canal. The previously untreated distobuccal canal was cleaned and the symptoms were resolved. C, Posttreatment radiograph.*

Fig. 4-16 *A, Mandibular molar with a two-canal morphology will have both orifices on the mesiodistal midline. B, If two canals are located in a mandibular molar and the mesial orifice is distinctly buccal or lingual to the mesiodistal midline, it is probable that there is a second canal in the mesial root, X.*

the instrument slightly into the orifice, and it will resist dislodgment, or "stick." To minimize perforation, reconfirm the location of the canal radiographically, leaving the explorer in place. At this point a fine instrument, usually a No. 8 or No. 10 K-file, is placed into the orifice, and an attempt is made to negotiate the canal. Some practitioners prefer to use a No. 6 K-file initially to negotiate the

canal; however, these instruments are very fine and lack stiffness in their shaft. If the canal is highly calcified or packed with necrotic debris, the No. 6 K-file will bend and curl instead of penetrating. An alternative option is to use instruments with reduced flutes, such as a Canal Pathfinder (JS Dental, Ridgefield, Conn.) or instruments with greater shaft strength such as the Pathfinder CS (Kerr Manufacturing Co, Romulus, Mich.), which are more likely to penetrate even highly calcified canals (Fig. 4-17).

When faced with trying to locate the position of the canal orifice, many dentists and endodontists have chosen to use magnification in the form of enhanced glasses or a microscope. Although it may be advantageous to be able to see the position of the orifice under magnification, this approach will not aid the clinician who does not know where to look for the orifice. Likewise it will not aid the clinician in the penetration of an instrument through the calcified canal space.

Because of curvature in the coronal 1 or 2 mm of many canals (Fig. 4-18, *A*), it is necessary to remove the cervical ledge or bulge (see Chapter 3,

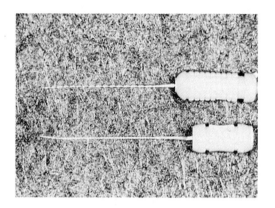

Fig. 4-17 *Pathfinder instruments.*

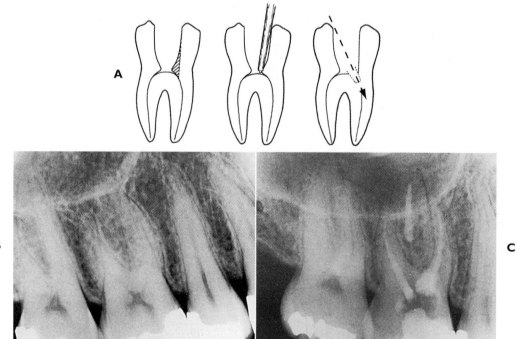

Fig. 4-18 *A,* Left, *shaded area represents the cervical ledge over the canal orifice.* Center, *Removal is performed by lateral cutting with a safe-ended diamond bur, which also flares the access opening.* Right, *Broken line with arrow indicates direction of penetration (countersinking) of a No. 2 round bur to facilitate canal location and negotiation.* **B,** *Preoperative radiograph showing a severe mesial curvature of the coronal third of the mesiobuccal canal.* **C,** *Posttreatment radiograph. Careful assessment of proper angulation and penetration is necessary to prevent furcation perforation (see Fig. 3-17, A).*

Fig. 3-16).[11] If the orifice still cannot be negotiated with a fine instrument, drill 1 or 2 mm into the center of the orifice with a No. 2 round bur on slow speed and use the explorer to re-establish the canal orifice (Fig. 4-18, *B* and *C*). When countersinking or troughing in an area where an orifice is located, *be sure the pulp chamber is dry.* The slow-speed rotating bur will remove whitish chips that then accumulate in the orifice. After a light stream of air is blown into the chamber, these chips appear as white spots on the dark floor of the chamber (Fig. 4-19) and serve as markers for exploration or further countersinking. This approach can be used if the fourth canal of the maxillary molar or a separation of the mesiobuccal and mesiolingual canals is anticipated in mandibular second molars. In some cases, however, it may be preferable not to penetrate the common orifice with a bur. These are cases in which the canals actually leave at a severely curved angle on the wall of the orifice, and bur penetration may risk perforation (Fig. 4-20). In these cases the use of sharply curved files may be appropriate to enter the canals initially (see Negotiating the Fine of Calcified Canal later in this chapter). Upon entry, the file is carefully rotated and teased apically around the canal curves. Chelating agents such as REDTA (Roth Drug Co, Chicago, Ill.), RC-prep (Premier Dental Products, Philadelphia, Penn.) and Canal (Septodont, Inc, New Castle, Del.) are seldom of value in locating the orifice but can be useful during canal negotiation.[14]

Problems in Management

Although the majority of attempts to locate canal orifices in the presence of severe calcification will be successful, there is always potential for perfora-

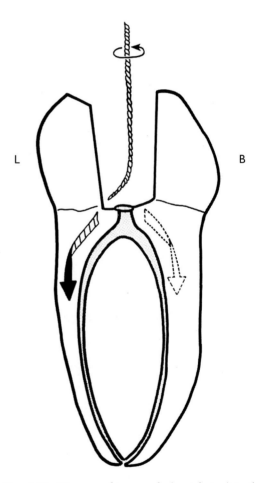

Fig. 4-19 *A, Excavation of chamber floor to locate the buccal canal orifices. Notice the white dentinal chips located in the projected orifices. Subsequent countersinking in these areas with a No. 2 round bur will enhance canal location. **B,** Canal orifices identified after countersinking.*

Fig. 4-20 *Diagram of two canals (mesial view) in the mesial root of a mandibular molar. Since the clinical view of the pulp chamber would reveal only one orifice and one canal, all such orifices should be explored for multiple canals with sharply curved, small instruments. L, Lingual; B, Buccal.*

tion. Probing with the explorer will yield the characteristic "stick" if, in fact, the excavation has come too close to the root surface and the explorer is actually penetrating a thin area of remaining dentin. This type of procedural accident must be detected as early as possible so that injury to underlying bone can be kept to a minimum. The most common sign of accidental perforation is bleeding, but bleeding may also indicate that the pulp in the calcified canal is vital. Likewise, it is not unusual to discover that accidental perforation has occurred and there is no bleeding.

If there is any question as to whether the orifice has actually been found, it is important to place as small an instrument as possible in the opening and expose a radiograph. A No. 6 or No. 8 K-file would not be suitable for length determination if the canal has been found, but it is much less traumatic if a perforation has occurred.

The prognosis for a perforation repair is good if the size of the perforation is small and the bone adjacent to it remains healthy.

Therefore the instrument should not be placed to the estimated canal working length. It is used only as a marker to identify the position of a possible deviation from the canal system.

When a perforation occurs, two problems arise that affect prognosis of the endodontic treatment: the perforation itself and the canal that remains to be located. The radiograph will be of great value in locating the canal. If, for example, the perforation has occurred on the furcation side of the mesial root in a mandibular molar, the orifices will be located more toward the mesial. The distance can be estimated from the file placed in the perforation.

After the perforation has occurred, studies have shown that healing is possible by covering the site with a hard-setting calcium hydroxide–containing cement such as Dycal (LD Caulk/Dentsply, Milford, Del.).[1] However, this is sometimes impractical if the orifice of the canal has yet to be located because of the limited space and visibility. If the perforation site is left exposed, only water should be used as an irrigant during subsequent procedures. If the tooth is closed at that appointment, no irritating medication such as paramonochlorophenol or formocresol should be placed in the pulp chamber. Presently, calcium hydroxide is the best medication for the perforation as well as an interim medication of the root canals. Rather than using a cement material, it is easier to mix plain calcium hydroxide powder with water and place the slurry in the pulp chamber. There is no chemical reaction between the water and powder, and so it will not set and will be easily removed from the pulp chamber. In lieu of this approach, commercial preparations such as Calasept (JS Dental Mfg, Inc., Ridgefield, Conn.) work very well and are easy to use.

Once the canal has been found and treated, the perforation should be sealed permanently (Fig. 4-21). If the perforation is very small, such as the size of an explorer tip or No. 10 file, the treatment of choice is a thin layer of calcium hydroxide cement covered by a permanent filling material (Fig. 4-21). If the perforation is larger than 1 mm, the treatment is the same, but the long-term prognosis is doubtful. When failure occurs, the lesion usually appears as a periodontal defect and is often treatable with standard periodontal surgical approaches.[8,16]

CLINICAL PROBLEM: A 43-year-old female presents with pain in the mandibular right first molar. The tooth is tender to percussion and hurts when

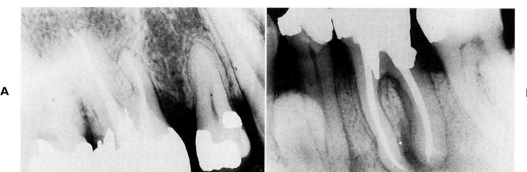

A　　　　　　　　　　　　　　　　　　　　　　　　　　　**B**

Fig. 4-21 *A* and *B*, *Repairs of a small perforation created with an endodontic explorer during excavation for canal orifices.*

cold is applied. The radiograph reveals periradicular lesions on the mesial and distal roots. The diagnosis is irreversible pulpitis with acute periradicular periodontitis, and root canal treatment will be necessary. However, what is also apparent on the radiograph is the presence of calcification in the coronal third of the mesial canals (Fig. 4-22, *A*). The initial access (Fig. 4-22, *B*) resulted in the location of the distal and mesiolingual canals. The orifice of the mesiobuccal canal was calcified at the level of the pulp chamber floor. Treatment was completed for the distal and mesiolingual canals; however, a perforation was suspected in the area of the mesiobuccal.

Solution: First the presence of a perforation must be identified if it exists. This was done in Fig. 4-22, *C* with the placement of a No. 10 K-file in the orifice created. The perforation was located slightly mesial to the true canal orifice. This

allowed for the location of the true orifice and management of the canal. The perforation was sealed with a calcium hydroxide–containing cement Fig. 4-22, *D, arrow*) and a zinc oxide-eugenol cement base and an amalgam restoration were placed in the access opening. A 9-month recall radiograph, coincident with the need for root canal treatment on the second molar, confirmed the presence of stable bone in the furcation region (Fig. 4-22, *E*). The patient was symptom free.

NEGOTIATING THE FINE OR CALCIFIED CANAL
Penetration and Negotiation

Once the orifice has been located, a 21-mm No. 8 K-file is the initial instrument of choice to negotiate the calcified canal. A No. 10 K-file is usually

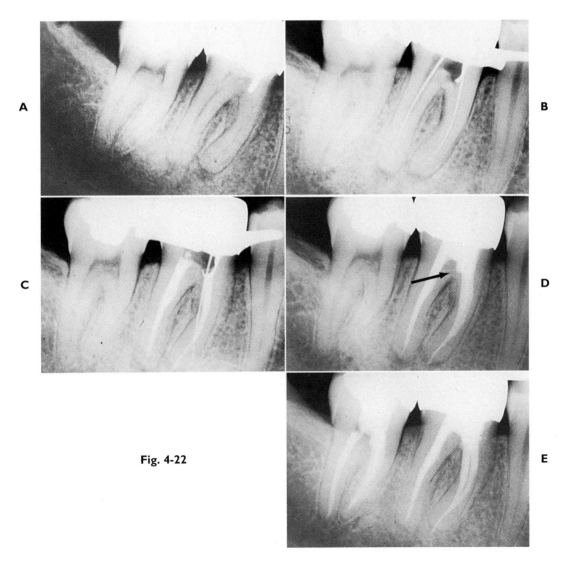

Fig. 4-22

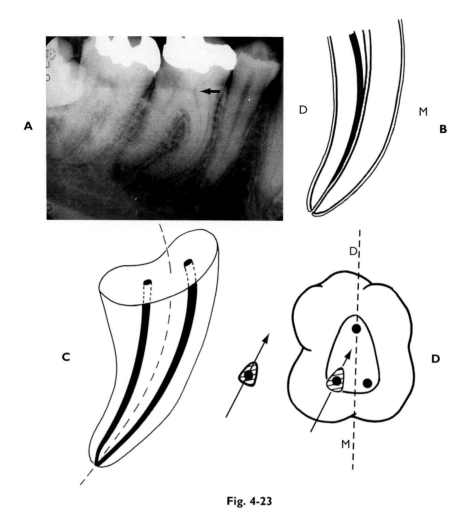

Fig. 4-23

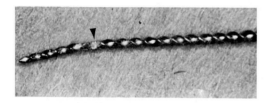

Fig. 4-24 *Shiny spot on shaft of file* (arrow) *indicates flute unwinding. These instruments must be identified and discarded.*

too large, and a No. 6 K-file is too weak to apply any firm apical pressure, particularly if precurved. Likewise, the use of nickel-titanium files is contraindicated for this purpose because of lack of strength in the long axis of the file. The 21-mm–long K-file is flexible enough to negotiate around curvatures of calcifications. If the canal is longer than 21 mm, it is simple to change to a 25

mm instrument once 21 mm of penetration has been achieved. It is essential to have a rubber stop on the shaft of the instrument, which has one directional point (see Chapter 5). Before the file is inserted into the canal, a small curve is placed in its apical 1 mm. The point on the rubber stop is then aligned with the curve. In negotiating the fine-curved canal, the precurved instrument must be directed along the pathway the canal is most likely to follow; consequently it is vitally important to know in which direction the curve in the instrument is pointed. This is easily accomplished by observing the rubber stop on the instrument shaft.

CLINICAL PROBLEM: The mandibular right first molar requires root canal treatment (Fig. 4-23, *A*). Notice the presence of a cervical bulge *(arrow)* and the severe curvature of the root. The canals in this root will also curve three dimensionally. The challenge in this case is to be able to penetrate easily to the full length of the canal and clean and shape it without deviating from its anatomic confines.

Solution: In preparing to negotiate the mesiobuccal canal of this mandibular molar, a review of the root morphology indicates that the canal will curve distally and either parallel to the mesiodistal midline of the tooth or slightly toward the midline, in a sense converging apically with the mesiolingual canal (Fig. 4-23, *B* and *C*). Thus, when the canal is successfully penetrated, the rubber stop should point directly distally or slightly distolingually (Fig. 4-23, *D*). There is no value in probing to the mesial or buccal side. Without the rubber stop providing visual control, it will be impossible to maintain a specific directional orientation. It may also be possible to use nickel-titanium files to achieve canal penetration and negotiation in this case because of the significant curvature present.

In most cases, the use of chelating agents is not necessary, though copious irrigation with NaOCl is important as the instrument is advanced. The file will tend to bind in the newly entered portion of the canal. Although forceful irrigation will not dislodge debris or calcified particles, it will follow the small instrument down the canal, aiding in keeping debris in solution and serving as a lubricant for the fine metal instrument. As the instrument is advanced farther and the coronal portion of the canal becomes more patent, the chance of apical penetration of the NaOCl is increased. During advancement, the file should not be rotated. This is especially true if nickel-titanium files are used because the combination of binding and rotating results in rapid and unanticipated fracture of the instrument. After irrigation of the access cavity, the stainless steel file is again precurved and passed to the previously established level. With a probing and very gentle "stem-winding" movement, the instrument is advanced another 1 to 2 mm. The newly penetrated space is filed until the instrument freely slides to that level. This technique continues with alternating irrigation and advancement in 1 to 2 mm increments. In extremely narrow canals, a No. 8 K-file should immediately be exchanged for a No. 6 K-file. If the No. 8 K-file is forced too vigorously, it may lead to blockage. It is also necessary frequently to inspect the apical curvature of the files. Any file that shows evidence of fatigue or irregularity of the spiral flutes should be replaced (Fig. 4-24). Once the estimated working length of the tooth has been reached, the No. 8 K-file should be used in a "filing-only" motion until a No. 10 K-file can be passed freely to within 1 mm of the

length. Once this length has been achieved, the file should be kept at that point in the canal and a radiograph obtained to verify the working length of the tooth.

CLINICAL PROBLEM: A 26-year-old male presents with a history of tooth trauma to his mandibular anterior teeth. His chief complaint was periodic pain to pressure in the right central incisor. The tooth was nonresponsive to sensibility tests, with a slightly abnormal response to palpation and percussion. A radiograph shows significant pulp chamber and coronal canal calcification (Fig. 4-25, *A*). The diagnosis was necrotic pulp with a subacute periradicular periodontitis, and root canal treatment was indicated. The question often facing the clinician in this situation is whether to attempt nonsurgical treatment or to go directly to surgical intervention because of the diminution of the visible canal space.

Solution: Because there is visible canal space in the apical half of the root and a periradicular lesion is present, an attempt at nonsurgical intervention is the treatment of choice. Initial penetration of the pulpal space (Fig. 4-25, *B*) shows a distal deviation of the file in the root. After a reorientation and an increase in the depth of the penetration into the tooth, the canal was located and penetration was achieved to the apex (Fig. 4-25, *C*). Fig. 4-25, *D,* shows the final canal obturation. Notice the deviation in the canal space in the coronal third (now obturated) that was created during aberrant penetration of the root. Recall radiograph (Fig. 4-25, *E*) indicates resolution of the periradicular lesion without surgical intervention.

As previously mentioned, use of a pathfinding instrument may also be indicated in an attempt to negotiate narrow canals. Since probing and penetrating can be accomplished without cutting the dentinal walls, this instrument may be preferable in highly calcified, tortuous canals.

CLINICAL PROBLEM: A 66-year-old male presents with periodic pain in the maxillary right lateral incisor. The tooth has a long history of decay and restorations. The tooth is very tender to percussion and palpation. Thermal sensibility tests are inconclusive and border on being nonresponsive. The diagnosis is irreversible pulpitis with acute periradicular periodontitis, and root canal treatment is indicated. However, the canal space is quite calcified, and the root is curved in the apical third (Fig. 4-26, *A*). The patient wishes to have nonsurgical treatment.

Solution: Initial attempts to locate the canal met with failure. As can be seen in Fig. 4-26, *B,*

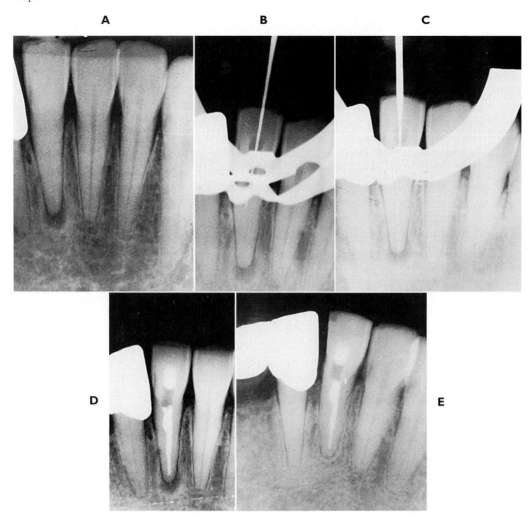

Fig. 4-25

deep penetration has been achieved without the canal being located. In fact there is a serious deviation in a distal (and clinically) buccal direction. Reorientation of the bur penetration and the use of a pathfinder instrument enabled the initial penetration into the true canal space (Fig. 4-26, *C*). Excessive use of irrigant and liquid EDTA was essential to penetrate slowly and carefully the partially calcified space to its apical extent (Fig. 4-26, *D*). If the canal had been calcified as seen in Fig. 4-5, *B*, penetration would not have been possible. Canal obturation is seen in Fig. 4-26, *E*.

The use of ultrasonic instrumentation to penetrate calcified or blocked canals passively has been advocated.[21] Coupled with the dissolving action of NaOCl,[3,23] ultrasonic systems can enhance the flow of an irrigant around the entire length of the file as it penetrates apically. With the physical action of the ultrasound dislodging calcifications and the NaOCl penetrating the dissolving collagen, the canal system becomes more amenable to file penetration. However, care must be exercised not to force the ultrasonic file apically, or ledging or new canal formation may result (see Chapter 5). In addition, for these systems to be effective in small calcified or blocked canals, penetration to the apex already must have been achieved with handheld instruments. Likewise, the ultrasonic instrument has never been shown to be an effective tool for negotiating any canal.

Perforation during Negotiation

Although it is reasonable to expect patent canal space on the apical side of a deep calcified blockage, success in penetration through the calcification and into the continuing canal is very limited. The fre-

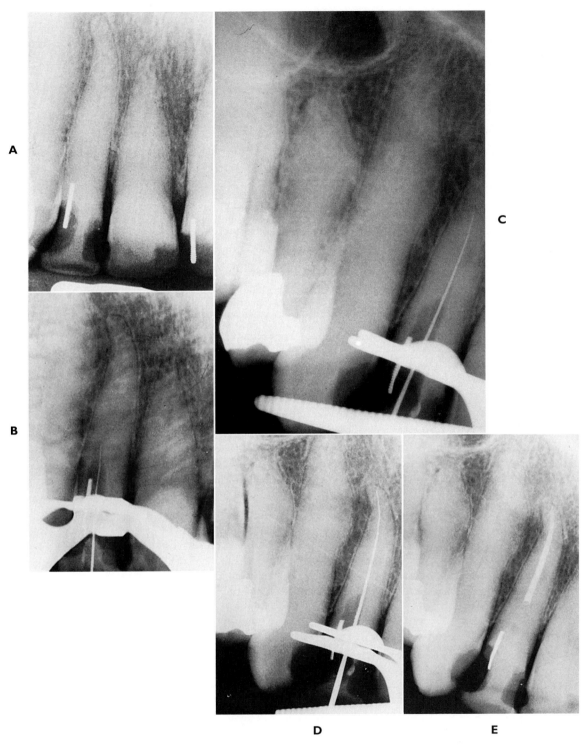

A

B

C

D

E

Fig. 4-26

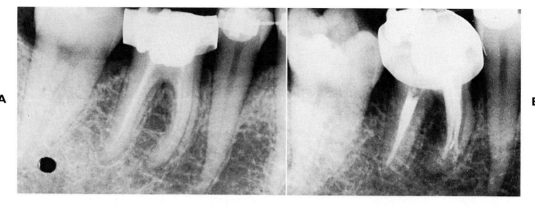

Fig. 4-27 *A, Symptomatic mandibular molar; retreatment is indicated. B, Posttreatment radiograph. After removal of paste fill, a file was broken in attempts to renegotiate the calcified mesiolingual canal. Further attempts to bypass the instrument resulted in a false canal and perforation along the mesial wall of the mesial root. The false canal was sealed with gutta-percha and sealer; the patient was prescribed a recall evaluation.*

quent result of vigorous probing with fine instruments and chelating agents is the creation of a false canal. In a calcified canal in which penetration is very slow, it is necessary to confirm the position of the instrument with a radiograph. Without close radiographic supervision, continued instrumentation in a false canal will result in perforation. If perforation does occur, it fortunately will be very small in diameter (if recognized early) and should be treated as a true canal by instrumentation and sealing of its orifice with gutta-percha (Fig. 4-27).[9,15,20] There is little value in renegotiating the canal in an attempt to locate its true continuation. However, if the false canal is identified before perforation, various procedures can be employed to attempt to relocate the true canal and negotiate it (see Chapter 5). If periradicular pathosis or symptoms develop, surgical intervention will probably be necessary (Fig. 4-28).

Complete Calcification and Obliteration

In the treatment of calcified canals it is common to find a total occlusion of the canal space at any level. Histologic studies reveal that these calcifications are seldom complete to the apex (Fig. 4-29). Consequently the prognosis of the root canal treatment will depend on the continued health of the pulp or the periradicular tissues on the apical side of the blockage. In the absence of symptoms or evidence of apical pathosis, it is clinically reasonable and acceptable to instrument and fill the canal to the level negotiated and continue to observe the tooth (Fig. 4-30). Evidence of apical pathosis and symptoms either at the time of treatment or during the

course of observation are an indication to consider periradicular surgery.[17,22]

CLINICAL PROBLEM: A 47-year-old female patient presents with a maxillary left first premolar that is fractured to the gingival margin. The tooth is symptom free, and radiographically there is no evidence of pathosis. However, there is no apparent canal space. Treatment planning includes root canal treatment for post placement before a core buildup. Neither canal was negotiable after deep excavation into both roots (Fig. 4-31, *A, arrows*). A decision was made to restore the canal excavations with posts, followed by a new core and crown. Three years later the patient presents with percussion tenderness and radiographic evidence of apical pathosis (Fig. 4-31, *B*).

Solution: It is obvious that there is untreated canal space in these roots. Even if the posts could be removed, further attempts to negotiate the canals would not be warranted. Two options are available to the clinician, periradicular surgery or tooth extraction.

TIPS IN NEGOTIATING CALCIFIED CANALS

1. Copious irrigation at all times with 2.5% to 5.25% NaOCl enhances dissolution of organic debris, lubricates the canal, and keeps dentin chips and pieces of calcified material in solution.
2. Always advance instruments slowly in calcified canals.
3. Always clean the instrument on withdrawal and inspect before reinserting it into the canal.

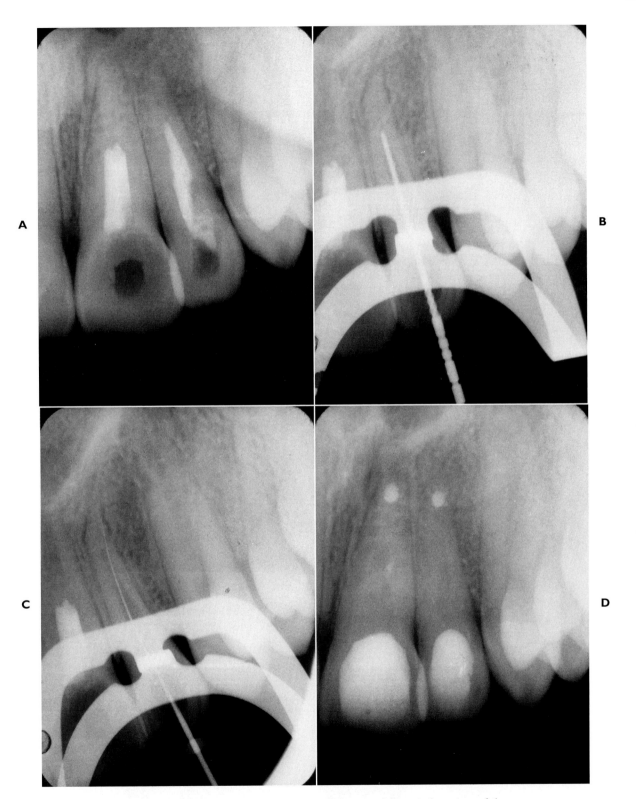

Fig. 4-28 *A, Maxillary incisors with apparent calcification of the apical portions of the roots. B, Attempts to locate and negotiate the canal in the lateral incisor were unsuccessful, with a perforation occurring in* **C. D,** *Because of symptoms, apical surgery was performed and root-end fillings were placed. The coronal portion of the roots was sealed with composite resin. (Case courtesy Dr. James Douthitt.)*

4. When a fine instrument has reached the approximate canal length, do not remove it; rather, obtain a radiograph to ascertain the position of the file.

5. Do not use acids (hydrochloric acid) or alkalis (sodium hydroxide) to aid in canal penetration.

6. Use chelating pastes or solutions to assist in canal penetration.

7. Use ultrasonic instruments in the pulp chamber to loosen debris in the canal orifices.

8. Flaring of the canal orifice and enlargement of any negotiated canal space will improve tactile perception in continued canal penetration.

9. The use of newer, nickel-titanium rotary orifice-penetrating instruments should be considered.

References

1. Beavers RA, Bergenholtz G, Cox CF: Periodontal wound healing following intentional root perforations in permanent teeth of *Macaca mulatta, Int Endod J* 19:36-44, 1986.

2. Bjorndal AM, Skidmore AE: *Anatomy and morphology of human teeth,* Iowa City, 1983, University of Iowa Press, p 59.

3. Cunningham WT, Balekjian AY: Effect of temperature on collagen dissolving ability of sodium hypochlorite endodontic irrigant, *Oral Surg Oral Med Oral Pathol* 49:175-177, 1980.

4. Dodds RN, Holcomb JB, McVicker DW: Endodontic management of teeth with calcific metamorphosis, *Comp Cont Educ Dent* 6:515-520, 1985.

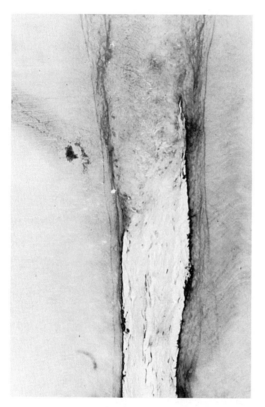

Fig. 4-29 *Calcification of the pulp space in the coronal portion with degenerating pulp apical to the calcifying front. (Hematoxylin and eosin, 100×.)*

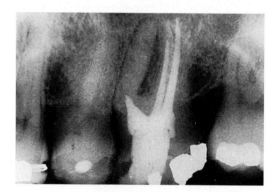

Fig. 4-30 *A nonnegotiable calcified canal in the mesiobuccal root of a maxillary molar was obturated to the calcification. Periodic recall is indicated, with surgery if pathosis develops or symptoms persist.*

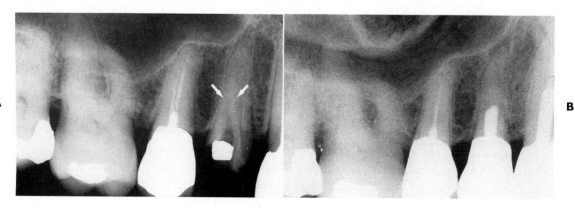

A

B

Fig. 4-31

5. Fahid A: Coronal root canal preparation. *Dental Student* 61:46-48, 1983.

6. Fava LRG: The double-flared technique: an alternative for biomechanical preparation, *J Endod* 9:76-80, 1983.

7. Goerig AC, Michelich RJ, Schultz HH: Instrumentation of root canals in molars using the step-down technique, *Endod* 8:550-554, 1982.

8. Gutmann JL, Harrison JW: *Surgical endodontics,* St. Louis, 1994, IEA [Ishiyaku EuroAmerica] Publications Inc, pp 409-448.

9. Ingle JI, Mullaney TA, Grandich RA et al: Endodontic cavity preparation. In Ingle JI, Taintor JF, editors: *Endodontics,* Philadelphia, 1985, Lea & Febiger, p 212.

10. Johnson WT: Instrumentation of the fine curved canals found in the mesial roots of maxillary and mandibular molars, *Quintessence Int* 17:309-312, 1986.

11. Leeb IJ: Canal orifice enlargement as related to biomechanical preparation, *J Endod* 9:463-470, 1983.

12. Marshall FJ, Pappin J: A crown-down pressureless preparation root canal enlargement technique. In *Technique Manual,* Portland, Ore, 1980, Health Sciences University.

13. Morgan LF, Montgomery S: An evaluation of the crown-down pressureless technique, *J Endod* 10:491-498, 1984.

14. Moss-Salaentijn L, Hendricks-Klyvert M: Calcified structures in human dental pulps, *J Endod* 14:184-189, 1988.

15. Nicholls E: Treatment of traumatic perforations of the pulp cavity, *Oral Surg Oral Med Oral Pathol* 15:603-612, 1962.

16. Oswald RJ: Procedural accidents and their repair. *Dent Clin North Am* 1979; 23:593-616.

17. Schindler WG, Gullickson DC: Rationale for the management of calcific metamorphosis secondary to traumatic injuries, *J Endod* 14:408-412, 1988.

18. Selden HS: Radiographic pulpal calcifications: normal or abnormal—a paradox, *J Endod* 17:34-37, 1991.

19. Serene TP: Technique for the location and length determination of calcified canals, *J Calif Dent Assoc* 4:62-65, 1976.

20. Sinai IH: Endodontic perforations: their prognosis and treatment, *J Am Dent Assoc* 95:90-95, 1977.

21. Stamos DG, Haasch GC, Chenail B et al: Endosonics: clinical impressions, *J Endod* 11:181-197, 1985.

22. Taintor JF, Ingle JI, Fahid A: Retreatment versus further treatment, *Clin Prev Dent* 5:8-14, 1983.

23. Trepagnier CM, Madden RM, Lazzari EP: Quantitative study of sodium hypochlorite as an in vitro endodontic irrigant, *J Endod* 3:194-196, 1977.

24. Wilcox LR: Pulpal anatomy and access preparations. In Walton R, Torabinejad M, editors: *principles and practice of endodontics,* ed 2, Philadelphia, 1995, WB Saunders, pp 531-547.

25. Wilcox LR, Walton RE: The shape and location of mandibular premolar access openings, *Int Endod J* 20:223-227, 1987.

26. Wilcox LR, Walton RE, Case WB: Molar access: shape and outline according to orifice locations, *J Endod* 15:315-318, 1989.

▼

Chapter 5

Problems in Canal Cleaning and Shaping

Gerald N. Glickman
Thom C. Dumsha

"In attempting to assign the success or failure of operations upon diseased teeth to their proper causes, factors of the greatest importance are frequently left out of account, and the results ascribed to some agent which may have been entirely indifferent. One of these factors, which forms the very foundation of successful root-treatment, is the *manner* in which the mechanical cleansing of the canal is carried out."*

Regardless of the instrumentation technique used for cleaning and shaping the root canal system, the objectives are to remove pulp tissue, debris, and bacteria, as well as to shape the canal for obturation.

As with access-opening preparations, failure to pay close attention to detail during canal cleaning and shaping will result in violations of the principles of biomechanical canal preparation. These procedural errors and their sequelae can adversely affect the prognosis of the treatment. This chapter describes the principal errors and means of preventing, identifying, and managing them. The errors that most often occur during canal preparation include:

1. Loss of working length
2. Deviations from normal canal anatomy
3. Inadequate canal preparation

In addition, various methods of cleaning and shaping curved canals, nickel-titanium instrumentation, and special problems encountered in the cleaning and shaping of canals with anatomic variations are addressed.

---

* From Hofheinz RH: *Dent Cosmos* 34:182–186, 1892.

LOSS OF WORKING LENGTH

Loss of working length during cleaning and shaping is a common and frustrating procedural error. The problem may be noted only on the master-cone radiograph or when the master apical file is short of the intended or initial working length. Assuming that there exists a clean, dry canal with proper shape and flare, the reestablishment of canal length becomes time consuming, tedious, and often hopeless.

The loss of working length is actually secondary to other endodontic procedural errors, since blockages, ledges, and fractured instruments can all result in loss of working length. However, these problems are usually recognized during cleaning and shaping procedures.

In most instances, loss of working length can be attributed to rapid increases in file size and the accumulation of dentinal debris in the apical third of the canal. Preventive measures include frequent irrigation with NaOCl, recapitulation, and periodic radiographic verification of working length. In other instances, lack of attention to detail, such as malpositioned instrument stops (Fig. 5-1), variations in reference points, poor radiographic technique, and improper use of instruments, will contribute to this problem.

To maintain proper working length during canal cleaning and shaping, adherence to the following specific guidelines is recommended:

1. Sound, reproducible reference points must be used.

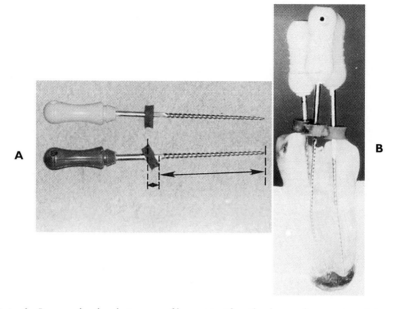

Fig. 5-1 *A, Improperly placed stop on a file can significantly change the accuracy of the working length. **B,** Cross-section of extracted tooth with files and stops in place. Stops are positioned at a proper angle with respect to the shaft of the file and the reference point on the tooth surface.*

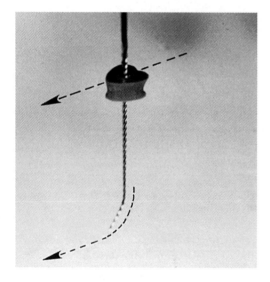

Fig. 5-2 *Directional rubber silicone stops should be used in all cases to ensure correct orientation of the precurved file with respect to the anatomy of the canal curvature.*

2. Use firm or secure rubber stops at right angles to the shaft of the instruments.
3. Precure all instruments with sterile 2 × 2-inch gauze, *overcurving* them in the apical third to compensate for some loss of curvature once in the canal.

4. Continually observe the instrument stops as they approach the reference points.
5. Directional instrument stops should be used. The direction of the stop must be constantly observed to maintain files in their proper relationship to the canal anatomy (Fig. 5-2).
6. When verifying the instrument position radiographically, use consistent radiographic angles.
7. Always maintain the original preoperative shape of the canal and clean and shape within these confines.
8. Use copious irrigation and recapitulation throughout cleaning and shaping procedures.
9. Always use sequential file sizes and do not skip sizes.

Blockage of the Canal System

A blockage is an obstruction in a previously patent canal system that prevents access to the apical constriction or apical stop. Blockages are commonly caused by the packing of dentin chips, tissue debris, restorative materials (Figs. 5-3 and 5-4), cotton pellets, paper points, or a fractured instrument in the canal. Canal blockages can be prevented by adherence to the following guidelines (see Chapter 3 for a more thorough discussion of items 1 to 6):

1. All caries and unsupported tooth structure must be removed before completion of the access opening.

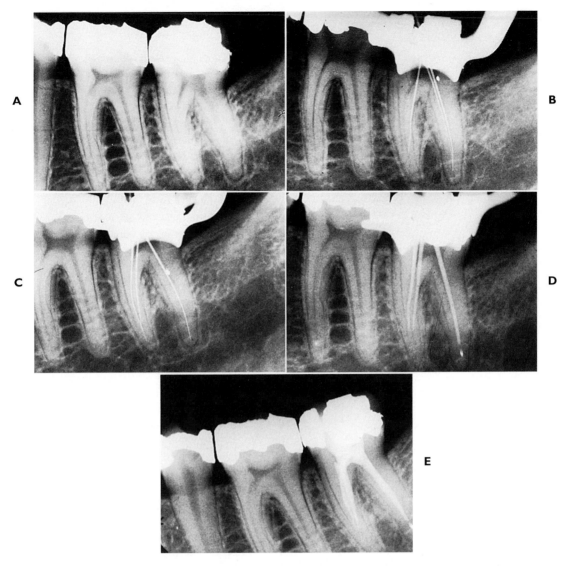

Fig. 5-3 *A, Preoperative radiograph showing a patent distal canal in the mandibular second molar. B, Working-length radiograph showing alloy particles on floor of the pulp chamber near the distal canal orifice. C, Second working-length radiograph and D, master cone radiograph shows that foreign material has worked its way down the canal. E, Final obturation radiograph showing alloy particle at the termination of the distal canal, limiting the length of the gutta-percha obturation. Blockage of the mesial canals with dentin chips limited further negotiation.*

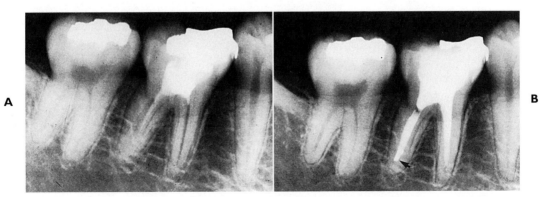

Fig. 5-4 *A, Preoperative radiograph of mandibular molar with gold inlay before access preparation for retreatment. B, Retreatment obturation radiograph shows gold particles (arrow) lodged at the apex of the distal canal.*

2. All loosened, weakened, or unsupported restorations must be removed before completion of the access opening.

3. The walls of the access opening must be flared occlusally or incisally. This is especially true when metallic or porcelain crowns are present.

4. Access openings must be modified to eliminate any structure that may impede direct canal entry and instrumentation procedures.

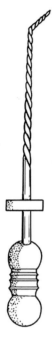

Fig. 5-5 *A 45-degree bend is placed in the last 3 mm of a file before attempting to bypass a blockage in the curved canal.*

5. When large restorations or crowns are present, water spray must be used to eliminate the accumulation of metallic or composite particles in the pulp chamber.

6. All temporary restorations around the outline of the access opening must be removed.

7. Copious irrigation must always be used during chamber and canal débridement, canal penetration, and canal cleaning and shaping.[15] Constant flushing and removal of debris reduces the amount of foreign material present in the canal system. Ultrasonics may also assist in this removal.

8. Intracanal instruments must always be wiped clean before they are inserted into the canal system.

9. K-files must always be used sequentially and should never bind excessively in the canal. This is also true for rotary instruments and Hedström files.

10. Recapitulation must be used during all instrumentation procedures. Recapitulation has been defined as the reintroduction and reapplication of instruments previously used throughout the cleaning and shaping process to create a well-designed, smooth, unclogged, evenly tapered, unstepped root canal preparation.[34]

11. Excessive pressure and rotation (especially counterclockwise) of intracanal instruments must be avoided.[5,21,29,33]

12. Never use instruments in a dry canal.[15]

13. Place a sound temporary filling.

Should a canal blockage of temporary restorative material or dentinal debris occur, a small but stiff

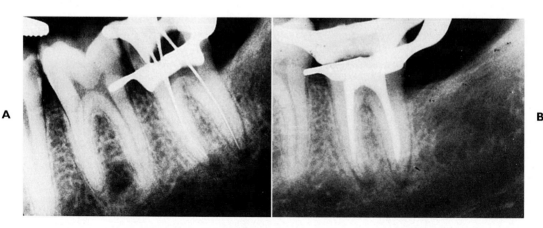

Fig. 5-6 *A, Original working length in mandibular molar demonstrating good length attainment in all three canals. B, After blockage of canal system, canals were obturated to the area of the block with a warm gutta-percha technique.*

instrument such as a No. 15 K-file or reamer is used to bore through the obstruction. In the case of metallic filings, especially if large particles are involved, use an instrument smaller than the last instrument that was placed into the canal system, preferably a No. 10. A 45-degree curve is placed at the apical 3 to 4 mm of the instrument (Fig. 5-5). The file is inserted into the canal and rotated circumferentially to detect a "catch" (the space between particles and canal). Once the catch is felt, the file is carefully rotated in a stem-winding fashion along with a slight in-and-out motion until the tip of the file bypasses the obstruction and negotiates the canal to length. Placement of a relatively straight file into a milieu of metallic filings or dentin debris may push the particles more apically into the canal or periradicular tissues, making them irretrievable. Once the file reaches the estimated working length, a radiograph is obtained to verify

the position of the file. *Do not remove the file.* It is essential that it be used circumferentially and with small amplitude to dislodge the packed debris.

Once sufficient space has been created through or along the side of the blockage, a smaller-sized Hedström file can be placed to length. Movement of this file on the outstroke will eliminate the debris. In cases of dense blockage with dentinal chips, chelating agents[28] such as RC-Prep (Premier Dental Products, Philadelphia, Penn.) or REDTAC (Roth Drug Co, Chicago, Ill.) may be used to soften the plug to facilitate penetration.

If the blockage cannot be penetrated or bypassed, instrumentation is completed at a new working length coronal to the blockage (Figs. 5-6 and 5-7). Variations in obturating techniques such as diffusion, thermoplasticized gutta-percha, or vertical compaction procedures (see Chapter 6) can be used to enhance penetration of the gutta-

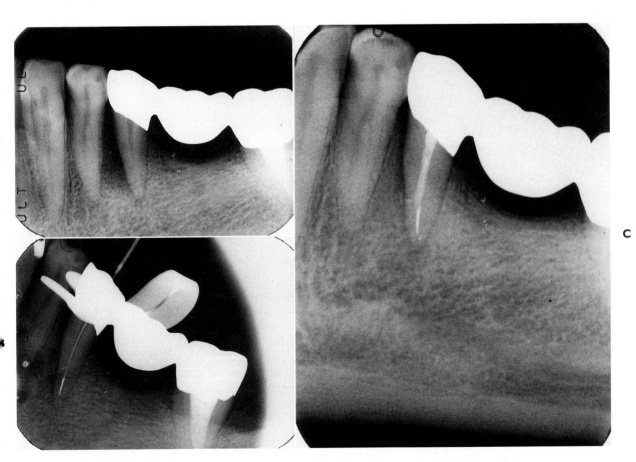

Fig. 5-7 *A, Preoperative radiograph of mandibular second premolar requiring root canal treatment. Tooth was the anterior abutment for a three-unit bridge. **B,** During cleaning and shaping, gold particles were inadvertently carried down the canal; ultrasonics could not remove the apical plug. **C,** Thermoplasticized gutta-percha technique was used to obturate the canal. Notice the filling of the lateral canal on mesial.*

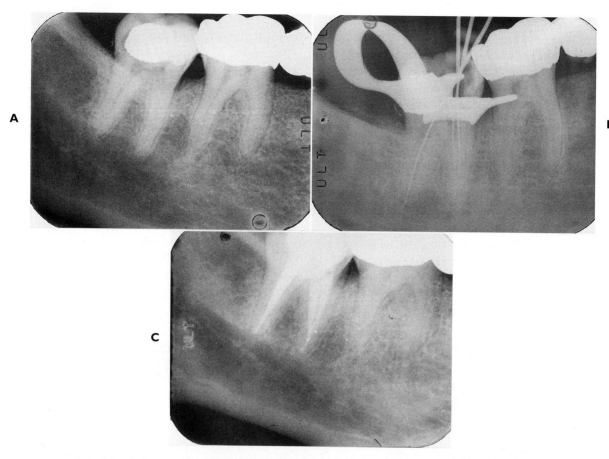

Fig. 5-8 *A, Preoperative radiograph of mandibular second molar demonstrating both temporary and alloy restorations. **B**, Working-length radiograph showing canals free of debris. **C**, Obturation radiograph with alloy particles in mesial canals; warm gutta-percha technique used to "encase" particles.*

percha and sealer around or through the blockage (Figs. 5-7 and 5-8). Periodic recall is mandatory after obturation. If further treatment is deemed appropriate, surgery may be necessary to correct the problem.

Ledging

A ledge is an artificially created irregularity on the surface of the root canal wall that prevents the placement of instruments to the apex of an otherwise patent canal (Fig. 5-9). Ledging is caused by insertion of uncurved instruments short of the working length with excessive amounts of apical pressure. The canal wall is gouged or a false canal is created, which results in ledge formation.

Prevention of ledges, especially in cases in which an accurate initial working length can be determined with a No. 15 K-file, is accomplished by adherence to the following guidelines.[15,16,25,37] Precurve or overcurve the apical 3 to 4 mm of the file

with the same curvature as the canal depicted in the radiograph. Do not force the file apically; rather, tease it to the most apical position.

Once inserted, each instrument is used sequentially in a filing motion (short, 1 to 3 mm amplitude in-and-out strokes) to the working length. Avoid excessive apical pressure until the instrument is *very loose* in the canal.

Rotating the file at the working length will cause a deviation from the natural canal pathway, straightening of the canal, and the creation of a ledge in the dentinal wall. Rapid advancement in file sizes or skipping file sizes can also result in ledge formation; therefore files must be used sequentially and must not bind excessively in the canal.

If binding is present, immediately return to a smaller file size, preferably a No. 8, 10, or 15, and use

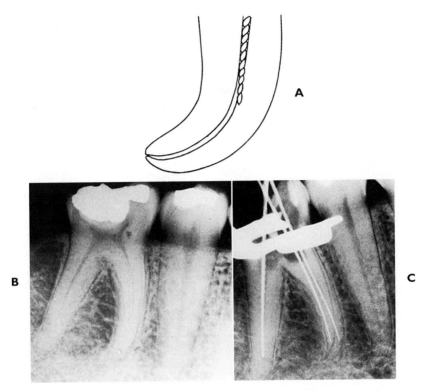

Fig. 5-9 *A, Canal ledge.* **B,** *Preoperative radiograph showing significant curvature of the mesial canals, which should warn the practitioner that ledging is more likely to occur if instrumentation is not cautiously performed.* **C,** *Master apical file radiograph shows that canals were instrumented larger than appropriate for size and curvature of mesial roots. Notice the loss of canal length and ledge formation.*

circumferential filing to remove any dentin irregularities or steps that may have begun to form during the placement of the larger-sized instrument. The effective use of circumferential filing, especially with Hedström files, will ensure smoothness and occlusal flaring of the canal walls and prevent the development of steps or irregularities (Fig. 5-10).

Instrumentation must always proceed with copious irrigation (2.5% to 5.25% sodium hypochlorite [NaOCl]) followed by recapitulation with smaller K-files.[3,15,36] Other lubricating agents recommended to enhance canal preparation include carbamide peroxide 10% in anhydrous glycerol (Gly-Oxide,[6,31] produced by Marion Laboratories, Inc., Kansas City, Mo.) and 3% hydrogen peroxide. Although chelating agents have also been advocated, they should be used with caution when one is attempting to negotiate curved canals. Since these agents soften the dentin walls,[11] a ledge can be begun anywhere along the root canal wall if excessive instrumentation pressure is used. Although self-limiting in their action,[28] chelating agents should be flushed from the canal with

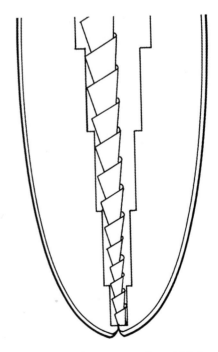

Fig. 5-10 *Method of removing "telescopic" ledges produced during a pure stepback canal preparation technique.*

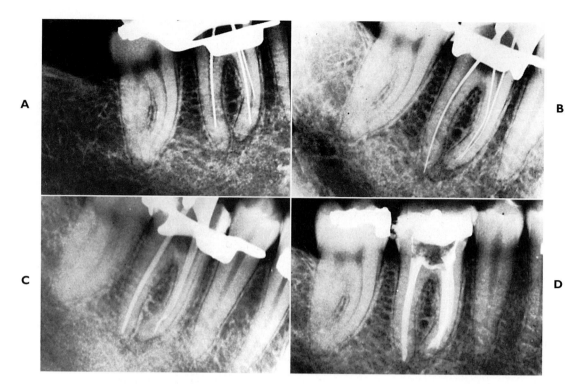

Fig. 5-11 *A,* Clinical example of ledge creation in each canal of a mandibular molar. *B,* After the negotiating files were bent 45 degrees they were carefully teased past the ledges to the original working lengths. *C,* Master cone radiograph shows that proper length was attained in two of three canals. In the third canal an instrument was separated but bypassed. *D,* Obturation of canals with lateral compaction.

NaOCl to remove debris, tissue tags, and any residual chelate present.

Prevention of ledges in small, fine, curved or calcified canals in which the working length cannot initially be determined should proceed in the following manner:

1. On an accurate periradicular radiograph, estimate the tooth length and subtract 1 mm from that length to determine the estimated working length.
2. Fill the pulp chamber with NaOCl.
3. Carefully tease a slightly curved No. 6, 8, or 10 K-file to the estimated working length. Do not force the file apically; rather, tease the instrument to the working length with a stem-winding action.
4. Once the initial file has reached the estimated working length, instrument the canal circumferentially until the file is loose and no longer binds against any of the canal walls. *Do not remove the file from the canal until this looseness is discernible.*
5. Remove the file, irrigate the canal, and proceed with the next larger file in a similar

manner. In tightly curved canals in which it is extremely difficult to advance from a No. 10 to a No. 15 file, customized files can be made to assist in instrumentation.[39] Cutting 1 mm from the tip of a No. 10 K-file converts the file to a No. 12 K-file. Subsequent filing with the No. 12 file will open the canal effectively to the next available standard size, a No. 15. Such half-step files are commercially available as FlexoFile Golden Mediums (LD Caulk/Dentsply, Milford, Del.) and are designed to aid canal negotiation and provide a more gradual increase in size.

6. Proceed until at least a No. 15 K-file will reach the estimated working length.
7. Obtain a radiograph and adjust the working length as necessary.
8. If the canal is extremely calcified and requires initial negotiation with a No. 6 or 8 K-file, refer to the instructions in Chapter 2.

Prevention of ledge formation also depends on the initial assessment of the canal size and type before active preparation. In small, curved canals with curvatures of 20 degrees or more, the working

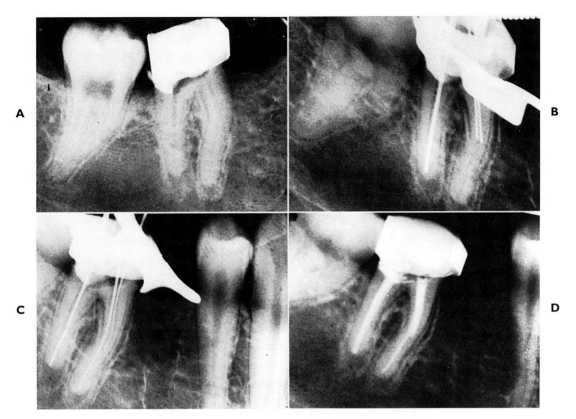

Fig. 5-12 *A, Preoperative radiograph showing previous instrumentation of canals. B, New working-length radiograph shows severe ledging in all canals. C, After a 45-degree bend was placed on all negotiating files, proper length was attained in one canal. D, Obturation of canals with warm gutta-percha technique.*

length can sometimes be determined with a No. 8 or 10 K-file. Subsequently, the extravagant use of smaller-sized K-files followed by similar-sized Hedström files will facilitate canal preparation to a final master apical size equivalent to a No. 25 or 30 file, without resorting to larger, stiffer files.

Early recognition of ledge formation will allow the potential management of this error. A ledge created by a No. 25 or 30 file is much more difficult to bypass than one created by a smaller file because the shelf created by the larger instrument is more likely to prevent penetration beyond the ledge. The smaller the width of the shelf, the less likely it is that the instrument will be prevented from reaching full canal length.

The technique used to bypass ledges is similar to that used to penetrate blockages caused by large particles or dentinal debris (Fig. 5-11); however, if ledges cannot be bypassed, a new working length is established immediately coronal to the ledge. The root canal system is obturated by use of softened gutta-percha and a thin mix of root canal sealer

(Fig. 5-12). Once the canal is filled, periodic recall is necessary for clinical and radiographic evaluation of the tooth. Evidence of failure may indicate the need for surgical treatment.

CLINICAL PROBLEM: A 39-year-old male patient was referred to an endodontist for completion of root canal treatment on a maxillary second molar. According to the referring dentist, there was a severe curvature of the mesiobuccal root and the end of the mesiobuccal canal was not completely negotiated; however, the palatal and distobuccal canals had been located and filed. The dentist stated that he used No. 20 and 25 K-files in an attempt to negotiate the mesiobuccal canal but was unsuccessful (Fig. 5-13, *A*). Because of the dilaceration of the root and fineness of the canal, it was likely that the canal was ledged with these files. The patient was symptom free.

Solution: After the patient was given an explanation of the proposed treatment plan, the tooth was isolated and the temporary was removed. Frequent irrigation and flushing were used to prevent

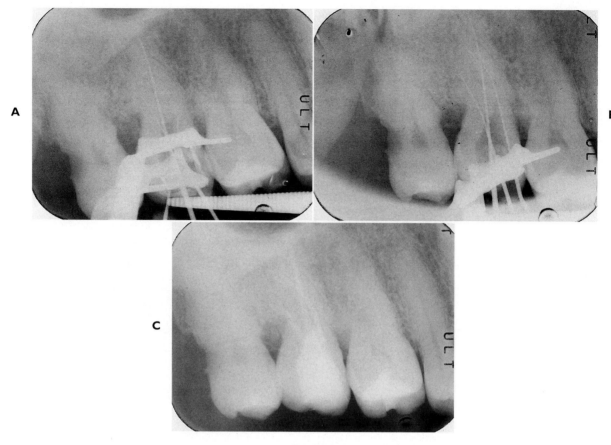

Fig. 5-13

any debris from obstructing any of the canals. The walls of the access cavity were modified with an Endo-Z bur (safe-ended carbide bur) (LD Caulk/Dentsply, Milford, Del.) to provide more straight-line access to the mesiobuccal orifice. Ultrasonic instrumentation was passively used to help open up the coronal third of the canal. A No. 10 K-file with a 45-degree bend was used to go around the ledge. After 30 minutes of file manipulation, a slight pop was felt, and the file was gently maneuvered down the canal. Without removal of the file, a radiograph was taken to confirm the file position and determine the working length. Once they were confirmed, the file was carefully and circumferentially worked until the ledge was smoothed and the file was loose in the canal (Fig. 5-13, *B*). The clinician must recognize that if the file had been prematurely removed reledging of the canal could have easily occurred. Canal cleaning and shaping were completed, and the canals were obturated using lateral compaction with nickel-titanium finger spreaders (Fig. 5-13, *C*). The patient was advised of the restorative needs of the tooth.

Breakage of Instruments in the Canal

Separated (broken) instruments within the root canal system are a potential hazard during root canal treatment. The possibility of instrument separation is remarkably enhanced when the instrument is incorrectly used. Hand instruments, including both stainless-steel and nickel-titanium K-files and Hedström files; rotary instruments such as Peeso reamers, nickel-titanium files, Gates-Glidden burs (Fig. 5-14), and lentulos; and compactors (Fig. 5-15) are commonly misused during root canal treatment. In most clinical situations the instrument fractures in the apical third of the canal, where it is almost impossible to remove or bypass, especially in cases of small, tight canals (see Chapter 7). However, some success in removal has been reported with the use of ultrasonic instrumentation.[26]

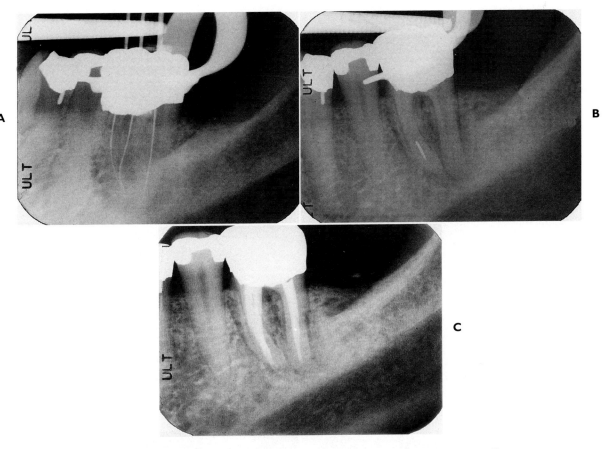

Fig. 5-14 *A, Working-length radiograph of a mandibular first molar depicting accurate file placement.* ***B,*** *Head of No. 2 Gates-Glidden drill separated and wedged in mesiolingual canal.* ***C,*** *Obturation with warm gutta-percha showing embedded "head." Notice the canal transportation that occurred during the cleaning and shaping.*

Prevention of instrument separation requires knowledge of the physical characteristics of the instruments and the guidelines for their proper use in the canal system.[15,33] The most common instruments to fracture are the K-files and Hedström files, but with the use of rotary systems on the rise, instrument separation is occurring in this arena as well. Generally, instruments should be discarded and replaced with new instruments in the following conditions:

1. Flaws, such as shiny areas or unwindings, are detected on the flutes (Fig. 5-16, *A*).
2. Excessive use has caused instrument bending or crimping (common with smaller-sized instruments). A major concern with nickel-titanium instruments is that they tend to fracture without warning; as a result, constant monitoring of usage is critical.
3. Excessive bending or precurving has been necessary.
4. Accidental bending occurs during file usage.
5. The file kinks instead of curving (Fig. 5-16, *B*).
6. Corrosion is noted on the instrument.
7. Compacting instruments have defective tips or have been excessively heated.

During canal cleaning and shaping, copious amounts of NaOCl should always be used with every instrument.

Once the file is placed to the working length, only a filing action should be used; short, 1 to 3 mm in-and-out circumferential strokes of the file are recommended. Rotation of the file, once it has reached the working length, is contraindicated; this can cause flute unraveling, especially if the file is rotated in a counterclockwise direction, with potential separation immediately above the point of binding.

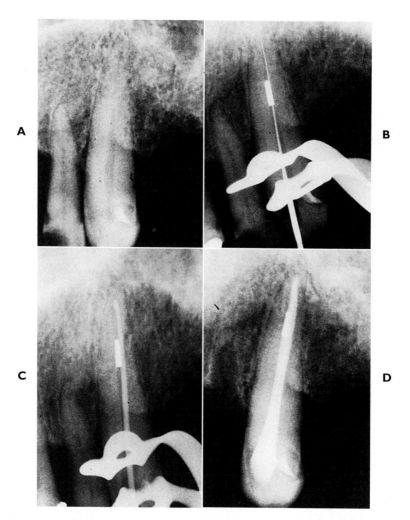

Fig. 5-15 *A, Maxillary canine for which root canal treatment is indicated because of patient symptoms. B, Small endodontic plugger, mistakenly used as a canal probe, was broken when it lodged in the canal. Because of the wide buccolingual dimensions of the canine canal system, a file could be negotiated past the broken fragment. C, Master cone fit to the correct length. D, Root canal obturation incorporating the fractured segment.*

Once the apical seat has been prepared with K-files, often Hedström files are used to facilitate the efficient removal of dentin to produce a continuously tapering funnel preparation. Hedström files are machined and not twisted and therefore are more likely to break. Hedström files should be loosely inserted into the canal and used only on the outstroke or pull stroke to remove dentin. For example, before a No. 25 Hedström file is used, the canal must be sufficiently instrumented with a No. 25 K-file. Since the K-files are a little larger, there will be less tendency for the No. 25 Hedström file to bind at the working length.

To prevent separation of instruments, do not advance too rapidly or skip file sizes during instru-

mentation. Any forcing of an instrument to length by rotation or boring with a large amount of apical pressure can weaken the file tip and may result in fracture. Guidelines for the management and retrieval of separated instruments are found in Chapter 7.

CLINICAL PROBLEM: A 29-year-old male patient presents with a maxillary first premolar requiring root canal treatment (Fig. 5-17, *A*). There had been decay on the mesial surface that had penetrated into the pulp. Although previously in pain, the patient was presently symptom free. The restorative plan for the tooth was post, core, and porcelain-fused-to-metal crown. After anesthesia, access was made, and working lengths were deter-

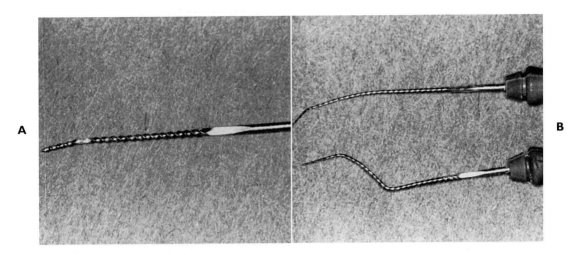

Fig. 5-16 *A,* Unraveling of file flutes before instrument fracture. *B,* Instruments that are bent, twisted, or kinked must be discarded.

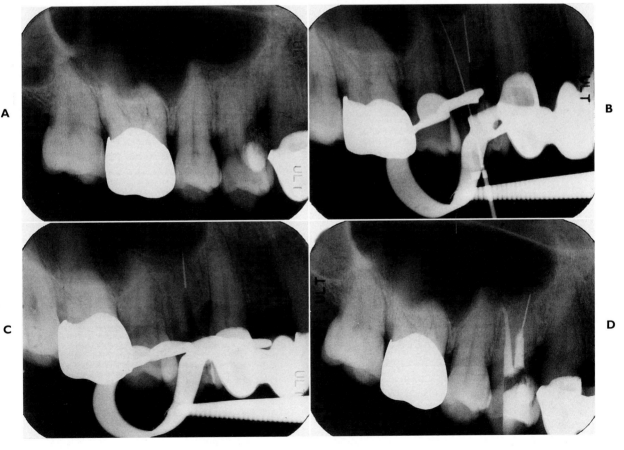

Fig. 5-17

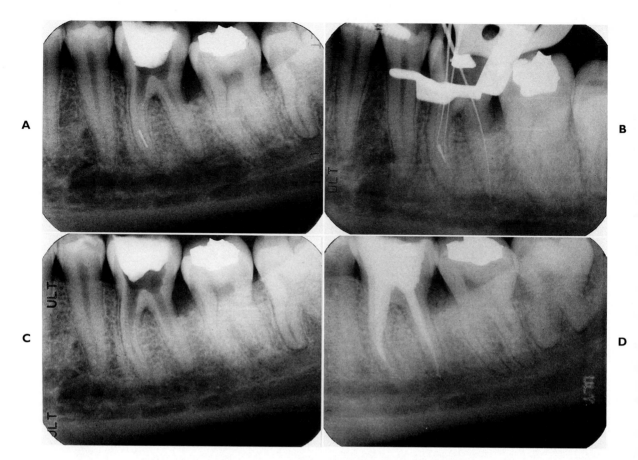

Fig. 5-18

mined. During cleaning and shaping using the balanced-force technique, a 5 mm segment of No. 30 FlexoFile separated in the apical half of the palatal canal (Fig. 5-17, *B*). The canals were irrigated and sealed until the following appointment.

Solution: At the conclusion of the first appointment, the patient was informed of the separated instrument along with the proposed plan of treatment, alternative treatments, and potential risks. At the subsequent appointment, the patient was symptom free and after anesthesia, an attempt was made to bypass and remove the instrument. The operating microscope was used to visualize the coronal extent of the file; a staging platform was made to the level of the file with a modified (the safe tip was removed with a diamond bur) Gates-Glidden bur (Fig. 5-17, *C*). With the aid of the microscope, a fine ultrasonic tip was used to trough around the file. The wedged file could not be removed or bypassed, since it had separated below the height of curvature of the palatal canal. All canals were subsequently obturated with thermoplasticized gutta-percha (Fig. 5-17, *D*). The patient

was informed of the outcome and that the tooth should be restored. Periodic reevaluation of this type of case is essential, especially since the fractured segment is beyond the end of the root and potentially penetrating into the maxillary sinus.

CLINICAL PROBLEM: A 26-year-old female patient was referred for root canal treatment of a mandibular left first molar. Previously there had been a pulp exposure that necessitated treatment. The referring clinician had separated an endodontic file in the mesiolingual canal and had appropriately informed the patient about the incident (Fig. 5-18, *A*). Although the patient was symptom free, she was informed of the potential risks involved in attempting to remove the instrument; these included unsuccessful removal with further wedging of the instrument, pushing the instrument beyond the apical constriction, and root fracture or perforation. The patient opted for treatment.

Solution: After rubber-dam isolation and removal of the temporary restoration, working lengths were determined for all canals (Fig. 5-18, *B*).

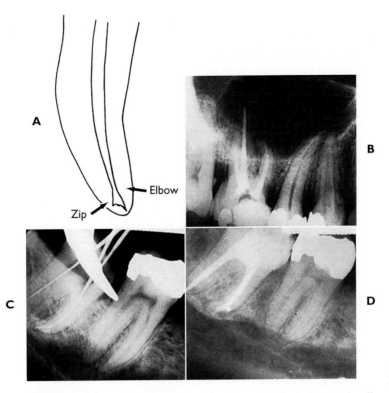

Fig. 5-19 *A, Zipped canal. Notice narrowing coronal to the zip, referred to as the elbow. **B**, Canal obturation showing a zipped mesiobuccal canal. The gutta-percha does not follow the root curvature. **C**, Initial working length; full length and curves negotiated. **D**, Obturation. Notice the zip and small perforation along the mesial wall.*

The mesiolingual canal was passively filed using a step-down approach to flare the coronal two thirds. The operating microscope was used to visualize the coronal extent of the file, and ultrasonic files were used to slightly bypass and loosen the instrument. After 10 minutes of vibration with the ultrasonic probe, the file loosened and was suctioned out of the canal. A radiograph was taken to confirm file removal (Fig. 5-18, *C*). Canal cleaning and shaping were completed, and the canals were obturated by means of lateral compaction (Fig. 5-18, *D*). The patient was informed of the result and was advised of the need to restore the tooth as soon as possible.

DEVIATIONS FROM THE NORMAL CANAL ANATOMY

Zipping (Ellipticarion)

Zipping, or ellipication, refers to transposition or transportation of the apical portion of the canal.[34,40] This phenomenon is characterized by a normally curved canal that has been straightened, especially in the apical third (Fig. 5-19). The main reasons for zipping are failure to precurve files, rotation of instruments in curved canals, and the use of large, stiff instruments to bore out a curved canal. In these situations, the apical foramen will tend to become teardrop shaped or elliptical and be transported from the curve of the canal. Files placed in curved canals will cut more on the outer portion of the canal wall at its apical extent, thus causing movement of the canal away from the curve and its natural path (Fig. 5-20). In contrast, the coronal third of the flutes will remove more on the innermost aspect of the canal wall, causing an uneven reduction of dentin in the coronal third. Excessive and uneven removal of dentin in the coronal part of the canal as well as in the apical third may result in actual perforations in roots having exaggerated external invaginations or severe apical curvatures.

When a file, precurved or not, is rotated in a curved canal, a biomechanical defect known as an *elbow* will form coronally to the elliptically shaped apical seat (Fig. 5-21; see also Fig. 5-19, *A*). This is the narrowest portion of the canal. In many cases the obturating materials terminate at the elbow, leaving an unfilled, zipped canal apical to the elbow. This is a common occurrence with laterally compacted gutta-percha. Use of vertical compaction or obturation with thermoplasticized gutta-percha would be ideal in these cases to compact a solid-core material into the apical preparation without using excessive amounts of sealer (see Chapter 6). Nevertheless, the apical seal will probably be less than optimal, since a zipped canal does not represent a continuously tapering funnel type of preparation.

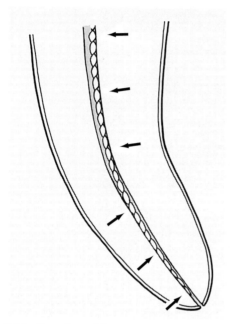

Fig. 5-20 *Curved canal being instrumented. The metal instrument contacts only certain walls (arrows) on the outward cutting stroke, mainly because of the resiliency forces of the files, which cause the files to straighten during cutting.*

To prevent zipping, files should be overcurved, especially in the apical 3 to 4 mm, and always worked in the direction of curvature with short, in-and-out strokes. Do not rotate the file or change its orientation. In preparing the apical seats of small, curved canals, the bulk of the cleaning and shaping is performed with smaller-sized files. Extensive use of small, flexible files to enlarge the apical seat will prevent the zipping that occurs with larger and stiffer instruments. In addition, sound radiographic techniques will disclose the presence of root curvatures and positions of the apical foramina.

In canals with root curvatures of 10 to 20 degrees, the flutes or cutting edges of the file may be removed at certain strategic areas with a diamond disk, fingernail file, or sharpening stone.[39] The portion of the file that makes contact with the outer dentinal wall at the apex (that is, away from the curve) and the portion that makes contact with the inner dentinal wall primarily in the midroot area (that is, toward the curve or toward the invagination) are the sites for flute removal. Reducing the flutes on each increasing file size decreases the tendency to zip and enhances maintenance of the original canal shape. Less tooth structure will be removed from the curve at the apical extent of the canal and less will be removed from the midroot area, where external root invaginations are common (see next section).

In root curvatures greater than 20 degrees, overcurvature of files is mandatory. Placing a precurved file into a noncompliant canal system will tend to reduce the curvature of the file, especially as file size increases. The curvature should generally represent the shape of the canal, with a greater degree of curvature in the apical 3 mm of the file.

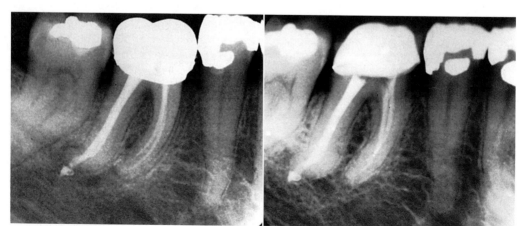

Fig. 5-21 *A, Clinical example of an elbow. B, Appearance at 1-year recall.*

Anticurvature, or reverse filing, should also be used in curved canals and in roots with deep proximal invaginations.[1] This filing variation prevents excess tooth removal in potentially dangerous areas of thin root structure. Heavier filing pressure is placed on tooth structure away from the direction of root curvature and away from the invaginations; it also prevents root thinning and possible fenestration of the root structure.

When a zip is present and there is no evidence of either an apical or lateral root perforation, any type of obturation technique may be used. However, techniques that soften the gutta-percha filling material are preferred. In some cases of zipping, a perforation may not be clinically evident. Therefore it may be judicious to use a root canal sealer containing calcium hydroxide (Sealapex, Kerr Manufacturing Co, Romulus, Mich., or Calciobiotic Root Canal Sealer, Hygenic Corp, Akron, Ohio). If a microscopic perforation does exist apically or in the midroot, the calcium hydroxide will be less irritating to inflamed tissue than a zinc oxide–eugenol sealer and may help to promote a hard tissue barrier when in contact with the periodontium (see Chapter 3).

If a created elbow prevents optimal compaction in the apical portion of the canal, the elbow essentially becomes the apical seat. The gutta-percha and sealer should be three-dimensionally compacted against the elbow, and the patient should be placed on periodic recall evaluation. Signs or symptoms of failure may necessitate surgical repair.

Stripping, or Lateral Wall Perforation

Stripping refers to thinning of the lateral root wall with eventual perforation. Stripping is primarily caused by overzealous instrumentation in the midroot areas of certain teeth, usually molars. Cross sections of these midroot areas reveal that the bulkiest portion of the root structure lies on the side opposite the invagination, away from the direction of root curvature (Fig. 5-22). Filing toward these bulkier regions with less pressure toward the area of the concavity or in the direction of the curvature (anticurvature filing) will prevent excessive removal of tooth structure.

Canals housed in this type of root, especially the mesiobuccal roots of maxillary molars and mesial roots of mandibular molars, are usually small and curved. Therefore it is necessary to clean and shape these canals using small files extravagantly and in a sequential manner. Avoid using large-diameter instruments as well as rotary instruments (Peeso reamers, Gates-Glidden burs) in the coronal half of the canal, especially during the step-back, or flare phase, of instrumentation. Excessive use of these instruments can lead to stripping of susceptible areas of the root wall. Small Hedström files (sizes 20 to 25) can be used to adequately flare the coronal half of the canal without placing excessive pressure on the canal wall adjacent to the concavity. However, Hedström files cut rapidly and efficiently; therefore, care must still be exercised

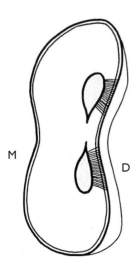

Fig. 5-22 *Buccolingual section of the midroot in a mesial root of a mandibular molar. Notice differences in root wall thickness on the mesial,* M, *and distal,* D, *surfaces when external invaginations are present.*

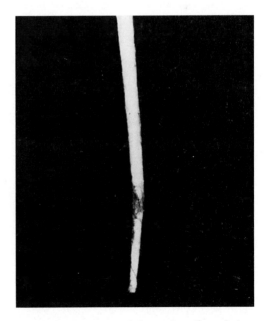

Fig. 5-23 *Paper point with hemorrhage located above the apical foramen. Lateral perforation was present at the level of the hemorrhage.*

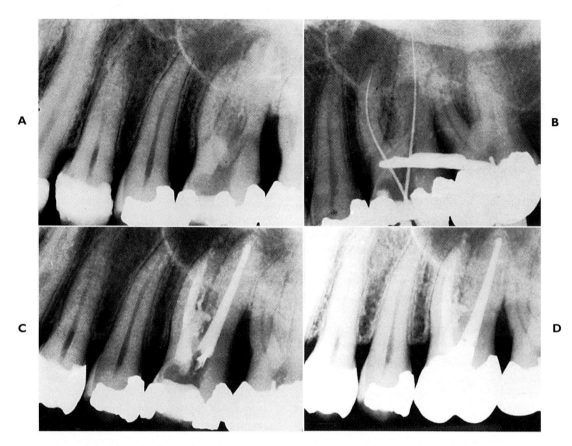

Fig. 5-24 *A, Maxillary molar with significantly curved roots. B, Initial working-length determination. C, Obturation shows zipping and stripping of the mesiobuccal canal system, along with a perforation into the furcation on the inner aspect of the coronal third of the mesiobuccal root. D, Recall radiograph obtained at 6 months. The patient was symptom free.*

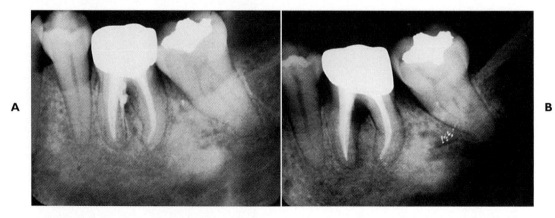

Fig. 5-25 *A, Osseous breakdown in furcation of mandibular molar caused by a strip perforation. Notice filling material leaving the site of the perforation. B, Postoperative radiograph after surgical repair of the strip perforation. Continual monitoring is necessary to assess the periodontium.*

even with anticurvature filing techniques. In roots that are especially thin in a mesiodistal direction, the canal flare may have to be compromised to avoid stripping of these roots.

If a strip is identified before canal cleaning and shaping have been completed, further damage to the defect must be prevented. When hemorrhage is evident in the canal, determine whether it is caused by a strip or an apical perforation. Dry the canal with paper points. If hemorrhage is located along the side of the point, it is likely that a lateral root perforation has occurred (Fig. 5-23). If hemorrhage is located primarily at the tip of the point, excessive instrumentation with perforation of the apex has occurred.

Once a strip has been identified, its management is identical to all forms of perforation repair (see Chapter 3). It is essential that the perforation be free from contamination and be sealed immediately. Although a variety of materials have been advocated for the repair of perforations, the most appropriate material for repairing lateral root perforations may be pharmaceutical-grade calcium hydroxide. The strip is usually difficult to seal with conventional compaction procedures. Calcium hydroxide is mixed to a thick paste with physiologic saline or local anesthetic solution and is carried to the canal system by means of the lentula, McSpadden compactor (see Chapter 10), or TLC burs (Brasseler USA, Savannah, Ga.) and vertically compacted against the strip. The calcium hydroxide will halt exudate or hemorrhage and promote healing with the potential for calcific barrier formation. The key factors for repair are immediate sealing of the perforation, which protects it from saliva and other contaminants, and preventing placement of sealing materials into the periodontium.

The calcium hydroxide paste should remain in the canal system for at least 4 to 6 weeks or until no symptoms are present. The paste is then carefully removed by copious irrigation of the canal and the use of anticurvature filing to minimize the pressure against the perforation site. Avoid penetrating the defect when removing the paste. There should be no evidence of hemorrhage or exudate in the canal. Irrigation with normal saline or 3% hydrogen peroxide is recommended. Once the canal system has been cleaned and the case is ready for obturation, a calcium hydroxide–containing root canal sealer such as Sealapex or Calciobiotic Root Canal Sealer is recommended. The patient is periodically evaluated (Fig. 5-24).

Attention must be paid to the development of any periodontal defects in the furcation region, especially in periodontally compromised teeth and those cases in which the strip occurred in the coronal third of the root surface. A perforation repair has the best prognosis when it is housed in bone. Thus the closer the perforation is to the oral environment, the more likely it is that a communication will develop between the perforation site and the oral cavity. This communication will result in periodontal destruction and eventual failure. Sealing the perforation or strip becomes extremely important, since most strips occur in furcation areas, which can readily give rise to salivary contamination. Therefore periodontal probing is mandatory at each recall examination to assess the integrity of the periodontal attachment in the area of the perforation. Once the canal system has been obturated, a "leakage-free" occlusal restoration is mandatory.

If symptoms persist or if there is periodontal destruction in the furcation area, surgical repair of the perforation or root resection of the involved root may represent a final effort to correct the problem (Fig. 5-25). However, the surgical repair of furcation perforations has had limited success. Access to the defect, the periodontal condition, and the strategic position of the tooth are all important factors to consider before resorting to a surgical approach to rectify the problem. In some situations root or tooth resection (see Chapter 8) or extraction may be indicated (Fig. 5-26).

INADEQUATE CANAL PREPARATION
Overinstrumentation (Excessive Instrumentation beyond the Apical Constriction)

Excessive instrumentation beyond the apical constriction violates the periodontal ligament and alveolar bone.

Many problems may arise from this error. Loss of the apical constriction creates an open apex with an increased likelihood of overfilling, lack of an adequate apical seal, and pain and discomfort for the patient. Excessive instrumentation beyond the constriction may be recognized when hemorrhage is evident in the apical portion of the canal, with or without patient discomfort. Thus it is imperative to perform all instrumentation within the confines of the root system.

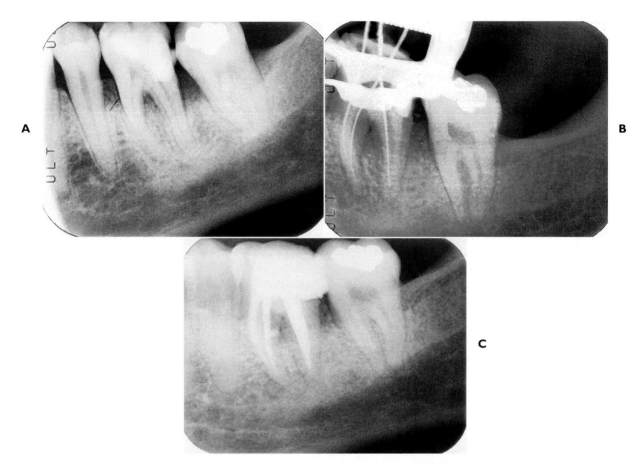

Fig. 5-26 *A, Preoperative radiograph of mandibular first molar requiring endodontic treatment. Notice constricted root anatomy on mesial root and furcation involvement. B, Angled working-length radiograph depicting midroot concavity on distal aspect of mesial root. C, Obturation radiograph demonstrating strip perforation on mesial root; patient developed swelling and severe furcation involvement within 6 weeks; tooth was subsequently extracted.*

Instrumentation beyond or through the constriction can be prevented by:

1. Using good radiographic techniques
2. Accurately determining the apical constriction of the root canal
3. Using sound reference points
4. Using stable instrument stops placed perpendicularly to the shaft of the instrument
5. Retaining all instruments within the confines of the canal system
6. Occlusal refinement or reduction before working-length determination and instrumentation
7. Periodic radiographic verification of the working length (when necessary)
8. Attention to detail during all cleaning and shaping procedures
9. Assessing the integrity of the apical stop with stiff paper points or files

When the apical constriction is lost, a new apical stop must be established within the confines of the root canal (Fig. 5-27). This position will be approximately 1 to 2 mm from the radiographic apex. The new apical stop should be equivalent to two to three sizes larger than the first file to bind at that position. In addition, since the canal is still patent apical to the new stop, a plug of dentin chips or pharmaceutical-grade calcium hydroxide should be placed apically to control the movement of gutta-percha and sealer during compaction procedures (Fig. 5-27, *A*). The dentin chips are obtained during canal shaping and flaring in the middle and coronal third of the canal by using a Hedström file short of the working length in a dry canal. The filings are then packed to the working length with a paper point or small plugger. However, this process is more difficult in curved canals, and caution must be exercised to prevent canal blockage, ledging, or perforation. The technique of packing dentinal chips at the apex and its effect on the seal of the canal and on the periradicular tissues remain controversial.[4,19,27,31,34] Continued research as to the efficacy of this procedure is warranted.

CLINICAL PROBLEM: A 52-year-old patient presents with severe pain to thermal changes and biting on a symptomatic mandibular left second molar. The pain started 2 weeks previously and had increased in severity over the past 3 days. Clinical examination revealed a large alloy restoration. There was exquisite pain to percussion on this tooth. Radiographically it appeared as though there may have been a previous pulp exposure, and there was loss of the lamina dura and periodontal ligament space apically. The tooth was diagnosed as having an irreversible pulpitis and acute periradicular periodontitis (Fig. 5-28, *A*). After anesthesia, an access cavity was made, the coronal pulp tissue was removed, working lengths were determined, and a pulpectomy was performed with K-files (Fig. 5-28, *B*). After rinsing the chamber with 5.25% sodium hypochlorite, a dry cotton pellet was placed on the pulpal floor, and the access was sealed with Cavit. The patient returned the following week, at which time the tooth was symptom free. After anesthesia, the three canals were completely cleaned and shaped using a step-back technique. Master apical files were seated to the recorded working lengths, and a radiograph was taken (Fig. 5-28, *C*). The radiograph demonstrated significant canal transportation in both mesial canals with perforations on the mesial aspect of the mesial root. In addition,

it is important to recognize that canal lengths had not changed even though canal shapes were significantly altered.

Solution: Since the mesial canals had been straightened and overinstrumented, the best treatment was to develop a three-dimensional obturation within solid root structure. Dry calcium hydroxide powder was first packed in the mesial canals to the level of the perforation. New apical seats were prepared with larger files 2 mm coronal to the perforation sites. A radiograph was taken to check master gutta-percha cone placement (Fig. 5-28, *D*). Depth of spreader penetration was closely monitored during lateral compaction to prevent the vertical movement of gutta-percha past the tenuous apical stops and calcium hydroxide plugs (Fig. 5-28, *E*). The patient was advised to have the tooth restored within a month.

Overpreparation (Excessive Removal of Tooth Structure)

Overpreparation is the excessive removal of tooth structure in a mesiodistal and buccolingual direction. During canal cleaning and shaping, the size of the apical preparation should correspond to the respective size, shape, and curvature of the root. For example, attempts to produce an apical seat equivalent to a No. 40 K-file in a moderately curved (10 to 20 degrees) mesiobuccal canal of a mandibular first molar is likely to cause not only zipping of the root apex but also perforation of the apical constriction. Adherence to the guidelines for the recommended range of size termination for each type

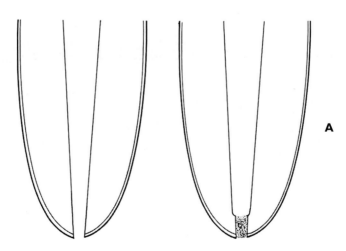

Fig. 5-27 *A, Apical constriction lost because of overinstrumentation. Plug of dentin chips or calcium hydroxide powder is placed before establishing a new apical stop.*

Continued.

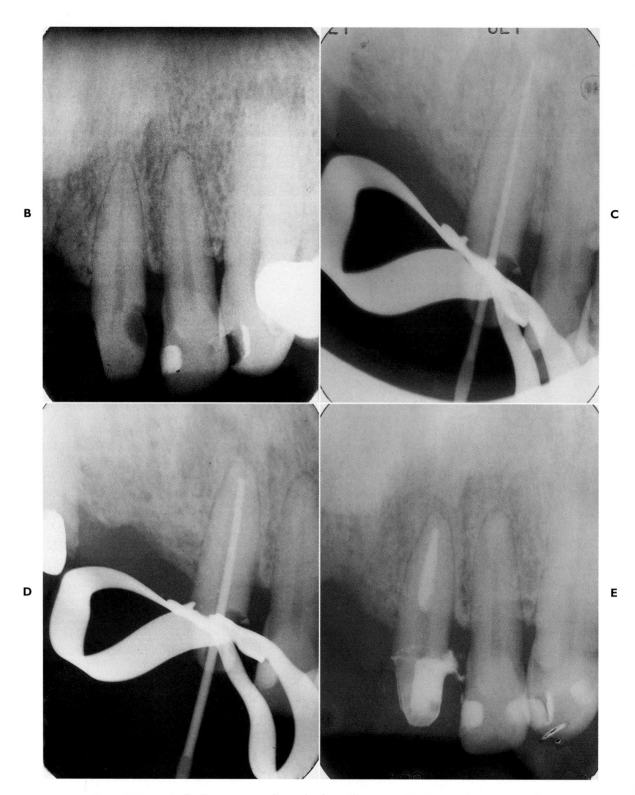

Fig. 5-27 cont'd. *B, Preoperative radiograph of maxillary central incisor requiring root canal treatment. C, Size No. 55 master gutta-percha cone extending beyond apex; loss of apical constriction is due to overinstrumentation. D, Size No. 80 master cone seated at established apical stop; calcium hydroxide powder packed apically and apical stop established by developing a mechanical seat within root structure, three sizes larger than the original master apical file. E, Completed obturation using lateral compaction.*

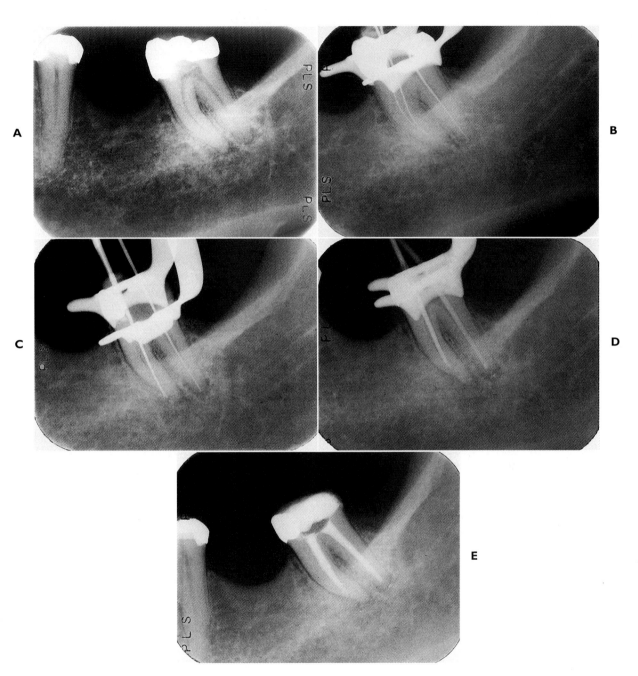

Fig. 5-28

▼ **Table 5-1** Recommended Sizes for Final Apical Preparation

TOOTH GROUP	FINAL APICAL SIZE*
Maxillary centrals	35-60
Maxillary laterals	25-40
Maxillary canines	30-50
Maxillary premolars	25-40
Maxillary molars	
MB/DB	25-40
Palatal	25-50
Mandibular incisors	25-40
Mandibular canines	30-50
Mandibular premolars	30-50
Mandibular molars	
MB/ML	25-40
Distal	25-50

DB, distobuccal; *MB,* mesiobuccal; *ML,* mesiolingual.
*With straight roots, anywhere in the range is acceptable. With curved roots (10 to 20 degrees), stay at the lower end of the range. Sizes may vary with stainless steel and nickel-titanium instruments.

of root is mandatory, with modifications made as necessary (Table 5-1).

Overpreparation is a special concern in the apical portion of the canal system, but it can easily occur in the middle and coronal portions of the canal as well. Excessive canal flaring increases the chances of stripping and perforation. When flaring the canal, a step-back or step-down procedure is recommended to create a continuously tapering funnel preparation for obturation with gutta-percha.[24] If necessary, careful and conservative use of rotary instruments, such as Peeso reamers and Gates-Glidden burs, can be considered to assist in refining the canal shape. However, excessive removal of tooth structure is not necessary because overprepared (overflared) canals are potentially weaker and subject to fracture during compaction and restorative procedures.

Underpreparation (Insufficient Canal Preparation)

Underpreparation is the failure to remove pulp tissue, dentinal debris, and microorganisms from the root canal system. In addition, the canal system is improperly shaped, and such a shape thus prevents three-dimensional obturation. Inadequate preparation of the canal system occurs in the following ways:

1. Insufficient preparation of the apical dentin matrix to control filling materials in the canal
2. Insufficient use of tissue-dissolving and bactericidal irrigants (NaOCl)

3. Inadequate canal shaping (flaring), which prevents depth of spreader or plugger penetration during compaction[2]
4. Establishing the working length short of the apical constriction, especially in cases of pulp necrosis
5. Creation of ledges and blockages that prevent complete canal cleaning and shaping

Inadequate canal preparation can generally be prevented by adherence to the principles of problem-solving already discussed in this chapter and in Chapters 4 and 6. The existence of this problem is determined by:

1. Inability to place compacting instruments to the working length without a master gutta-percha cone in place (see Fig. 6-15); instrument must not bind on canal walls
2. Inability to place compacting instruments close to the working length with a master cone in place (see Fig. 6-15)
3. Binding of the master apical file at the working length or inability of the file to reach the full working length
4. Failure of the master apical file to fall within the lower end of the suggested ranges for final apical preparation (see Table 5-1)
5. Penetration of the master apical file beyond the established working length, with subsequent apical perforation (lack of apical stop and constriction)

Underprepared canals are best managed by adherence to sound principles of proper length determination, canal cleaning and shaping, and recapitulation. Copious irrigation and attention to detail during instrumentation will ensure a properly cleaned canal. Before obturation, spreaders and pluggers must be prefit to determine their depth of placement and to ensure proper canal shape. A critical assessment of the preparation can often be made only by evaluation of the final obturation (Fig. 5-29).

Parameters for this evaluation and its relationship to canal preparation are reviewed in Chapter 6. In some situations, immediate retreatment is indicated to correct the discrepancies in canal preparation (see Chapter 7). In others, recall evaluation is warranted before a course of action is considered.

GUIDELINES FOR CONTEMPORARY METHODS OF CLEANING AND SHAPING CURVED CANALS

Complex root anatomy, such as canal curvatures greater than 20 degrees, inherent limitations of endodontic instruments, and operator variability render any "instrumentation technique" its own technical nuances, each not without its problems. To overcome some of these liabilities, new methods continuously evolve. The recent advent of nickel-titanium alloy and the resurgence of mechanized instrumentation are contemporary approaches to instrumentation, conceptually designed to help reduce some of the inherent problems associated with stainless steel instruments and conventional methods of canal cleaning and shaping.[35] The following guidelines are basic principles to consider during various instrumentation techniques for canal curvatures greater than 20 degrees.

Step-Back (Telescopic) Technique (Apical-to-Coronal Preparation)[25]

1. Determine working length and serially develop an apical stop to a size 25. Precurve (overcurve) stainless steel files in apical 2 to 3 mm and insert in the same orientation as the canal curvature. Consider using a K-file before using a same-sized Hedström file to facilitate the serial preparation (for example,. use 15 K-type, then 15 H-type, then 20 K, then 20 H, and so forth).
2. Recapitulate with smaller files and irrigate frequently during the serial preparation.
3. Achieve step-back (flare) by shortening the No. 30, 35, 40 files or larger by 1, 2, and 3 mm or more (or 0.5, 1, and 1.5 mm or more if more apical taper is desired) to produce the desired taper.
4. Recapitulate and circumferentially file with a 25 K-file.
5. Use a No. 2 and No. 3 Gates-Glidden bur to flare and shape the preparation coronally.
6. Recapitulate and smooth preparation with master K-file.

Step-Down Technique (Coronal and Radicular Access are Established First to Aid in Achieving Direct Access to the Apical Third)[14]

1. Passively use No. 15, 20, and 25 Hedström files with light apical pressure in coronal two thirds of canal. Files must not be forced and should be placed to a point short of binding. If the canal is extremely curved or calcified, establish patency first with No. 8 or No. 10 K-file. The rasping of the canal with Hedström files eliminates dentinal interferences and gross pulpal tissue and sufficiently enlarges the canal before Gates-Glidden burs are used.

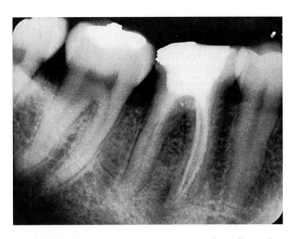

Fig. 5-29 *Obturation radiograph shows that all canals were inadequately prepared. Notice that the filling material is only in the coronal third of the distal canal.*

2. After irrigation, use No. 2 and No. 3 Gates-Glidden burs with light apical pressure, directing them laterally away from the furcation to avoid stripping and perforation.
3. Establish working length and develop an apical seat by standard serial filing.
4. Develop step-back preparation to blend the coronal shape with the apical preparation.
5. Recapitulate and circumferentially file with a master K-file to smooth the entire preparation.

Crown-Down Pressureless Technique (Similar in Concept to Step-Down Technique)[14,24]

1. Rotate straight files two times in a clockwise direction, from a larger to a smaller sequence, without apical pressure, until a depth of 16 mm is reached.
2. Passively use No. 2 and No. 3 Gates-Glidden burs.
3. Establish a provisional working length 3 mm short of radiographic apex by rotating successively smaller files. Take a radiograph to establish working length.
4. Rotate straight files two times in a clockwise direction, from larger to smaller, without apical pressure, until working length is achieved.
5. Complete crown-down preparation with a file size two times larger than first file to reach working length.

Balanced Force Technique[20,30]

1. With this technique, use a Flex-R file (Moyco Union Broach, Emigsville, Penn.),

FlexoFile, or any other flexible triangular file with a modified noncutting tip.

2. Establish radicular access by step-down or crown-down techniques before preparing the apical third of the canal.

3. Rotate the uncurved file clockwise from 90 to 180 degrees with light apical pressure to engage dentin. If apical force is excessive, file may lock, predisposing it to fracture upon counterclockwise rotation.

4. Rotate file counterclockwise at least 120 degrees with apical force, flexing it to conform to the canal curvature, to cut the engaged dentin. This cut is often tactilely felt as a "pop." The clinician must press apically to prevent outward movement of the file and to obtain cutting.

5. Use a combination of threading clockwise turns and unthreading counterclockwise turns with apical loading until adequate enlargement to working length is achieved.

6. Use precurved files in canals with severe curvatures and do not enlarge beyond a size 35 in curved canals.

7. Inspect files frequently and discard those showing any defects or signs of unwinding.

The modified tip of the Flex-R file allows it to follow canal anatomy without cutting dentin. The balanced-force technique has been shown to reduce canal transportation and ledging but requires an extended learning curve to master.

Double-Flared Technique[10]

1. Use straight files in a larger to a smaller sequence, progressively and passively, moving them further into the canal (until the apical third is reached). No binding of instruments should occur.

2. Use frequent irrigation to remove contents and to aid in cleaning apical third.

3. Establish working length with small K-file.

4. Continue to use larger to smaller files until full working length is reached.

5. Serially prepare apical stop and step-back apical preparation to blend with the coronal step-down flare.

6. Circumferentially file with master K-file.

Passive Step-Back Technique[38]

1. Establish working length with small K-file.

2. Use passive instrumentation with progressively larger K-files. This establishes a minimally flared canal before insertion of Gates-Glidden burs.

3. Use No. 2, 3, and possibly 4 Gates-Glidden burs to flare the coronal third.

4. Confirm working length, since flaring and removal of curvatures reduce the working length.

5. Carefully rework Gates-Glidden burs or Peeso reamers to provide more straight-line access.

6. Serially prepare the apical stop and step-back the apical preparation to blend with the coronal step-back flare.

In contrast to the conventional step-back technique, each of these aforementioned techniques results in a coronal pathway for early debris removal, allows for a deeper penetration of irrigating solutions, reduces procedural accidents such as ledging and zipping, permits straight-line access to the apical third, and causes less extrusion of debris apically.[10,14,20,24,30,38] However, during any coronal-to-apical preparation, frequent irrigation is critical, and any forceful penetration of instruments could result in canal blockage, instrument separation, or deviations in anatomy.

NICKEL-TITANIUM INSTRUMENTATION
Concepts

The recent introduction of nickel-titanium (Ni-Ti, niti) alloy to endodontics is purported to have "problem solved" many of the negative features that have been associated with stainless steel instruments. Endodontic files made from this "superelastic" alloy are significantly more flexible and are highly resistant to fracture and corrosion.[35] The advantages of Ni-Ti files for canal cleaning and shaping seem to be enhanced canal negotiation, especially in curved canals; decreased canal transportation and ledging; reduced chance for breakage; faster and more efficient instrumentation; and no precurving.[7,9,12,13,17,22] However, some of these purported advantages are clinical impressions and have yet to be substantiated. Although many of these characteristics of Ni-Ti indicate that cleaning and shaping skills may be less forgiving, on the contrary, the clinician must understand that nickel-titanium is not without its problems, that there is a long learning curve with Ni-Ti instrumentation, and that there are still many unknowns. For example, when stressed, the metal undergoes a crystalline (microscopic) phase transformation and can become structurally weaker; however, there is usually no visible or macroscopic indication that the metal has become fatigued; thus a Ni-Ti file may break without warning (unwinding), especially if used improperly.[35]

Considerations and Problem Solving

K-files, Hedström files, S-files, Flex-R files, reamers, and compactors (see Chapter 6) are available in nickel-titanium alloy. However, because of their extreme flexibility, Ni-Ti instruments are not designed for pathfinding, negotiating small calcified, curved canals, or bypassing ledges. Stainless steel instruments should be used initially for pathfinding because of their enhanced stiffness. Once the canal has been negotiated or the ledge has been bypassed and removed, Ni-Ti instruments can then be used. Since there may be a reduced tactile sensation when Ni-Ti hand instruments are used, the clinician may feel that the file is not cutting. On the contrary, Ni-Ti files can be as aggressive as stainless steel files, and overpreparation can occur if filing pressures and instrumentation times are not carefully monitored.[35] If Ni-Ti hand files, especially K-files and S-files, are used in a conventional push-pull, or filing, motion, deviations in anatomy may occur with a tendency of the outer wall of the preparation to "belly out" below the height of curvature. This is probably attributable to the file's tendency to "unflex," or straighten out. Recent research suggests that Ni-Ti files may function best and cause less transportation and deviation in anatomy when used in a reaming or rotary motion.[12] In turn, the evolution of mechanized or rotary instrumentation using specially designed Ni-Ti files in gear-reduction, high-torque handpieces, has recently revolutionized endodontics because of their speed and efficacy in canal shaping and maintaining canal curvature.[13] Although such variably shaped Ni-Ti files are quite flexible, Ni-Ti metal, like any other metal, will eventually fail when rotated in a curved canal. Strict monitoring of instrument usage should be maintained so that Ni-Ti files can be periodically disposed of before failure. In addition, care must be taken to use these systems per the manufacturer's instructions (for example, a crown-down approach with light pressure is essential when using most Ni-Ti rotary instruments). It should also be noted that these systems require a significant learning curve to achieve mastery.

SPECIAL ANATOMIC PROBLEMS IN CANAL CLEANING AND SHAPING

C-shaped Canals

Although the prevalence of C-shaped canals is low, those requiring treatment present a diagnostic and treatment challenge to the practitioner. Some C-shaped canals are difficult to interpret on radiographs and often are not identified until an endodontic access is made. These anatomic variations occur primarily in mandibular second molars and maxillary first molars.[8] When roots in these teeth appear very close or fused, a C-shaped canal anatomy should be anticipated.

The C-shaped canal in the mandibular second molar is usually ribbon shaped and includes the mesiobuccal and distal canals. It may or may not also include the mesiolingual canal if present (Fig. 5-30). In maxillary molars, the C-shaped canal can encompass the mesiobuccal and palatal canals or the distobuccal and palatal canals. In any of these cases, canal orifices may be found within the C-shaped trough or the C-shape may be continuous throughout the length of the canal.

The key problems encountered during cleaning and shaping C-shaped canals are difficulty in removing pulp tissue and necrotic debris, excessive hemorrhage, and persistent discomfort during instrumentation. Because of the large volumetric capacity of the C-shaped canal system, often housing transverse anastomoses and irregularities, continuous circumferential filing along the periphery of the C with copious amounts of 5.25% NaOCl is necessary to ensure maximum tissue removal and cessation of bleeding. Hedström files are especially effective for efficient tissue removal. If hemorrhage persists, ultrasonic removal of tissue or placement of calcium hydroxide between appointments may be used to enhance tissue removal and control hemorrhage. Further ultrasonic instrumentation should be considered to remove tissue and debris in inaccessible areas. Overpreparation of C-shaped canals should be particularly avoided, since there are only minimal amounts of dentin between the external root surface and the canal system in these teeth.[23] In some cases, even with adequate local anesthesia, pain persists during canal cleaning. Frequent administration of intrapulpal anesthesia may be necessary (see Chapter 9) to keep the patient comfortable until all remnants of pulp tissue have been removed.

Once the canals have been properly cleaned and shaped, a cold or warm gutta-percha or a thermoplasticized gutta-percha obturation technique should be used to manage the complex three-dimensional nature of the C-shaped system (Fig. 5-30, C).

S-shaped Canals

S-shaped, or bayonet-shaped, canals can be troublesome and challenging, since they involve at least

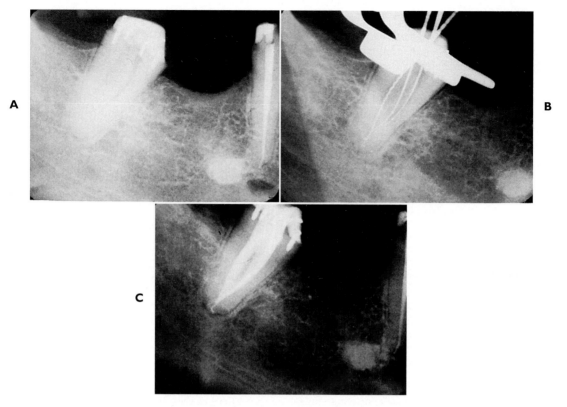

Fig. 5-30 *A, Radiograph of a mandibular molar with a C-shaped canal. Notice root fusion and apical orientation of canals toward the distal side.* ***B,*** *File placement in tooth. In this case there was a C-shaped trough connecting the mesiobuccal and distal canals. There was a separate mesiolingual canal. Notice centering of files, which gives the radiographic appearance of a furcation perforation.* ***C,*** *Obturation using lateral compaction. Notice the creamy appearance of the filled C-shaped trough.*

two curves, with the apical curve being the most vulnerable to deviations in anatomy and loss of working length. These double-curved canals are usually identified radiographically if they traverse in a mesiodistal direction; if in a buccolingual direction, they may be identified with multiple-angled radiographs, or when the initial apical file is removed from the canal and it simulates multiple curves. S-shaped canals are found in maxillary lateral incisors, maxillary canines, maxillary premolars, and mandibular molars.[18] They occur most often in maxillary second premolars (Fig. 5-31, *A*).

To prevent problems during cleaning and shaping of these types of canals, the three-dimensional nature of the S-shaped canal must be visualized with special attention and assessment to the multiple concavities along the external surfaces of the root. Failure to recognize these may lead to stripping of the canal along the inner surface of each curve (Fig. 5-32). During initial canal negoti-

ation, it is essential that there be an unrestricted approach to the first curve. To accomplish this, the access preparation is skewed to allow for a more direct entry (Fig. 5-31, *B*). Once the entire canal is negotiated, passive shaping of the coronal curve is done first, to facilitate the cleaning and shaping of the apical curve. However, constant recapitulation with small files and frequent irrigation is necessary to prevent blockage and ledging in the apical curve. As in the instrumentation of any curved canal, overcurving the apical 3 mm of the file will aid in maintaining the curvature in the apical portion of the canal as the coronal curve becomes normally "straightened out" during the later stages of cleaning and shaping. In most cases the practitioner should not use a master apical file size larger than 25. Gradual use of small file sizes with short-amplitude strokes is essential to manage these canals effectively and to prevent stripping and ledging in the apical curve. To prevent stripping in the coronal

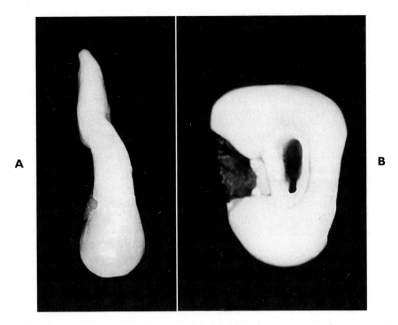

Fig. 5-31 *A, Maxillary second premolar with an S-shaped root. **B,** Divergent and skewed access opening to allow for unimpeded entry to the coronal curvature.*

curve, anticurvature or reverse filing is recommended, with primary pressure being placed away from the curve of the coronal curvature.

Once loss of working length or deviations in anatomy are identified, the same principles of error management apply as those with a straightforward canal system. However, focusing on a problem that has occurred in the apical curvature can easily produce an additional problem in the coronal curvature. Thus the astute practitioner must render careful clinical judgment when managing problems in the apical curve. Once cleaning and shaping have been completed, use of finger condensers with either a cold or warm gutta-percha technique is suggested to obturate these delicate canal systems (Fig. 5-33).

SUMMARY OF GUIDELINES FOR PROPER CANAL CLEANING AND SHAPING

The following step-by-step guidelines summarize the key points discussed in this chapter and highlight the cognitive awareness required of the practitioner when biomechanically cleaning and shaping the root canal system.

1. Knowledge of root and root canal anatomy is essential.
2. Use good radiographic technique. Periradicular areas must be viewed as well as total root structure.

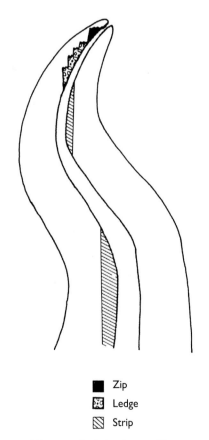

■ Zip

▨ Ledge

▨ Strip

Fig. 5-32 *Diagram depicting key problem areas in S-shaped canal systems. Notice that stripping can occur in areas where external root concavities exist.*

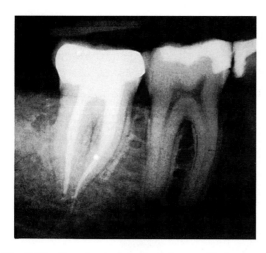

Fig. 5-33 *Completed obturation of a mandibular second molar with S-shaped canals in the mesial root. Finger spreaders were used during lateral compaction.*

3. Always use clean, flawless instruments. Monitor clinical usage of nickel-titanium instruments.

4. Use files that correspond to working lengths. For example, do not use 25 mm files in canals that measure 21 mm or less. The working end of the file will be closer to the fingers, enhancing tactile sensation. In addition, files that are too long, especially in posterior teeth, may be difficult to manipulate, and the patient may close the jaws, forcing the files apically.

5. Precurve stainless steel instruments to simulate canal curvature; overcurve in the apical 3 to 4 mm.

6. With conventional radiographic techniques, working-length films should be obtained with a minimum of a No. 10 K-file in the canal.

7. If any doubt exists about the true working length, verify it with a new radiograph.

8. Use all intracanal instruments sequentially.

9. Use small instruments extravagantly, especially sizes 8 to 20.

10. Use copious irrigation, preferably NaOCl.

11. Recapitulate throughout *all phases* of cleaning and shaping.

12. Never rotate files at the working length unless the particular instrumentation technique so dictates (such as balanced force).

13. Use a K-file *before* using the same-sized Hedström file.

14. Use short amplitude (1 to 3 mm) circumferential in-and-out strokes to clean and shape the canal.

15. Use stable, properly positioned silicone stops on files to ensure orientation and length maintenance during preparation.

16. Use sound, reproducible reference points.

17. The working end of the intracanal instruments must contact only the canal wall and not the walls of the access opening preparation.

18. Never advance instrument sizes too fast. Before advancing to the next-sized instrument, see that each previous file fits *loosely* in the canal at the appropriate length.

19. Use anticurvature filing when indicated.

20. Avoid large-sized files or rotary instruments in small, curved canals and in roots with external invaginations.

21. Always pay attention to detail during cleaning and shaping procedures.

Most of these guidelines are not new, yet their violation results in a significant number of procedural errors that could be prevented. As with many other things in life, the lessons of history go unheeded, lessons for which guidelines have been with us for many years.

"After the pulp is removed, canals must be enlarged so as to remove shreds of tissue adhering to uneven walls. This step should be given most careful attention, for the average root canal presents many irregularities, and a delicate instrument may be readily broken off in the tooth. Such an accident almost invariably means failure, as the broken part is wedged at some inaccessible point. New and tested instruments should be used. When a reamer or file binds, it should be gently pulled out of place and not twisted further. The larger size reamers should not be used until the canal has been thoroughly explored with the smaller ones. This will prevent the formation of ledges, so readily caused by the larger and less flexible instruments, and over which it is often very difficult to proceed."[†]

References

1. Abou-Rass M, Frank A, Glick D: The anticurvature filing method to prepare the curved root canal, *J Am Dent Assoc* 101:792-794, 1980.

2. Allison DA, Weber CR, Walton RE: The influence of the methods of canal preparation and the quality of apical and coronal seal, *J Endod* 5:298-304, 1979.

3. Baker NA, Eleazer PD, Averbach RE et al: Scanning electron microscopic studies of the efficacy of various irrigating solutions, *J Endod* 1:127-135, 1975.

4. Brady JE, Himel VT, Weir JC: Periapical response to an apical plug of dentin filings intentionally placed after root canal overinstrumentation, *J Endod* 11:323-329, 1985.

[†]From Jasper EA: *Dent Cosmos* 75:823-829, 1933.

5. Chernick LB, Jacobs JJ, Lautenschlager EP et al: Torsional failure of endodontic files, *J Endod* 2:94-97, 1976.

6. Cohen S, Stewart G, Laster L: The effects of acids, alkalies, and chelating agents on dentin permeability *Oral Surg Oral Med Oral Pathol* 29:63-634, 1970.

7. Coleman CL, Svec TA, Rieger MR et al: Stainless steel vs. nickel-titanium K-files: analysis of instrumentation in curved canals, *J Endod* 21:221, 1995.

8. Cooke HG, Cox FL: C-shaped canal configurations in mandibular molars, *J Am Dent Assoc* 99:836-839, 1979.

9. Diandreth M, Ellis RA, Fagundes D: The effectiveness of hand and rotary files to maintain canal curvature: a comparison, *J Endod* 21:236, 1995.

10. Fava LRG: The double-flared technique: an alternative for biomechanical preparation, *J Endod* 9:76-80, 1983.

11. Fraser JG: Chelating agents: Their softening effect on root canal dentin, *Oral Surg Oral Med Oral Pathol* 37:803-811, 1974.

12. Gambill JM, Alder M, del Rio CE: Comparison of niti and stainless steel hand files using computed tomography, *J Endod* 21:220, 1995.

13. Glosson CR, Haller RH, Dove SB et al: A comparison of root canal preparations using ni-ti hand, ni-ti engine-driven, and K-flex endodontic instruments, *J Endod* 21:146-151, 1995.

14. Goerig AC, Michelich RJ, Schultz HH: Instrumentation of root canals in molar using the step-down technique, *J Endod* 8:550-555, 1982.

15. Grossman LI: Guidelines for the prevention of fracture of root canal instruments, *Oral Surg Oral Med Oral Pathol* 28:746-752, 1969.

16. Heuer MA: The biomechanics of endodontic therapy, *Dent Clin North Am* 7:34-359, 1963.

17. Himel VT, Ahmed KM, Wood DM et al: An evaluation of nitinol and stainless steel files used by dental students during a laboratory proficiency exam, *Oral Surg Oral Med Oral Pathol* 79:232-237, 1995.

18. Ingle JI, Taintor JF: *Endodontics,* ed 3, Philadelphia, 1985, Lea & Febiger, pp 138-141, 152-153, 162-163.

19. Jacobsen EL, Bery PF, Begole EA: The effectiveness of apical dentin plugs in sealing endodontically treated teeth, *J Endod* 11:289-293, 1985.

20. Kyomen SM, Caputo AA, White SN: Critical analysis of the balanced force technique in endodontics, *J Endod* 20:332-337, 1994.

21. Lautenschlager EP, Marshall GW: Brittle and ductile torsional failures of endodontic instruments, *J Endod* 3:175-178, 1977.

22. Luiten DJ, Morgan LA, Baumgartner JC et al: A comparison of four instrumentation techniques on apical canal transportation, *J Endod* 21:26-32, 1995.

23. Melton DC, Krell KV, Fuller MW: Anatomical and histological features of C-shaped canals in mandibular second molars, *J Endod* 17:384-388, 1991.

24. Morgan LF, Montgomery S: An evaluation of the crown-down pressureless technique, *J Endod* 10:492-498, 1984.

25. Mullaney TP: Instrumentation of finely curved canals, *Dent Clin North Am* 23:575-592, 1979.

26. Nagai O, Tani N, Kaybaya Y et al: Ultrasonic removal of broken instruments in root canals, *Int Endod J* 19:298-304, 1986.

27. Oswald RJ, Friedman CE: Periapical response to dentin fillings: a pilot study, *Oral Surg Oral Med Oral Pathol* 49:344-355, 1980.

28. Patterson SS: In vivo and in vitro studies of the effect of the disodium salt of ethylenediamine tetra-acetate on human dentine and its endodontic implications, *Oral Surg Oral Med Oral Pathol* 16:83-103, 1963.

29. Roane JB, Sabala C: Clockwise or counterclockwise, *J Endod* 10:349-352, 1984.

30. Roane JB, Sabala CL: The balanced force concept for instrumentation of curved canals, *J Endod* 11:203-211, 1985.

31. Rome WJ, Doran JE, Walker WA: The effectiveness of Gly-oxide and sodium hypochlorite in preventing smear layer formation, *J Endod* 11:281-288, 1985.

32. Safavi K, Horsted P, Pascon EA et al: Biologic evaluation of the apical dentin chip plug, *J Endod* 11:18-24, 1985.

33. Sampeck A: Instruments of endodontics: their manufacture, use and abuse, *Dent Clin North Am* 11:579-601, 1967.

34. Schilder H: Cleaning and shaping the root canal, *Dent Clin North Am* 18:269-296, 1974.

35. Serene TP, Adams JD, Saxena A: *Nickel titanium instruments: applications in endodontics,* St. Louis, 1994, [Ishiyaku EuroAmerica] IEA.

36. Stewart GG: The importance of chemomechanical preparation of the root canal, *Oral Surg Oral Med Oral Pathol* 8:993-997, 1955.

37. Tidmarsh BG: Preparation of the root canal, *Int Endod J* 15:53-61, 1982.

38. Torabinejad M: Passive step-back technique, *Oral Surg Oral Med Oral Pathol* 77:398-401, 1994.

39. Weine FS, Healey HG, Gerstein H et al: Precurved files and incremental instrumentation for root canal enlargement, *J Can Dent Assoc* 4:155-157, 1970.

40. Weine FS, Kelly RF, Lio PJ: The effect of preparation procedures on original canal shape and on apical foramen shape, *J Endod* 1:255-262, 1975.

41. Weisenseel JA, Hicks ML, Pelleu GB: Calcium hydroxide as an apical barrier, *J Endod* 13:1-5, 1987.

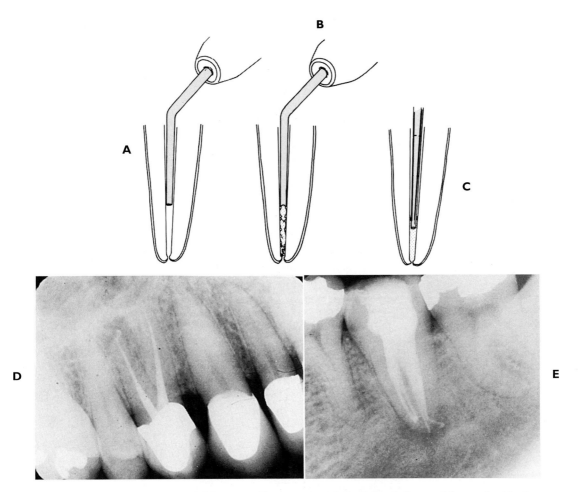

Fig. 6-3 *A, Placement of delivery needle into prepared canal. B, Delivery of thermoplasticized gutta-percha into the prepared canal. C, Condensation of softened gutta-percha with plugger. D and E, Clinical examples of obturation with injectable thermoplasticized gutta-percha.*

With this technique a small amount (2 to 3 mm) of the viscous, softened gutta-percha (SuccessFil, produced by Hygenic Corporation, Akron, Ohio) is extruded onto a metallic K-file carrier and delivered to the apical portion of the canal system. The carrier is counterrotated so that the softened gutta-percha is left in the apical portion of the canal. This material is condensed apically with a small plugger. The remainder of the canal is filled with gutta-percha injected from the Ultrafil system. The efficacy of this technique has been shown to be equivalent to if not better than lateral compaction[26] (Fig. 6-4).

Thermoplasticized Core-Filler Techniques

Gutta-percha that has been previously coated on a metallic or plastic core (carrier), corresponding to standardized instrument sizes (Fig. 6-5, *A*), is heated in a preset system (ThermaPrep Oven, Thermafil, produced by Tulsa Dental Products, Tulsa, Okla.). When properly softened, the gutta-percha–coated core is placed to the working length with the harder core being used as a plunger to carry the softened material apically and laterally (Fig. 6-5, *B* and *C*). Root canal sealer is an intimate and essential part of this system. Intracanal vertical compaction of the softened material around the core is recommended. Once complete, the core is cut off with a bur at the orifice (Fig. 6-5, *D*). Variations on this theme consist of placing the softened gutta-percha on the core (Successfil, Hygenic Corp., Akron, Ohio; Alpha Seal–The Cutting Edge, Chattanooga, Tenn.) before placement in the canal. Radiographic and laboratory evaluations of these

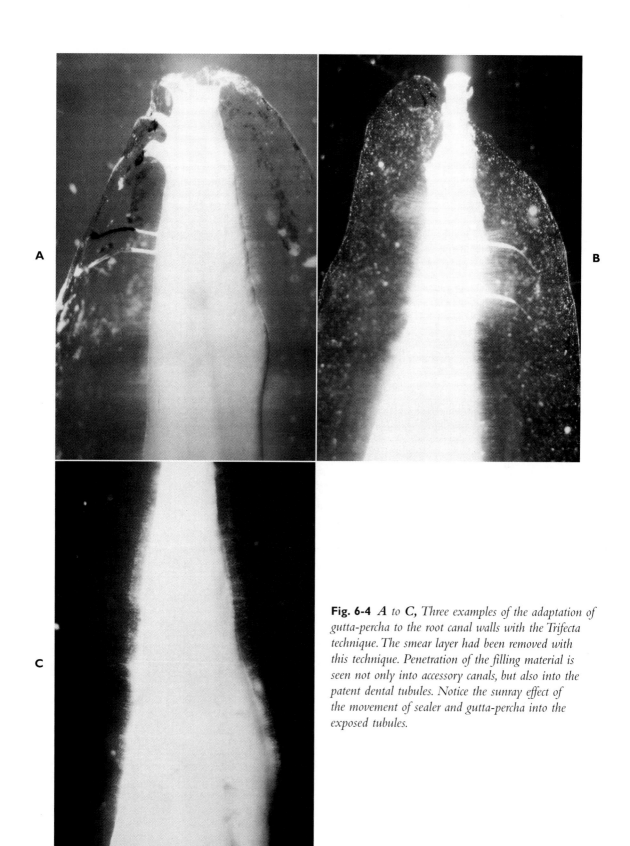

Fig. 6-4 *A to C, Three examples of the adaptation of gutta-percha to the root canal walls with the Trifecta technique. The smear layer had been removed with this technique. Penetration of the filling material is seen not only into accessory canals, but also into the patent dental tubules. Notice the sunray effect of the movement of sealer and gutta-percha into the exposed tubules.*

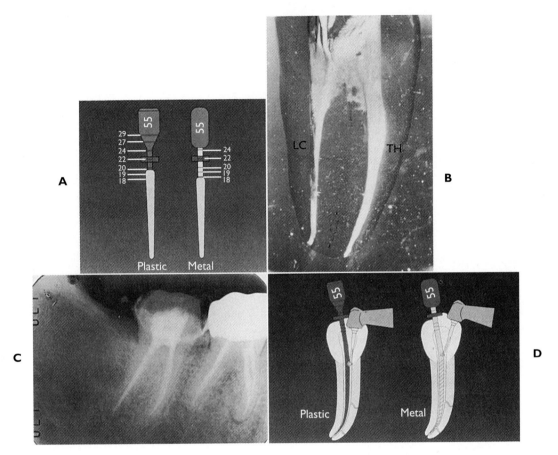

Fig. 6-5 *A, Drawing of Thermafil core fillers. Both metal and plastic carriers have a silicone stop and specific markings for length control. **B**, Mesial root of mandibular molar from a proximal view.* LC, *lateral compaction;* TH, *Thermafil. Notice the smooth adaptation of the alphaphase gutta-percha with the Thermafil (plastic carrier).* **C**, *Mandibular second molar obturated with the Thermafil plastic core filler.* **D**, *The core must be stabilized before cutting with a bur or heat.*

Continued.

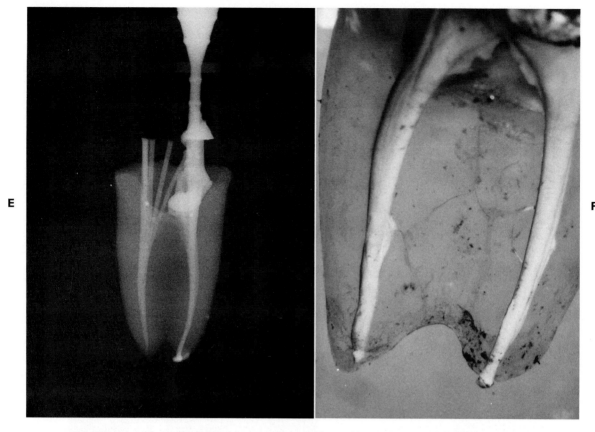

E

F

Fig. 6-5 cont'd. E, *Radiographic appearance of Thermafil obturation on the right compared with lateral compaction on the left. Both techniques provide dense, well-adapted fillings.* **F,** *Demineralized cleared specimen of the tooth in* **E.** *Notice the adaptation with both techniques.* (**A** *and* **D,** *Courtesy Thermafil, Tulsa Dental Products, Tulsa, Okla.*)

techniques demonstrate well-filled canals with three-dimensional adaptation of the gutta-percha to the intricacies of the canal (Fig. 6-5, *E* and *F*).

Modifications in and combinations of these techniques yield numerous possible ways to obturate the prepared root canal space. For example, recent attempts to enhance the adaptation of the gutta-percha delivered in the thermoplasticized state to the intricacies of the canal walls have shown an intimate adaptation and penetration into the dentinal tubules when the smear layer is removed[17] (Fig. 6-6). As long as gutta-percha is the primary material of canal obturation, efforts should continue to explore these avenues of enhanced delivery and canal filling.

Regardless of the technique chosen and modifications introduced in the obturation of the root canal, there are basic principles that must be understood to achieve success.

Attention to these principles during obturation procedures often negates the need for problem solving.

1. The success of any root canal–obturating technique depends largely on the care exercised in the canal preparation.
2. Canals should be prepared with a definite apical matrix (seat, stop, or constriction in sound dentin) to retain the filling material within the canal space.
3. Gutta-percha filling material that is manufactured in the beta phase (after being heated, it shrinks considerably upon cooling) will definitely require compaction if the material is heated as a part of the compaction technique. However, even the alpha-phase gutta-percha techniques (with material shrinkage) (Thermafil, Successfil, Ultrafil–regular and firm set, and Alpha Seal) can benefit from compaction during material hardening.

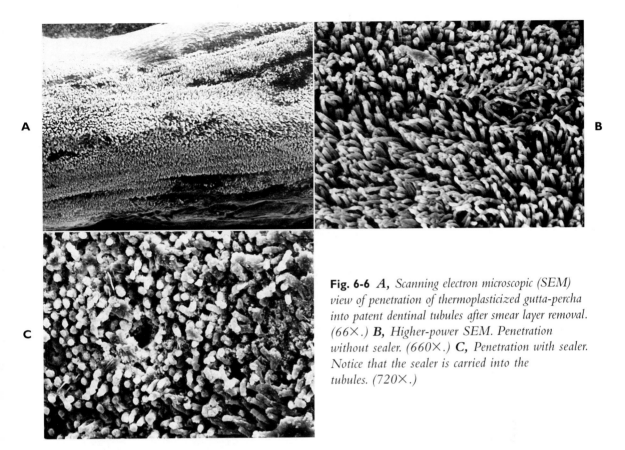

Fig. 6-6 *A, Scanning electron microscopic (SEM) view of penetration of thermoplasticized gutta-percha into patent dentinal tubules after smear layer removal. (66×.)* **B,** *Higher-power SEM. Penetration without sealer. (660×.)* **C,** *Penetration with sealer. Notice that the sealer is carried into the tubules. (720×.)*

4. A complete and appropriate armamentarium to accomplish the chosen technique must be readily available to the practitioner.
5. The practitioner must be ready to modify the obturating technique to meet the needs of an individual case. Multiple techniques are often required to obturate properly a single canal because anatomic challenges dictate the need to practice problem solving during this phase of treatment.

The discussion of problem solving during canal obturation focuses on three general areas: problems encountered in preparing to obturate the canal, problems encountered during active obturation procedures, and problems identified in the postobturation evaluation. Where appropriate, a specific obturation technique will be mentioned.

PROBLEMS ENCOUNTERED IN PREPARING TO OBTURATE THE CANAL

Failure to Seat the Master Gutta-Percha Cone to Full Working Length

Failure to seat the master cone to full working length is a common problem in root canal obturation during lateral compaction and generally can be attributed to the following causes:

1. Dentin chips are packed in the apical third of the canal, preventing full penetration of the master cone to the prepared working length. Likewise, packed dentin chips may also prevent the movement of gutta-percha in other techniques.
2. The canal has been ledged coronally to the working length (see Chapter 5).
3. The canal lacks proper taper and smoothing in the transition from the middle to the apical third of the canal (see Chapter 5). *This is a major problem in the delivery of gutta-percha with all obturation techniques.*
4. A false canal has been created or a curved canal has been straightened, resulting in loss of the original working length (see Chapter 5).
5. A master cone too large for the canal preparation has been selected, or the cone is not a standard cone and its taper is irregular.
6. Any combination of the above.

Packing of dentin chips, which potentially affects all gutta-percha techniques, results from a failure to use copious irrigation with sodium hypochlorite (NaOCl) and failure to recapitulate during canal cleaning and shaping (see Chapter 5).

Radiographically, chip packing may appear as the absence of a canal space apical to the tip of the master cone (Fig. 6-7, *A*). To rectify this situation, removal of the packed chips with small K-files (Nos. 10 to 20) with curved tips in small, curved canals or stiff reamers (Nos. 20 to 30) in larger canals is recommended, along with vigorous irrigation of the canal with NaOCl (Fig. 6-7, *B* and *C*). The instrument is placed to the area of blockage and given small, quarter- to half-turns clockwise while slight apical pressure is applied to the instrument. Avoid full rotation of the instrument to prevent penetrating deeper than desired, pushing of debris past the apical constriction, and unwinding or breaking of the fluted instrument. Ledging may also occur when dentin chips are packed apically, as may the creation of a false canal or the straightening of a curved canal. These errors and their management are discussed in Chapter 5.

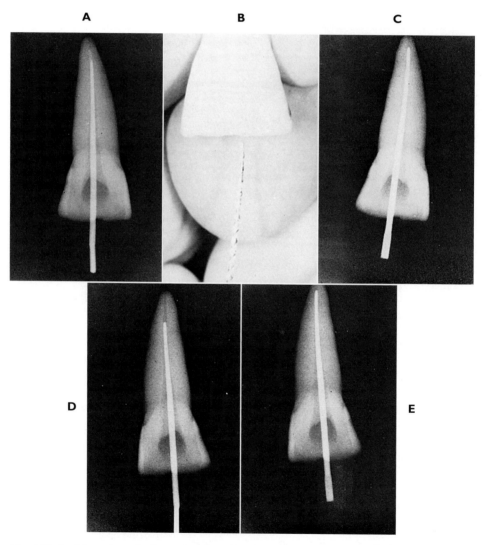

Fig. 6-7 *A, Master cone fit short of working length because of canal blockage with dentin chips. B and C, After recapitulation, chip removal, and confirmation of working length, master cone fit to correct length. D, Binding of master cone in tight underprepared canal. E, Repreparation and seating of master cone to proper length.*

Probably the most common reason for failure to seat the master gutta-percha cone fully is improper shaping of the canal in the apical and middle thirds.

All canals to receive gutta-percha by any technique require a continuously tapering funnel preparation.[18] Failure to prepare canals in this manner will result in binding of the master gutta-percha cones coronally to the working length (Fig. 6-7, *D* and *E*), in addition to preventing proper apical placement of spreaders or pluggers. The problem is compounded because contact of the canal wall with the compacting instruments in narrow constricted areas of the canal can result in root fractures (see Chapter 11).

Additional reasons for failure to reach the working length with the master cone are an incorrectly sized master cone, an incorrect working length, and canal blockage (primarily packed dentin chips). When a master cone binds in the canal short of the full working length, the following procedure is recommended:

1. Recapitulate with the last K-file to the apex (master apical file). Precurve all files as appropriate for the canal shape.
2. Verify radiographically that the working length is correct and no ledges, blockages, or false canals have been created.
3. Use the same size Hedström file as the master apical file and carefully shave the canal walls in a step-back circumferential fashion.[18]
4. Use copious irrigation to enhance instrumentation and dentin chip removal.
5. After reestablishing length with the file and drying the canal with paper points, recapitulate once more to remove any dry packed chips from the apical dentin matrix.

Vertical compaction techniques do not necessarily require placement of the master cone to the full working length unless technique modifications are employed. If placement of the master cone to the full working length is chosen with vertical compaction, the same problems and solutions cited for lateral compaction will apply. Provided that chips are not packed and the canal is not ledged, this problem by itself does not occur with vertical compaction.

With thermoplastic injection techniques, the narrow, constricting canal prevents proper flow of the softened gutta-percha, which prevents filling material from reaching the apical matrix. With thermoplastic core-filler techniques the harder core penetrates through the softer gutta-percha,

thereby stripping the material from its core matrix at the position of canal constriction. In these cases, core materials will be evident apically with little or no surrounding gutta-percha (Fig. 6-8).

Failure to Achieve "Tugback," or "Snugness of Fit"

Tugback has been defined as the resistance felt when a master gutta-percha cone is removed from the canal.[30] However, this is an often misunderstood concept because it is nothing more than the tactile perception of the amount of surface contact between the gutta-percha cone and the surface of the dentin wall. In apical sizes 25 to 40, tugback is hard to achieve. Therefore it is recommended that the largest-sized master cone that fits to the full working length and that produces a perceptive feel of a "snugness of fit" be used. Although desirable, resistance to removal is not necessarily a requirement.

When tugback cannot be achieved, most practitioners will choose the next larger-sized cone. However, this cone will often not reach the desired working length, even though tugback may be felt. When this situation occurs, the following procedure should be considered:

1. File the apical portion of the canal to the next larger size. However, this is not always feasible, especially in curved canals.
2. Develop additional canal flaring with step-back circumferential filing.
3. Cut small increments (0.5 to 1 mm) from the smaller master cone. Be aware that using scissors may result in lateral flanges on the master cone[21] that will also prevent full penetration to the working length (Fig. 6-9, *A* and *B*). If this is the case, cold rolling of the cone on a glass slab with a spatula will reshape the shaft of the cone (Fig. 6-9, *C*), or sections can be removed with a No. 11 or 15 scalpel blade (Fig. 6-9, *D*). A smooth-cut circular surface at the apex of the cone (Fig. 6-9, *E*) is created by rolling the cone on a glass slab while cutting.

Other causes of lack of proper fit of the master gutta-percha cone may include improper consistency in the taper of the gutta-percha cone, a prepared canal that has no taper from the apex to the orifice or that has excessive flare in these dimensions, tissue or dentin debris left in the canal, the choice of too small a master cone, and irregular canal preparation, such as zipping (see Chapter 5). To correct these problems, the practitioner must be able to identify their presence and plan an appropriate course of action. However, most of these

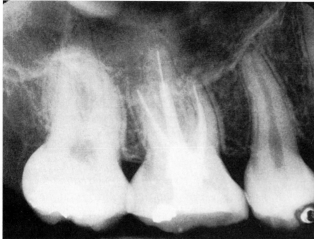

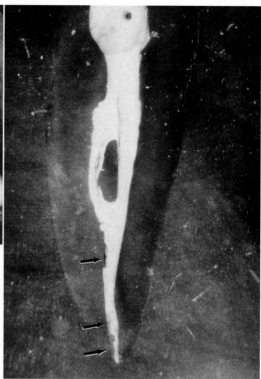

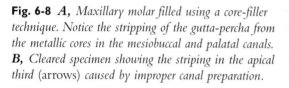

Fig. 6-8 *A, Maxillary molar filled using a core-filler technique. Notice the stripping of the gutta-percha from the metallic cores in the mesiobuccal and palatal canals. B, Cleared specimen showing the striping in the apical third* (arrows) *caused by improper canal preparation.*

problems, especially the lack of tugback, do not occur with the thermoplasticized gutta-percha technique.

Various techniques can be used to enhance the adaptation of the master gutta-percha cone to the prepared apical portion of the canal. These include customizing the apical portion of the cone with methylchloroform (Aldrich Chemical Co, Milwaukee, Wisc.), rectified white turpentine (Lorann Oils, Lansing, Mich.), Endosolv E (Septodont, New Castle, Del.), eucalyptol, or heat.[2,22,23,30,42] These methods can also be used to adapt the master cone to irregularly prepared apices, to resorbed apices (see Chapter 10), and to irregularly developed apices (apexification) (Fig. 6-10).

Chemical Solvents

The apical 2 to 3 mm of a slightly oversized master cone is placed in a solvent such as methylchloroform, rectified white turpentine, or eucalyptol for about 3 to 5 seconds (Fig. 6-11, *A*), removed, and placed into the canal until the working length is achieved with a good apical fit (Fig. 6-11, *B* and *C*). Be sure to mark the position of the cone in the canal with regard to depth of placement and orientation to curves. This can be done by scoring the cone with either a cotton for-

ceps or an explorer (Fig. 6-12). It is always best to fit the cone in a canal when an irrigant is present to prevent the adherence of the gutta-percha to the canal walls and to moderate the action of the solvent. Once properly fit, the cone is checked radiographically and then removed and thoroughly irrigated with sterile water to eliminate any residual solvent. Alcohol can also be used to remove the solvents. Let the master cone dry for 1 or 2 minutes before cementation and compaction.

Heat Softening

In place of a chemical solvent, heated water can be used to soften the apical portion of the master cone before it is placed in the canal. The cone is dipped into the water (100° to 120° F) for 2 to 4 seconds to soften only the outer layers of the apical portion of the cone (Fig. 6-13, *A*). The coronal portion of the cone will remain firm and will serve as a mechanical plunger to seat the softened cone into the prepared apical matrix. Again, radiographic verification of the position of the cone (Fig. 6-13, *B*) and scoring of the cone for orientation are necessary before the cone is removed from the canal. Normal compaction procedures are then instituted.

It may be possible to soften the master cone and adapt it to the apical matrix after placement with

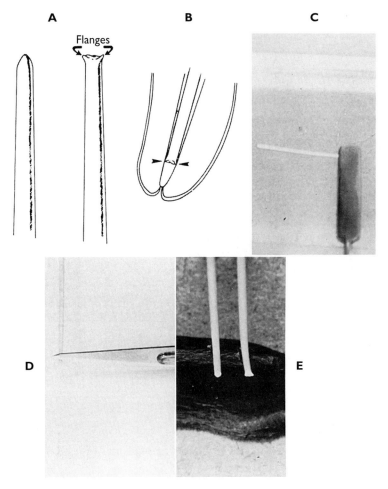

Fig. 6-9 *A,* left, *Normal gutta-percha cone;* right, *flanges on gutta-percha cone cut with scissors.* *B,* *Binding of flanges on canal wall may prevent attainment of full working length with the master cone.* *C,* *Cold rolling on glass slab to eliminate flanges.* *D,* *Gutta-percha cut with sharp scalpel to avoid irregularities.* *E,* *Gutta-percha master cones cut with scalpel* (left) *and scissors* (right). *Notice flanges on right cone.*

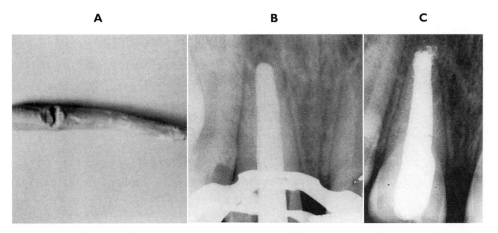

Fig. 6-10 *A,* *Custom-rolled and adapted gutta-percha cone for irregular apex following apexification.* *B,* *Cone fit in tooth. Notice large canal and irregular apical formation.* *C,* *Obturation of canal space. There is slight porosity of apical matrix.*

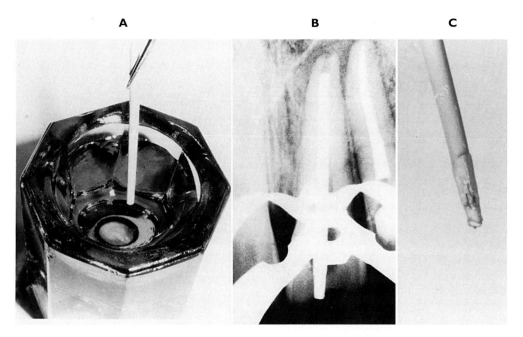

Fig. 6-11 *A, Apical 2 to 3 mm of master cone dipped in solvent.* **B,** *Cone fitted into canal and adapted to canal anatomy.* **C,** *Adapted cone demonstrating canal wall irregularities.*

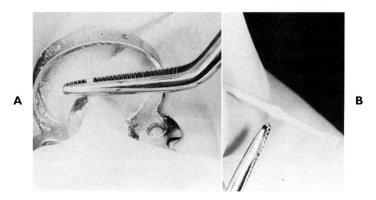

Fig. 6-12 *A, Pinch master gutta-percha cone with forceps at working length to score position of cone in tooth.* **B,** *Orientation of cone marked with forceps.*

sealer. This can be accomplished with EndoTec (LD Caulk/Dentsply, Milford, Del.). Likewise, sealers with solvents may be used.

Breakage of the Master Cone during Trial Placement

If a gutta-percha cone becomes aged and brittle, there is an increased likelihood of breakage on removal from a canal in which it has been snugly fit. This is caused by a transformation of the gutta-percha to a more highly crystalline form, which makes it more brittle.[36] This problem is easily prevented by constantly rotating stock, by keeping the gutta-percha in frozen storage, or by testing a cone in a seldom-used package to determine its freshness. The last is easily accomplished by pulling the cone between the forefinger and thumb of each hand. If the cone stretches, it is fresh. If it snaps, it is brittle, and the gutta-percha must either be discarded or rejuvenated (Fig. 6-14). The following procedure can be used to clinically rejuvenate brittle gutta-percha cones.‡

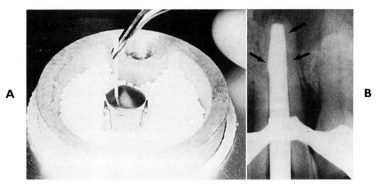

A

B

Fig. 6 **1,** *Place master gutta-percha cone in heated*
wate *n the outer surface.* **B,** *Master cone*
adap *in the confines of the canal. Notice adapta-*
tion *s) in the apical third.*

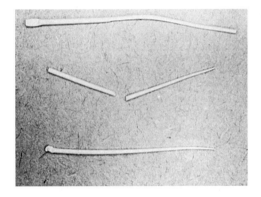

Fig. 6-14 Top, *Stretched gutta-percha cone.* Middle,
Broken gutta-percha cone. Bottom, *regular gutta-*
percha cone.

1. Hold the cone with a cotton forceps.
2. Immerse the cone vertically in hot tap water (130° F) until the compressive force of the pliers indents the cone (1 to 2 seconds).
3. Remove the cone and immediately immerse it vertically in cold tap water (60° F) or in alcohol (that is, 70% isopropyl alcohol) for 5 to 10 seconds.
4. Disinfect the cone as usual and insert it into the prepared canal.

If a brittle cone breaks when it is trial fitted into the canal, normal procedures for retreatment of gutta-percha are initiated (see Chapter 7). Proper storage (cold) and projected usage of fresh materials will prevent breakage.

---

‡Bear in mind that this technique will not always work and depends on the age and composition of the gutta-percha.

PROBLEMS ENCOUNTERED DURING ACTIVE OBTURATION PROCEDURES

Failure to Place the Compacting Instrument to the Prepared Apical Seat

The achievement of an apical seat with the lateral or vertical compaction technique is predicated on the placement of either a spreader or a plugger into a position in the apical third of the canal, which allows for compaction of the apical segment of gutta-percha.[1,32] Failure to achieve this level of penetration may result from the following:

1. Lack of proper canal shape and taper
2. Use of compacting instruments that are too large
3. Use of a straight compacting instrument in a curved canal
4. Any combination of the above

When lateral compaction is used, a properly shaped spreader must be prefit into the canal to ascertain that it will penetrate freely to the apical matrix without contacting the dentin walls (Fig. 6-15). The same is true of pluggers used in the vertical compaction technique, which should penetrate to within 1 to 2 mm from the apical matrix. If the compacting instruments do not freely penetrate the canal to the desired depth, the following steps are recommended:

1. Evaluate the shape and flow of the canal with the master apical file.
2. Use Hedström files to give the canal a better shape and flow.
3. Recapitulate to remove any packed debris.
4. If the instrument binds in the middle or coronal portion of the canal, either change the compacting instrument or provide a greater

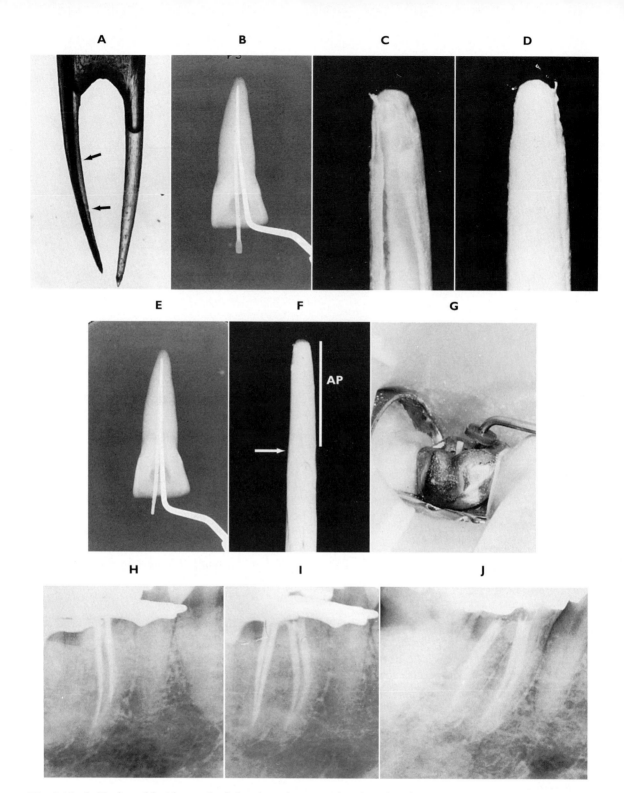

Fig. 6-15 *A,* Tooth model with spreader fit loosely to the prepared working length. Notice space (arrows) around the spreader in the middle and coronal thirds of the canal. *B,* Spreader fit to the apical extension of the canal adjacent to the master cone. *C* and *D,* Adaptation of master cone in which the spreader was placed to the full working length. Notice the reproduction of the canal details. *E,* Spreader placed 2 to 3 mm short of the depth of the master cone. *F,* Master gutta-percha cone in which the spreader penetrated only to within 2 to 3 mm of the apical extent (arrow). Notice the lack of adaptation and condensation of the cone in the apical portion (AP). *G,* Clinical photograph showing depth of spreader penetration adjacent to master cone. *H,* Spreader penetration adjacent to master cones in mesial root of mandibular molar. Spreader penetration in the mesiobuccal canal is approximating the correct depth. Depth of penetration in the mesiolingual canal is inadequate because of larger-sized spreader. *I,* Penetration of two spreaders adjacent to master cones in distobuccal and distolingual canals (same case as in *H*). *J,* Obturation of four canals in molar from *H* with lateral compaction.

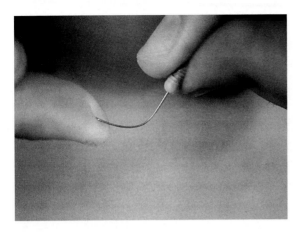

Fig. 6-16 *Flexibility of nickel-titanium finger compactor. (Courtesy Texceed Corp, Costa Mesa, Calif.)*

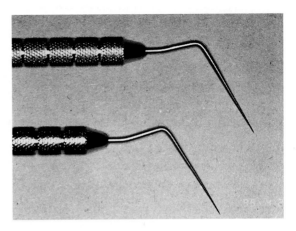

Fig. 6-17 *Nickel-titanium hand spreaders: D-11T (above) and 4-SP (below). (Brasseler USA, Savannah, Georgia.)*

coronal flare with careful use of Gates-Glidden burs or sonic or ultrasonic preparation systems.

5. Precurve the compacting instruments to conform to the coronal shape of the canal. This is not necessary when using nickel-titanium spreaders.

6. Use instruments that have a taper similar to that of the prepared canal. For example, not all D-11T spreaders have the same thickness and tapered shape because there are differences among the various manufacturers. In smaller prepared canals, such as a size 25 to 35 at the apical extent, a D-11TS spreader is appropriate. In larger canals a D-11T will work. In long canals, that is, greater than 23 mm, these spreaders will not work. In these cases a GP-3 (Hu-Friedy Co., Chicago, Ill.) is recommended.

Finger spreaders and hand spreaders are also available in nickel-titanium alloy (Figs. 6-16 and 6-17). Compared to stainless steel spreaders, these highly flexible condensers can more easily negotiate properly shaped curved canals[2]; this is essential for adequate apical compaction. In addition, no precurving is necessary, and recent research suggests that there is decreased stress on root structure when one is compacting with Ni-Ti finger spreaders, thus potentially decreasing the chance of vertical root fracture[12] (Fig. 6-18). Potential disadvantages of using these compactors include buckling of the instrument during compaction and limited accessibility to some canals because the spreader cannot be precurved. Present findings indicate that the flexible Ni-Ti finger spreaders

should be used to compact the gutta-percha in the apical third followed by stiffer stainless steel finger spreaders to compact the gutta-percha in the remaining coronal two thirds[37]; use of stainless steel finger spreaders in the more flared portion of the canal may compensate for the buckling that would occur if Ni-Ti compactors were used for the entire obturation procedure (Fig. 6-19).

When a canal is obturated with the injectable thermoplasticized gutta-percha techniques, similar solutions as mentioned above are recommended. However, vertical pluggers do not have to be fit to within 1 to 2 mm from the apical dentin matrix. Pluggers are fit loosely only to within 3 to 5 mm from the apical dentin matrix.[38] Likewise, the shape and flow of the canal in this area must be a smooth, continuously tapering funnel. With core-filler techniques, it is very important to seat the core to the depth of the prepared canal.

Pulling the Obturating Material Out of the Canal on Removal of the Compacting Instrument

In lateral-compaction techniques, this problem is caused by one of the following:

1. Too much canal wall divergence and lack of a snugly fit master gutta-percha cone
2. Too much sealer
3. Failure to wipe the tacky sealer from the spreader before reinsertion
4. A bent spreader or a hooked, curled tip on the spreader
5. Moisture in the canal other than from the root canal sealer

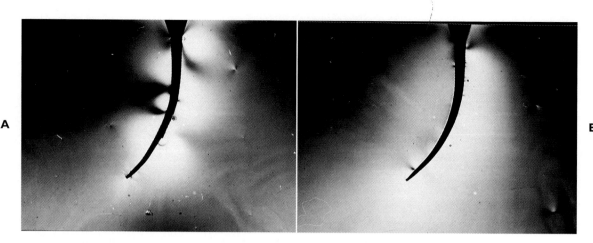

Fig. 6-18 *Photoelastic stress patterns during lateral compaction of gutta-percha in simulated curved canals in photoelastic resin. **A,** Compaction of master gutta-percha cone and two accessory cones using a stainless steel finger spreader under a constant load. Notice areas of heavy point stress along inner wall. **B,** Same conditions as in **A** except a nickel titanium finger spreader is placed under a similar load; notice even distribution of stress and no areas of point stress.*

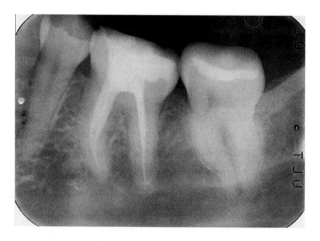

Fig. 6-19 *Radiograph of endodontically treated mandibular molar, obturated using nickel-titanium finger spreaders, apically followed by stainless steel finger spreaders coronally.*

6. Too small a master cone with the spreader penetrating past the apex of the cone
7. Failure to passively loosen the spreader before withdrawal from the canal
8. Trying to rotate a curved spreader

To rectify this problem, the circumstances of each situation must be assessed. If the canal walls are too divergent, a customized cone adapted to the apical 1 to 3 mm by means of a solvent or heat may be necessary. Moderate use of sealer is always recommended to provide a seal between the interface of gutta-percha and dentin.

Always introduce a clean spreader (wipe sealer off with an alcohol sponge) adjacent to the master gutta-percha cone, making sure that there are no flanges, hooks, or severe kinks in the instrument (Fig. 6-20).

Canals must always be dry before compaction. Since there may be some residual moisture in the root canal from previous irrigation, medications, or exudate from the ingress of tissue fluids, it may be necessary to dehydrate the root canal before obturation. Sterile paper points are the best devices for moisture removal. If necessary, the canal may be

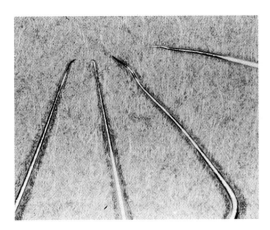

Fig. 6-20 *Various spreaders with irregularities at the tip that will tend to interfere with thorough canal obturation. Instruments should either be discarded or cut off and used as pluggers.*

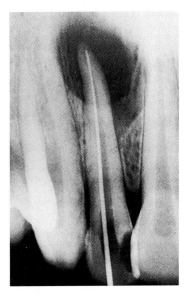

Fig. 6-21 *Improper master cone size for canal preparation. Cone should contact canal walls in the apical third.*

irrigated with 2 to 3 ml of either 70% or 95% isopropyl alcohol. Allow the alcohol to remain in the canal for 3 to 4 minutes and then dry with sterile paper points.

The presence of too small a master cone must be determined before compaction. Radiographically the cone will appear to float in the canal, while clinically there will be no snugness of fit (Fig. 6-21). Properly fit master cones will penetrate to within 0.5 mm of the working length, and there will be space on either side of the cone from the junction of the apical third and middle third to the coronal orifice (Fig. 6-22, *A* to *C*).

When removing a spreader from a canal during compaction, the instrument should be rotated in a 180-degree curve until it becomes loose within the canal (Fig. 6-23). Gradually during this movement a retracting force can be applied to allow the spreader to passively "walk" out of the canal without dislodging the compacted gutta-percha. However, if the canal is curved and the spreader is curved, rotation will have to be limited to approximately 90 degrees while the practitioner exerts a continuous, gradual, coronal retracting force.

Gutta-percha can also be pulled from the canal when vertical compaction, thermoplasticized gutta-percha, or core-carrier techniques are used (Fig. 6-24). This may also be caused by canal moisture, but primarily it is caused by failure to use a separating medium on the plugger (zinc oxide or zinc phosphate powder for vertical compaction, alcohol for thermoplasticized gutta-percha procedures) or by allowing the plugger to stay in the warmed gutta-percha while it cools. When heated gutta-percha is to be compacted, firm and thorough yet rapid compaction is recommended. With the core-filler techniques, it is possible to pull the core from the softened gutta-percha, if the core is twisted during or after placement. Also, during the cutting of the core (metallic carrier with a bur or plastic carrier with a bur or a controlled heat source, such as Touch 'N Heat [Analytical Technology, Redmond, Wash.]), the handle of the core must be stabilized to prevent removal of the core (carrier) (see Fig. 6-5, *D*). Failure to stabilize the top of the core may significantly disrupt the previously placed gutta-percha.

Popping or Cracking during Compaction

This problem may occur at any time during compaction of gutta-percha with any of the techniques mentioned, and may be a result of:

1. Cracking of the root caused by excessive compaction pressure, contact of the root dentin walls with the metal compactor, or using a compactor too large in both cross-sectional diameter and taper[29]
2. Cracking of septa, which may be located between closely placed multiple canals such as the mesiobuccal root in the maxillary first molar or the distal root of the mandibular first molar

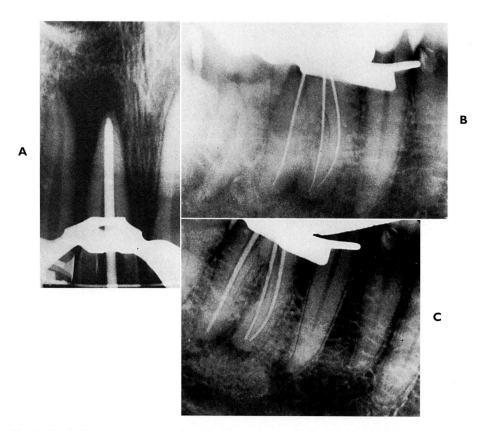

Fig. 6-22 *A, Proper master cone adaptation in anterior tooth. B, Working length in mandibular molar. C, Proper master cone adaptation demonstrating good adaptation to the walls in the apical segment with a tapering space around the cone in the coronal two thirds.*

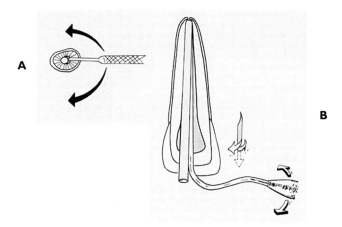

Fig. 6-23 *A, Rotation of spreader in a 180-degree arc will loosen the instrument in the canal without dislodging the filling material. B, During the rotation, force is gradually exerted in a coronal direction to allow passive removal of the spreader.*

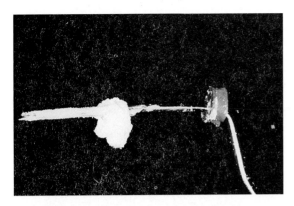

Fig. 6-24 *Removal of the gutta-percha filling that adhered to the spreader during compaction. When this occurs, the obturation process should begin with new filling materials.*

The fracturing of a septum is most often unanticipated and does not present a clinical problem. However, root fractures can occur during compaction procedures and can best be prevented by not overpreparing canals through the excessive use of Gates-Glidden burs or Peeso reamers, by always prefitting compacting instruments to avoid instrument wedging in the canal, by using compactors of appropriate size for the shape of the canal, by precurving stainless compacting instruments when necessary, or by using Ni-Ti compaction instruments (see Chapter 11).

Since thermoplasticized core-filler techniques involve minimal compaction or wedging, if the canal is properly prepared and the gutta-percha is properly heated, their use may be more favorable in cases that exhibit cracks or craze lines. Also, since canal preparation for these obturation techniques does not have to be excessive, the use of these core fillers in roots that are narrow and amenable to fracture may be warranted.

PROBLEMS IDENTIFIED DURING POSTOBTURATION EVALUATION
Overfilling of Canals or Overextension of the Obturating Material

For a proper understanding of the nature of the problem of overfilling or of overextension, an important distinction must be made between them. Overfilling implies that a root canal system has been filled in three dimensions and a surplus of filling material extrudes beyond the confines of the canal (Fig. 6-25, *A* to *C*). However, an overex-

tended root filling is limited solely to the vertical dimension of the root canal filling material relative to the apical foramen. An overextended fill does not imply that the root canal has been three-dimensionally obturated, rather that the filling material has been placed beyond the confines of the canal but does not necessarily seal the apical foramen (Fig. 6-25, *D*). The major causes of placing the root canal filling material beyond the apical constriction in either overfilling or overextension when lateral or vertical compaction techniques are used are the following:

1. Excessive instrumentation (overinstrumentation) beyond the apical constriction, resulting in the lack of an apical dentin matrix
2. Unanticipated communicating resorptive defects anywhere in the canal system (see Chapter 10)
3. Defects incorporated into the canal system during cleaning and shaping, such as zips, perforations, strips, and so on (see Chapter 5)
4. Excessive compaction force
5. Excessive amounts of sealer
6. Use of too small a master cone
7. Excessive penetration of the compacting instrument
8. Any combination of the above

Intentional placement of gutta-percha beyond the confines of the root canal system is not considered an acceptable technique because there are no long-term prospective or retrospective studies to justify this approach to canal obturation.

However, many techniques used in canal obturation predispose to this possibility, and their use should be modified to produce predictable control of the obturating material. The following guidelines will assist in retention of the gutta-percha filling material within the canal during obturation:

1. All instrumentation should be retained within the root canal system, coronal to the dentin-cementum junction.[19]
2. Thorough radiographic evaluation in the treatment-planning phase will usually disclose abnormal anatomic or pathologic entities. In the case of periradicular resorption, the apical termination of instrumentation may often have to be 1 to 2 mm or more from the resorptive defect (see Chapter 10).[19,40]
3. To avoid stripping, limit the use of rotary instruments (Gates-Glidden burs, Peeso

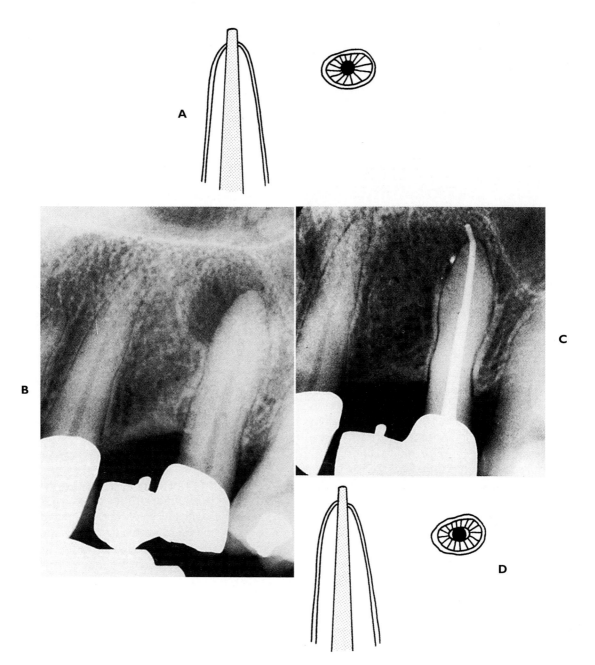

Fig. 6-25 *A, Longitudinal and cross-sectional appearance of an overfilled canal. **B,** Clinical case before obturation. **C,** Appearance at 1-year recall. Healing is evident; the patient was symptom free. **D,** Longitudinal and cross-sectional appearance of an overextended root canal fill. There are voids adjacent to the gutta-percha in the cross section.*

reamers, and so forth) in the root canal system, especially where roots are curved or very thin in a mesiodistal dimension, (see Chapter 5).

4. Use limited force and a limited amount of sealer during compaction. Always prefit compacting instruments and mark their depth of penetration with either a rubber stop or a notch on the instrument. The same applies to

thermoplastic core fillers, which will have either stops or notches indicating the appropriate length (see Fig. 6-5).

5. Properly fit the master gutta-percha cone, making sure that it fills the bulk of the prepared canal space.

In thermoplasticized gutta-percha techniques many of the same causes for overfilling exist. The major ones are lack of an apical dentin matrix to control the material, the use of excessive amounts of sealer, excessive compaction forces, or the stripping and placement of the core filler beyond the apical matrix. Failure to prevent these causes will result in routine overfilling or overextension beyond the apical foramen.

Occasionally, even though proper technique has been followed, gutta-percha or root canal sealer may be unintentionally pushed beyond the confines of the root canal system. However, gutta-percha is a bacteriostatic substance that is generally tolerated by the periradicular tissues. Although sealers may provoke an initial inflammatory response, to a greater or lesser degree, over a short period of time, the macrophage scavenger system eliminates the excessive material from the periradicular tissues. In either case, the mere placement of filling material outside the canal system is not a major cause for alarm if the canal space is three-dimensionally obturated.

In cases of overextension with the lateral compaction technique, the filling material can often be teased back through the foramen, provided that the sealer has not hardened. If the sealer has hardened it may still be possible to retrieve the gutta-percha provided that it is an intact cone. The gutta-percha is softened with one of the previously mentioned solvents in the apical third of the canal.[28] While the gutta-percha is soft, a Hedström file is inserted into the softened mass. The excess solvent is flushed from the root canal, and in a few minutes, the gutta-percha will harden around the Hedström file. The file is carefully teased out of the canal as parallel as possible to the long axis of the canal.

In cases of overextension with the vertical compaction or an injectable thermoplasticized gutta-percha technique, retraction of the filling material through the apical foramen is impossible. While some authors may cite this situation as an indication for periradicular surgery,[35] the routine and immediate use of surgical intervention is neither indicated nor justified.[16] In most cases the periradicular tissues will heal and the patient will be symptomless. If, however, the patient exhibits signs or symptoms of periradicular inflammation, surgery may be indicated.[16] In cases of thermoplastic core-filler overextension, it is necessary to remove the core from its overextended position. Concomitantly, it may be possible to retrieve small amounts of gutta-percha from beyond the confines of the apical matrix if they remain attached to the core.

Failure to Achieve Adequate Apical Density (Underfills)

Failure to achieve adequate apical density is a common problem in root canal obturation that only too often goes unnoticed by the practitioner. In essence, the apical third of the canal is filled with a sea of root canal cement and a single uncondensed master cone or poorly condensed mass of previously softened gutta-percha. Radiographically the apical third of the canal appears less radiodense. An ill-defined outline to the canal wall is evident, along with obvious gaps or voids in the filling material or its adaptation to the confines of the canal.

CLINICAL PROBLEM: A review of the final obturation in Fig. 6-26, *A,* reveals a poorly compacted gutta-percha filling in the apical half of the canal. The coronal third appears densely packed. What is the major reason why this occurs?

Solution: The first aspect that should be addressed is the shape of the canal. In this case the shape appears sufficient to obtain a well-compacted filling. This leaves the most likely problem as being the failure to obtain proper depth of penetration with the compacting instrument. One can surmise that the waving shape of the master gutta-percha cone is due to a coronal compaction as opposed to compaction at the depth of the material in the canal. Retreatment of the canal and achievement of penetration to the working length are seen in Fig. 6-26, *B.* Notice the degree of apical density.

The major cause for lack of apical density is similar in all obturation techniques (Fig. 6-27), that being the lack of canal patency and sufficient taper to allow for spreader penetration to the apical seat in the lateral-compaction technique,[1] plugger penetration in the vertical-compaction technique,[31] and flow of gutta-percha in thermoplasticized gutta-percha injection and core-filler techniques.[38,39] In particular, this lack of proper shape and taper will accentuate the wiping or removal of the gutta-percha from the carriers in the thermoplasticized core-filling techniques. Secondary causes of this problem include the following:

1. Failure to coat the accessory cones with a thin layer of root canal sealer (lateral compaction)
2. Failure to insert accessory cones to the full length of spreader penetration (lateral compaction)
3. Use of accessory cones with very fine tips that curl up or kink on placement (lateral compaction)

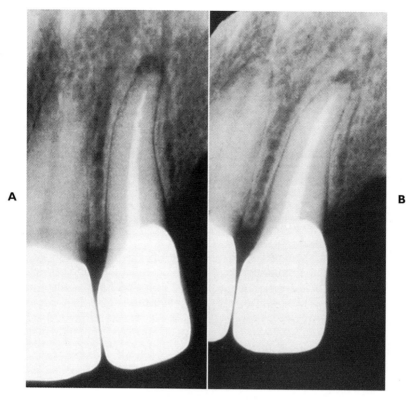

Fig. 6-26

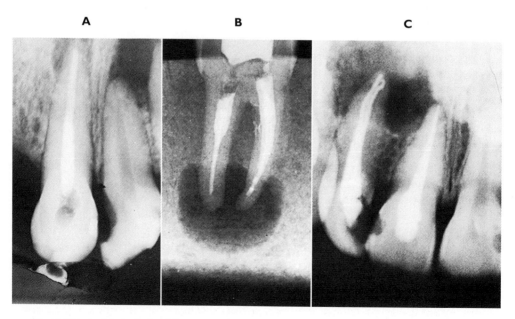

Fig. 6-27 *A,* Notice lack of density in the apical half of the root compared with the coronal half. *B,* Apical half of these canals are insufficiently prepared to allow for thorough compaction of the filling material. *C,* Placement of two cones apically without any apparent compaction in the maxillary lateral incisor.

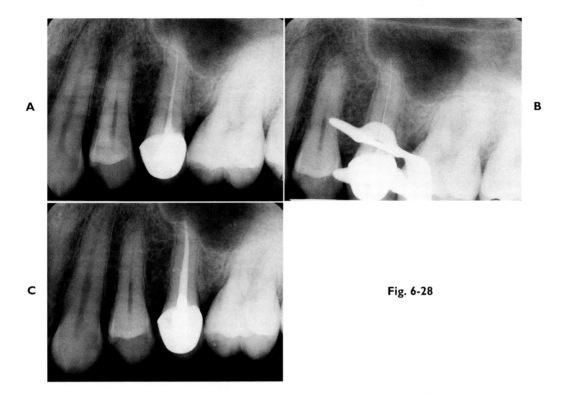

A

B

C

Fig. 6-28

4. Use of too large a spreader (lateral compaction) or plugger (vertical compaction, thermoplasticized gutta-percha injection techniques)
5. Too much root canal sealer (all techniques)
6. Use of a rapidly setting root canal sealer or an improperly mixed sealer that may set up too fast (all techniques)
7. Failure to achieve depth of compaction and flow of softened gutta-percha (vertical compaction, all thermoplasticized gutta-percha techniques)
8. Failure to soften the apical segment of the gutta-percha before compaction (vertical compaction)
9. Excessive packing of dentin chips in the apical 1 to 3 mm
10. Failure to seat the core-filler to the apical seat or stripping of the core-filler at its apical extent
11. Inconsistent heating, too little or too much, with the core-filler techniques. This is easily prevented by use of the manufacturer's heating systems. The heating of the core filler over an open flame is subject to too many discrepancies and should be avoided.

> To obturate the prepared root canal system as densely as possible throughout its entire length, attention must be paid to canal preparation, proper fit of compacting instruments, and effective use of not only root canal sealer, but also accessory gutta-percha cones or segments to fill the prepared canal space.

CLINICAL PROBLEM: A 27-year-old male patient presents with severe pain to biting on a maxillary premolar that had had root canal treatment 2 weeks earlier. The tooth had never felt comfortable, and the patient had requested that the practitioner not put the new crown on the tooth until it felt better. The patient had been informed that the crown was needed to not only protect the tooth but also to "help the tooth feel better." Now the patient is disgruntled, in pain, and wants to know what has happened. The maxillary left second premolar is painful to percussion andpalpation, and the placement of ice on the tooth stimulates an abnormal response. The patient wants to know how this can happen becausehe was told the tooth was dead. A radiographreveals the tooth has had previous root canal treatment and a crown (Fig. 6-28, *A*). The filling material is short of the ideal length and there is canal space visible along the mesial aspect of the filling material. The adjacent teeth respond normally to all testing and reveal no abnormal radiographic findings.

Solution: Based on the patient's symptoms and clinical findings, there is pulp tissue remaining in the apical portion of the root and possibly in a second canal that may be commonly present in this tooth. Needless to say, the root canal treatment is a practitioner failure, and nonsurgical root canal retreatment is indicated. The old filling material was removed along with the remaining pulp tissue. A new working length was determined (Fig. 6-28, *B*) and the canal was reprepared and obturated in one visit (Fig. 6-28, *C*). Within 24 hours the patient was symptom free. Attention to detail in a problem-solving format to working-length determination and canal cleaning, shaping, and obturation would have prevented this problem. This case highlights the major effect that treatment below the standard of care can have on the patient, both psychologically and financially, and that the treatment rendered lacked any quality assurance assessment.

Radiographic Voids in the Final Root Canal Obturation

The causes for voids in the root canal filling (Figs. 6-29 and 6-30) are numerous; however, these potential gaps or irregularities in obturation have never been shown to lead directly to failure in treat-

ment. It is true that classic studies[13,20] identified poor obturation as the major cause of failure of root canal treatment. However, these findings were based on cases in which cleaning and shaping were not performed as is done today. Also, obturation was performed with little compaction, using single gutta-percha or silver cones. In addition, occlusal leakage may have contributed to many of the failures, especially in the single gutta-percha cone fills or when silver cones were used, and corrosion products initiated adverse periradicular tissue responses (Fig. 6-31).

Modern approaches to root canal cleaning, shaping, and obturation minimize the likelihood of voids. In addition, if proper apical compaction is performed, any voids are usually limited to the middle and coronal canal segments and pose no threat to prognosis. As with problems encountered with lack of apical density (see previous section), voids have similar causes and similar solutions:

1. Proper apical penetration of spreader, plugger, or compactor is necessary.
2. Whenever a void is created by a compacting instrument, that space should be obturated with additional gutta-percha or softening and additional compaction.
3. Spreaders and pluggers must be clean and require some type of separating medium to prevent the gutta-percha from sticking and to ensure proper depth of placement for increased obturation density.
4. Excessive use of root canal sealer should be avoided.

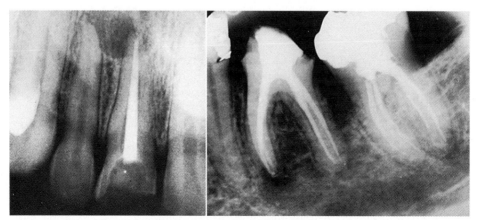

Fig. 6-29 *A, Obvious voids along the whole length of the gutta-percha fill. **B,** Comparing the obturation in the first molar with the second molar. Notice the voids and lack of density and adaptation of the gutta-percha in the second molar.*

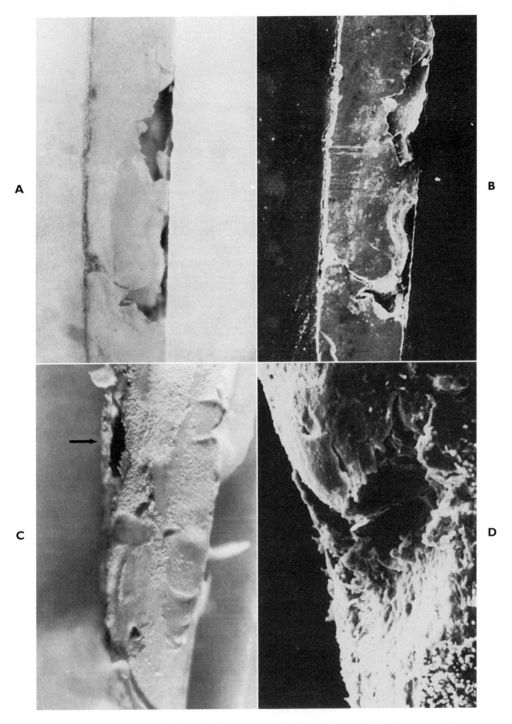

Fig. 6-30 *A, Cross-sectional view of obturated canal with voids created during compaction.
B, Scanning electron microscopic (SEM) photograph shows incomplete compaction of the softened material deep in the canal. (240×.) C and D, Multiple voids in the root canal obturation
resulting from failure to achieve consistent depth of plugger penetration while the thermoplasticized material was soft.* Arrow in **C** *indicates void depicted in* **D** *(SEM 44×).*

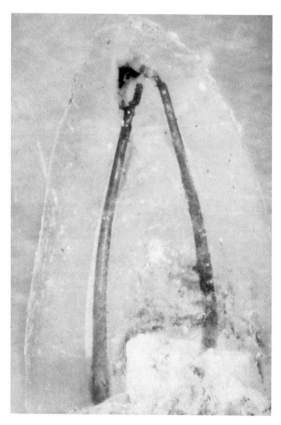

Fig. 6-31 *Extracted maxillary premolar that had been obturated with silver cones 20 years earlier. The specimen has been demineralized and cleared. Notice the corrosion products and lack of adaptation to the root canal walls.*

5. Placement of root canal sealer with an ultrasonic instrument (ENAC, Osada Electric Co, Los Angeles, Calif.) enhances distribution of the sealer along the canal walls.

6. In softened gutta-percha techniques (vertical compaction, thermoplasticized gutta-percha) (see Fig. 6-30):
    (a) Fold the material over on itself to fill voids made by the plugger.
    (b) Compact centrally, folding the material along the walls into the central core of the gutta-percha.
    (c) Make sure that the material is sufficiently softened for adequate compaction.
    (d) Use pluggers that compact the material en masse instead of just piercing the material and creating voids.

7. Minimal voids with lateral compaction can be eliminated through the use of properly shaped spreaders and matching-sized accessory cones. For example, the D-11TS spreader matches very well with both extra-fine and fine-fine accessory cones. With the D-11T, fine-fine or medium-fine may be appropriate, depending on the shape of the canal and depth of spreader penetration. Considerations should be given to using Ni-Ti compaction instruments in curved canals.

If voids are present, the gutta-percha can be removed with chemical solvents, heated instruments, files, Peeso reamers, or Gates-Glidden burs to the level of the void (see Chapter 7). Then compact the coronal section with the technique of choice.

GUIDELINES FOR ROOT CANAL OBTURATION

The following guidelines are basic tips to consider during various compaction techniques.

Lateral Compaction

1. Match accessory cones with the spreader or use a slightly smaller cone.
2. Cut off small fragile ends of accessory gutta-percha cones.
3. Use a scalpel and glass slab to cut off the apical segment of master cones to ensure their roundness.
4. Always wipe the spreader clean with alcohol before entering the canal during compaction.
5. Use a stop on the spreader to observe proper depth of penetration during compaction.
6. The spreader must be less tapered than the shape of the canal.
7. Always prefit the spreader, curving it if necessary in the case of a stainless steel instrument, to ensure depth of placement without contact with the dentin wall. The availability of nickel-titanium spreaders will undoubtedly enhance penetration in curved canals, and their use should be considered.
8. The spreader must be long enough to penetrate to the apical dentin matrix.
9. Do not use spreaders with kinks or curled tips. Cut off the tips and smooth the spreader with a sharpening stone.
10. Always loosen the spreader passively before removing it from the canal to prevent dislodgment of the filling material.
11. Always use a root canal sealer judiciously and place a light coating on the accessory cones. Initial placement with an ultrasonic instrument may aid in sealer dispersion.
12. Avoid excessive wedging of the spreader in the canal.

13. Consider using finger spreaders to achieve greater depth of placement plus a concentrated force during compaction.[34]

Vertical Compaction

1. Always prefit pluggers to ensure their depth of penetration to the apical 1 to 2 mm.
2. Pluggers must fit freely and not contact the dentin walls. Precurve the pluggers if necessary. If using nickel-titanium pluggers, precurving will not be necessary.
3. Do not place a large amount of root canal sealer in the apical portion of the canal.
4. If instruments are heated to soften the gutta-percha, make sure that they are hot enough to transfer sufficient heat to the material so that it will flow when compacted. Use of instruments such as the Touch 'N Heat (Analytical Technology, Redmond, Wash.) are recommended.
5. Avoid excessive vertical compacting pressures.
6. Radiographically verify apical movement and compaction of the gutta-percha as necessary.
7. Always use a separating medium on the plugger to prevent it from sticking to the gutta-percha.

Thermoplasticized Injection

1. Pluggers must be prefit into the apical third of the canal 3 to 5 mm from the apical dentin matrix in canals with a master apical file of size 50 or less. With larger canals, fit to within 5 to 8 mm. Precurve the pluggers as necessary.
2. Use very small amounts of a slow-setting root canal sealer placed no deeper in the canal than the depth of the plugger placement.
3. Do not wedge injection needles against the canal walls. Similarly the needles must be able to reach the junction of the apical and middle thirds of the prepared canal.
4. Inject gutta-percha slowly and steadily without exerting any apical pressure on the injection needle. Allow the flowing gutta-percha to lift the needle out of the tooth.
5. Avoid excessive vertical compacting pressures.
6. During compaction, fold the softened material over on itself as previously discussed.

Thermoplastic Core Fillers

1. Proper heating of the gutta-percha on the core is essential. The use of the manufacturer's heating device, such as the ThermaPrep Oven (Thermafil, Tulsa Dental Products, Tulsa, Okla.) is recommended.
2. The heated core filler must be inserted to working length *without* rotation or twisting. This prevents wedging, failure to seat to the full depth, or stripping of the softened gutta-percha (see Fig. 6-8).
3. Once seated, the top of the carrier is stabilized, and a bur or heat is used to resect it from the radicular core (see Fig. 6-5, *D*). Leave 1 to 2 mm of core above the canal orifice.
4. Do not use the core or carrier as a root canal post.
5. Compaction after placement is optional but recommended to enhance adaptation. In canals with wide buccolingual dimensions, lateral compaction followed by the insertion of accessory cones is recommended. Not only does this aid in the obturation of the space, but it also allows the movement of the previously softened material into the intricacies of the canal space that are often located in this dimension (fins, webs, invaginations, and so forth).

Regardless of the type of compaction technique chosen, the ultimate quality of the obturation will be no better than the canal preparation.[6]

Modern tenets of root canal treatment dictate the need for a canal that is prepared to a smooth, tapered, three-dimensional funnel from the dentin-cementum junction to the canal orifice and located within the anatomic confines of the root (Fig. 6-32).

CLINICAL PROBLEM: A 47-year-old female patient presents with severe pain to biting or touching on her maxillary right lateral incisor. There is a history of root canal treatment approximately 1 month previously. Clinically there is slight swelling in the soft tissue overlying the lateral incisor. Percussion and palpation both give acute, abnormal responses. A radiograph reveals a poorly obturated root canal and the presence of a periradicular lesion (Fig. 6-33, *A*). A diagnosis of previous inadequate root canal treatment along with acute periradicular periodontitis is appropriate. Nonsurgical retreatment is indicated with the possible need for surgical intervention. Clinically the solution appears straightforward. However, the problem-solving approach demands an assessment of what went wrong, why it happened, and what implications it creates for the practitioner providing

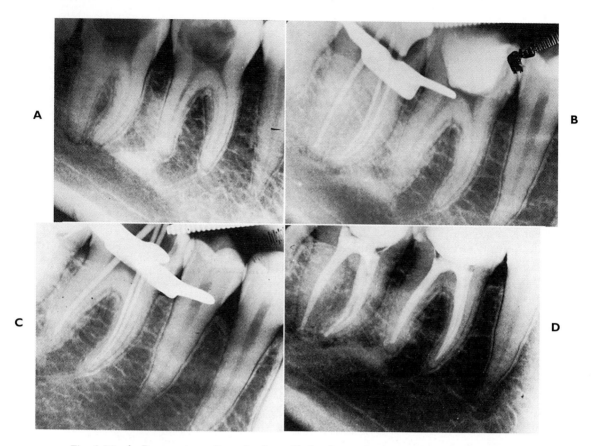

Fig. 6-32 *A, Preoperative radiograph of mandibular first and second molars requiring root canal treatment. **B,** Radiograph showing fit of master cones in second molar. Notice proper depth of placement, proper adaptation, and space around the cones in the coronal half for spreader penetration and compaction. **C,** Fit of master cones in the first molar with same result as in **B. D,** Obturation of both molars. Notice smooth, tapered canal shape, dense canal obturation, and maintenance of filling material within the anatomic confines of the canals.*

the retreatment. For the astute, problem-solving professional it also helps to prevent future problems.

Solution: Reflecting on the treatment rendered, an examination of all the facts is essential. Initially, the patient had had an acute episode of pain and swelling with this tooth 6 months previously. She had been seen on an emergency basis, and the tooth was endodontically accessed and left open for drainage (Fig. 6-33, *B*). Within 48 hours the patient felt better and failed to return for the timely completion of treatment. Three months later she returned to have the root canal completed. The tooth working length was determined, and the canal was cleaned (Fig. 6-33, *C*). However, because the tooth had been open for a long period of time, a temporary was not placed for fear on the part of the practitioner that a flare-up would ensue. Within the next 2 months the root canal was completed (Figs. 6-33, *A* and *D*).

Key issues that must be addressed deal primarily with the prevention of problems. First, leaving a tooth open for drainage is rarely warranted and is often done for the convenience of the practitioner, not the patient (see Chapter 9). Second, failure to close the tooth in a timely manner allows bacteria easily to establish themselves in the canal system and periradicular tissues. Third, although the working length film is quite good (Fig. 6-33, *C*), it is obvious in the master cone film (Fig. 6-33, *D*) that the apical portion of the canal is either ledged or blocked. This occurs when the distopalatal curvature of the canal, common in this tooth, is not considered. Fourth, it is also obvious that there was poor placement of both the compacting instruments and accessory filling materials (Fig. 6-33, *A*). Such placement is often due to poor canal preparation. The acceptance by the practitioner of this final outcome as being the standard of care probably raises the most concern

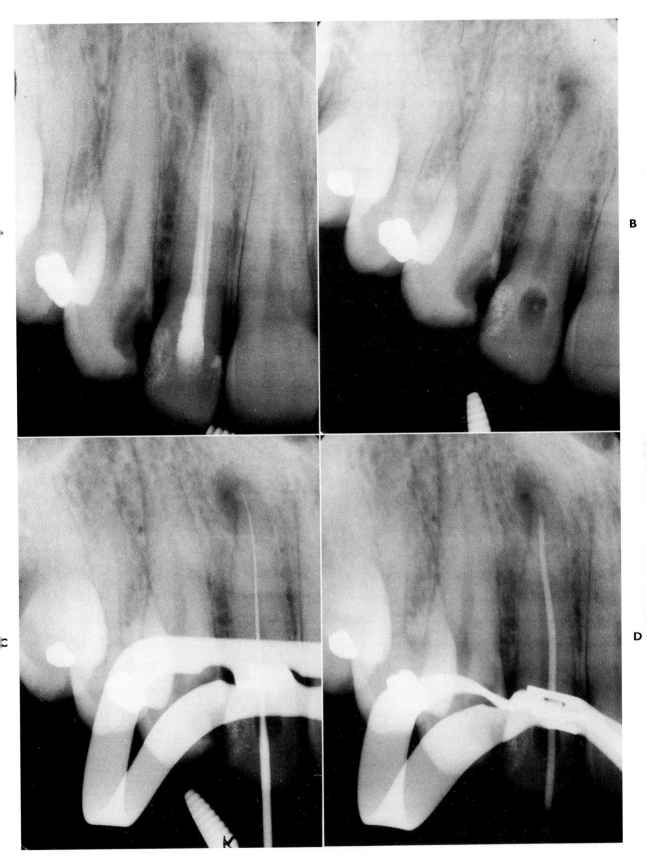

B

C

D

Fig. 6-33

153

regarding this case. The inherent problems in this case point to the need to practice continuously a problem-solving approach to assessment and treatment. Although this case can be managed as a straightforward nonsurgical retreatment, introspection as to the causes, their prevention, and achievement at or above the standard of care is essential for all practitioners who integrate quality assurance assessments into their practice.

This case also raises a very important point regarding its ultimate management. If surgical intervention is chosen instead of nonsurgical retreatment, the major cause for surgical failure will not be addressed, that being failure to clean, shape, and obturate properly the root canal system. As can be seen from many perspectives, this case highlights and epitomizes the need to practice a problem-solving approach in the delivery of endodontic therapy.

References

1. Allison DA, Weber CR, Walton RE: The influence of the method of canal preparation on the quality of apical and coronal obturation, *J Endod* 5:298-304, 1979.
2. Berry KA, Primack PD, Loushine RJ et al: Nickel-titanium versus stainless steel finger spreaders in curved canals, *J Endod* 21:221, 1995.
3. Beatty RG, Zakariasen KL: Apical leakage associated with three obturation techniques in large and small root canals, *Int Endod J* 17:67-72, 1984.
4. Block RM, Lewis RD, Sheats JBet al: Antibody formation to dog pulp tissue altered by "N2" paste within the root canal, *J Endod* 3:309-315, 1977.
5. Block RM, Lewis RD, Sheats JB: Cell mediated immune response to dog pulp tissue altered by "N2" paste within the root canal, *Oral Surg Oral Med Oral Pathol* 45:131-142, 1978.
6. Block RM, Lewis RD, Sheats JBet al: Cell mediated immune response to dog pulp tissue altered by 6.5 percent paraformaldehyde via the root canal, *J Endod* 4:346-352, 1978.
7. Block RM, Lewis RD, Hirsch J et al: Systemic distribution of N2 paste containing 14c paraformaldehyde following root canal therapy in dogs, *Oral Surg Oral Med Oral Pathol* 50:350- 360, 1980.
8. Brady JM, del Rio CE: Corrosion of endodontic silver cones in humans: A scanning electron microscope and x-ray microprobe study, *J Endod* 1:205-210, 1975.
9. Budd CS, Weller RN, Kulild JC: A comparison of thermoplasticized injectable gutta-percha obturation techniques, *J Endod* 17:260-264, 1991.
10. Callis PD, Paterson AJ: Microleakage of root fillings: Thermoplastic injection compared with lateral condensation, *J Dent* 16:194-197, 1988.
11. Cohler CM, Newton CW, Patterson SS et al: Studies of Sargenti's technique of endodontic treatment: Short-term response in monkeys, *J Endod* 6:473-478, 1980.
12. Dwan JJ, Glickman GN: 2-D photoelastic stress analysis of niti and stainless steel finger spreaders during lateral condensation, *J Endod* 21:221, 1995.
13. Dow PR, Ingle JI: Isotope determination of root canal failure, *Oral Surg Oral Med Oral Pathol* 8:1100-1104, 1955.
14. England MC, West NM, Safavi K et al: Tissue lead levels in dogs with RC-2B root canal fillings, *J Endod* 6:728-730, 1980.
15. Grossman LI, Oliet S, del Rio C: *Endodontic practice,* ed 11, Philadelphia, 1981, Lea & Febiger, p 242.
16. Gutmann JL: Principles of endodontic surgery for the general practitioner, *Dent Clin North Am* 28:895-908, 1984.
17. Gutmann JL: Adaptation of thermoplasticized gutta-percha in the absence of the dentinal smear layer, *Int Endod J* 26:87-92, 1993.
18. Gutmann JL, Dumsha TC: Cleaning and shaping the root canal system. In Cohen S, Burns R, editors: *Pathways of the pulp,* ed 4. St Louis, 1987, Mosby, pp 156-182.
19. Gutmann JL, Leonard JE: Problem solving in endodontic working length determination, *Comp Contin Educ Dent* 16:288-304, 1995.
20. Ingle JI, Luebke RG, Zidell JD et al: Obturation of the radicular space, in Ingle JI, Taintor JF, editors: *Endodontics,* Philadelphia, 1985, Lea & Febiger, pp 223-307.
21. Jacobsen EL: Clinical aid: adapting the master gutta-percha cone for apical snugness, *J Endod* 10:274, 1984.
22. Kaplowitz GJ. Evaluation of gutta-percha solvents, *J Endod* 16:539-540, 1990.
23. Kaplowitz GJ: Evaluation of the ability of essential oils to dissolve gutta-percha, *J Endod* 17:448-449, 1991.
24. LaCombe JS, Campbell AD, Hicks LM, Pelleu GB: A comparison of the apical seal produced by two thermoplasticized gutta-percha techniques, *J Endod* 14:445-450, 1988.
25. Lares C, ElDeeb ME: The sealing ability of the Thermafil obturation technique, *J Endod* 16:474-479, 1990.
26. Lloyd A, Thompson J, Gutmann JL, Dummer PMH: Evaluation of the sealability of the Trifecta technique in the presence and absence of a smear layer, *Int Endod J* 28:35-40, 1995.
27. Luks S: Guttapercha versus silver points in the practice of endodontics, *NY State Dent J* 31:341-350, 1965.
28. Metzger Z, Ben-Amar A: Removal of overextended gutta-percha root canal fillings in endodontic failure cases, *J Endod* 21:287-288, 1995.
29. Newton CW, Patterson SS, Kafrawy AH: Studies of Sargenti's technique of endodontic treatment: six-month and one-year responses, *J Endod* 6:509-517, 1980.
30. Patterson SS, Newton CW: Preparation of root canals and filling by lateral condensation techniques. In Gerstein H, editor: *Techniques in clinical endodontics,* Philadelphia, 1983, Saunders, pp 42-75.
31. Pitts DL, Matheny HE, Nicholls JI: An in vitro study of spreader loads required to cause vertical root fracture during lateral condensation, *J Endod* 9:544-550, 1983.
32. Schilder H: Vertical compaction of warm gutta percha. In Gerstein H, editor: *Techniques in clinical endodontics,* Philadelphia, 1983, Saunders, pp 76-98.
33. Seltzer S, Green DB, Weiner N et al: A scanning electron microscope examination of silver cones removed from endodontically treated teeth, *Oral Surg Oral Med Oral Pathol* 33:589-605, 1972.

34. Simon J, Ibanez B, Friedman S, Trope M: Leakage after lateral condensation with finger spreaders and D-11-T spreaders, *J Endod* 17:101-104, 1991.

35. Siskin M: Surgical techniques applicable to endodontics, *Dent Clin North Am* 11:745-769, 1991.

36. Sorin SM, Oliet S, Pearlstein F: Rejuvenation of aged (brittle) endodontic gutta-percha cones, *J Endod* 5:233-238, 1979.

37. Speier MB, Glickman GN: Volumetric and densitometric comparison between nickel titanium and stainless steel condensation, *J Endod* 22:195, 1996.

38. *Technique manual: obtura II heated gutta-percha system,* Costa Mesa, Calif, Texceed Corp, 1991.

39. *Thermafil endodontic obturators technique manual,* Tulsa, Tulsa Dental Products, 1991.

40. Weine FS: *Endodontic therapy,* ed 4, St Louis, 1989, Mosby, pp 287-295.

41. West NM, England MC, Safavi K et al: Levels of lead in blood of dogs with RC-2B root canal fillings, *J Endod* 6:598-601, 1980.

42. Wourms DJ, Campbell AD, Hicks ML, Pelleu GB: Alternative solvents to chloroform for gutta-percha removal, *J Endod* 16:224-226, 1990.

Chapter 7

Problems in Nonsurgical Root Canal Retreatment

Paul E. Lovdahl
James L. Gutmann

"Whenever a pulp is removed and the canal treated and filled in a manner that is compatible with or favorable to a physiologic reaction, we may expect a satisfactory percentage of success. Also, whenever treatment is carried on in such a way as to antagonize biologic processes of repair, we will continue to have many failures."*

"If by accident, the instrument used should break—and this is an accident careful handling should make very rare—it will sometimes be found difficult, and it may be impossible, to remove. If not jammed in the fang so as to be immovable, it may, in many cases, be withdrawn by rendering a small instrument magnetic, and passing gently up till it comes into contact with the fragment to be removed. The use of a magnetized instrument was suggested some time ago by the late Dr. John Harris, for a similar purpose. Once or twice during my practice I have found it impossible to remove the broken fragment of the instrument from the fang, and was obliged to fill without regard to it. I have observed no unfavorable results in these cases which I could attribute to this cause."†

The retreatment of a previously treated root canal is very common in today's practice of endodontics. Most retreatments can be eliminated, however, if adherence to the principles of success and prevention provided in this book are a priority for the practitioner during the initial endodontic treatment. Likewise, if retreatments are to be eliminated and replaced with initial quality treatment, there is no room for quick or magical techniques in canal cleaning, shaping, or obturation.

The purpose of this chapter is to address the multiplicity of issues involved in problem solving retreatments. These cases are more difficult and usually involve compromised circumstances.[2,10] Also, teeth requiring retreatment usually have undergone extensive restorations, and techniques not commonly used for initial treatment are indicated.[11,36] As with normal treatment cases, retreatment cases may present with or without symptoms. In those cases in which symptoms are present, in particular acute periradicular periodontitis, retreatment in one visit is not recommended because of the high potential for flare-ups in these cases.[41] By the very nature of the need for retreatment, the major focus of this chapter is on the identification and management of retreatments, and supporting chapters provide the preventive aspects.

COMMON CAUSES FOR FAILURE OF ROOT CANAL TREATMENT
Untreated Contaminated Canal Space

Because failure of initial root canal treatment may have multiple causes, retreatment planning must cover all bases. That is, the practitioner must start from the assumption that all possible causes are present.[1] As indicated in Chapter 1, failure to débride the canal system of its irritating contents is the prime cause for failure. When coupled with other identifiable entities such as ineffective three-dimensional sealing of the canal space both apically and coronally, incomplete fills using only sealers or medicated pastes, gross overextension of filling

---
*From Blayney JR: *J Am Dent Assoc* 15:1217-1221, 1928.
†From Arthur R: *J Dent Sci* 2:505, 1852.

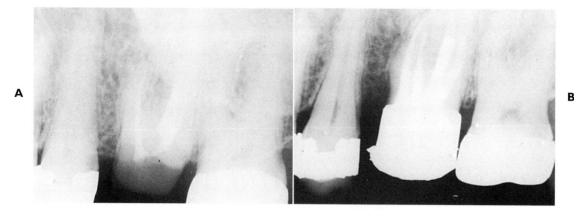

Fig. 7-1 *A, Symptomatic maxillary first molar at initial examination. B, Retreatment included the cleaning, shaping, and obturation of a previously undiscovered second mesiobuccal canal.*

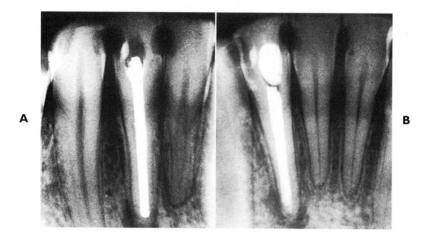

Fig. 7-2 *A, Apparent failure of previous root canal treatment with single silver cone. B, Postoperative radiograph. A previously untreated second canal on the lingual aspect is evident, with two distinct canal terminations at the apex.*

materials, or the presence of a cyst that fails to heal, the percentage of failures will increase.[19] However, the common thread in these failures is primarily the incomplete removal of tissue debris and bacteria from the canal system and the lack of a radicular seal.[4,18]

Failure can almost always be anticipated in an untreated root canal containing necrotic or inflamed tissue.

The canals most commonly left untreated in clinical practice are the second distal canal in mandibular molars (see Fig. 1-4, *B*), the second canal in the mesiobuccal root of maxillary molars (Fig. 7-1), and the second canal (invariably lingual)

in mandibular anterior teeth. Methods of locating and negotiating canals are described in Chapters 3 and 4.

Fig. 7-2, *A,* shows a failing silver-cone root-canal treatment on a mandibular incisor. When the cone was retrieved, it was found to be corroded, and such corrosion is evidence of canal leakage. Failure to seal the canal contributed to breakdown of the periradicular tissues with subsequent treatment failure; however, what is not apparent radiographically is a second canal. Close inspection of the apex of the posttreatment film (Fig. 7-2, *B*) discloses the radiopaque outline of the larger root canal preparation (which previously held the silver cone), which could not be renegotiated further, and the apical extension of the second, lingual

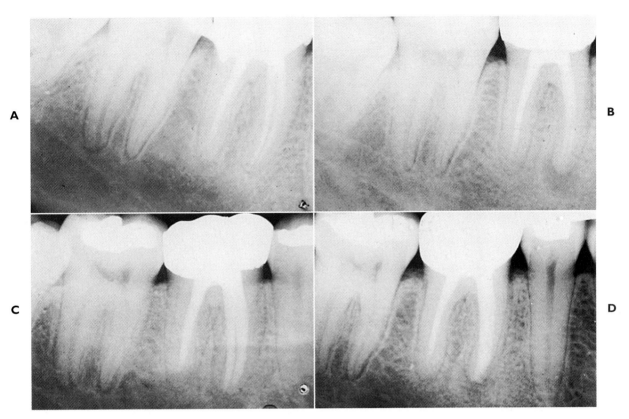

Fig. 7-3 *A, Completed root canal treatment on a mandibular first molar. The tooth was symptomless and there was no radiographic evidence of pathoses. B, Five years later the patient presented with mild pain to percussion and radiographic evidence of a lesion on the mesial root. Retreatment was initiated. C, Immediately after retreatment of the mesial root only. D, Four-year recall film showing apical healing.*

canal. Simply reinstrumenting and refilling the buccal canal would have resulted in a second failure because the source of the irritation, necrotic tissue in the lingual canal, would not have been removed and the canal would not have been sealed.

Canal Leakage Resulting from Inadequate Canal Seal

Fig. 7-3 presents a relatively uncomplicated endodontic case. No periradicular lesions were present at the time of treatment. The tooth remained comfortable but evidenced a periradicular rarefaction 3 years later. Two years later, the lesion was larger and the tooth was sensitive to percussion. The patient was referred for retreatment, which was completed only on the mesial root. A subsequent 4-year recall demonstrates healing of the periradicular tissues. This case typifies the main causes for failure and supports the initial nonsurgical correction of the inadequacies in root canal treatment.

Fig. 7-4 presents an obvious case of an inadequate radicular seal with silver cones. The cone in the distal canal is both too short and too narrow. Radiographically the canal appears to be filled principally with root canal sealer. In the mesial root, the mesiobuccal canal is instrumented short of optimal length. The silver cone in this canal barely extends to the midroot, whereas the remaining 2 mm of prepared canal is filled with sealer. The mesiolingual silver cone extends beyond the apex, suggesting the possibility of inadequate adaptation to the canal wall circumferentially. In addition, corrosion products from the silver cone have produced an inflammatory response in the periradicular tissues. These corrosion products are cytotoxic and may contribute to ultimate failure and to patient symptoms.[3,35] Fig. 7-4, *B,* shows the immediate postoperative retreatment result with gutta-percha. In this case, it was possible to prepare all the canals to within 1 mm of the radiographic apex. This is essential to thorough

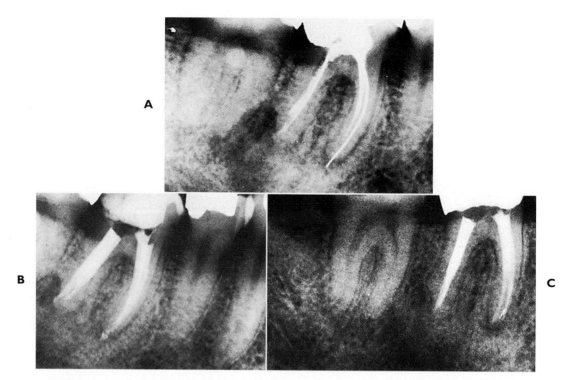

**Fig. 7-4 *A,* *Root canal treatment failed because of inadequate sealing of canal spaces.*
B, *Appearance immediately after nonsurgical retreatment.* *C,* *Appearance at 1-year recall. Notice*
*the healing of periradicular tissues.***

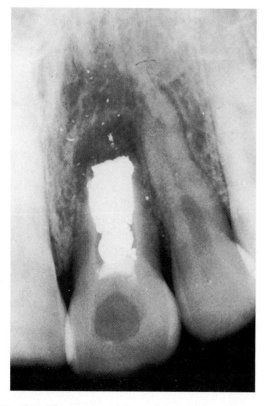

Fig. 7-5 *Thirteen-year failure after surgical treatment of*
a central incisor with an open apex.

canal débridement of the silver-cone corrosion products. A radiograph obtained at the 1-year recall visit revealed healing of the periradicular tissues (Fig. 7-4, *C*). It was also significant that a second, previously untreated canal was found in the distal root.

Failure resulting from canal leakage is also common in attempts to complete nonsurgical root canal treatment on nonvital open-apex teeth. Without apexification techniques,[9] the sealing of these canals is very difficult because of the divergency of the canal walls without an apical barrier. Although periradicular surgery (Fig. 7-5) has been used to treat these cases, calcium hydroxide apexification techniques are preferable.[9] Fig. 7-6 illustrates a failed case of nonsurgical management of an open-apex tooth. It was possible to retrieve the gutta-percha using Gates-Glidden burs and large Hedström files. Treatment time for apexification on the 35-year-old patient shown was 2 years and 9 months. This is essentially the same time as that for the young patient.

Fig. 7-7 shows a similar case in which it was necessary to remove a cast gold post and a porcelain veneer crown before retreatment. Esthetics,

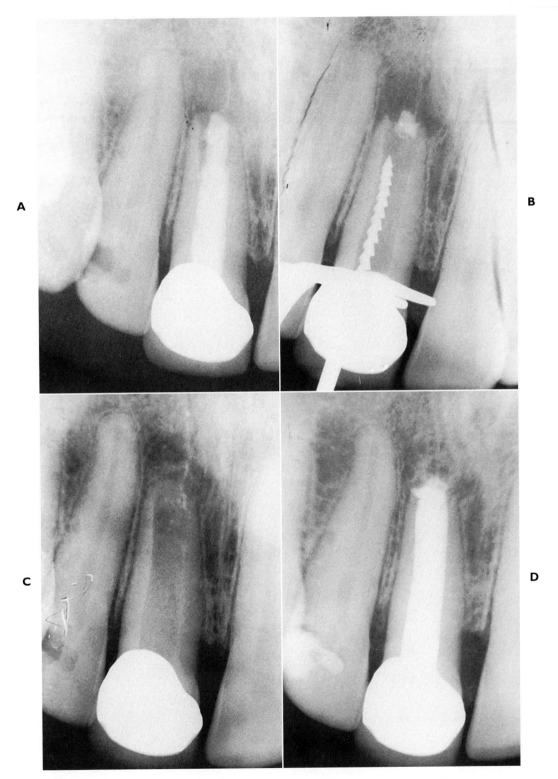

Fig. 7-6 A, *Nonsurgical root canal treatment without attempts at apexification, failing 28 years after original treatment. Patient was 35 years of age.* **B,** *Retreatment was initiated by removing the old gutta-percha filling with Gates-Glidden burs and large Hedström files.* **C,** *Apical barrier formed after treatment with calcium hydroxide for 2 years, 9 months.* **D,** *Completed retreatment.*

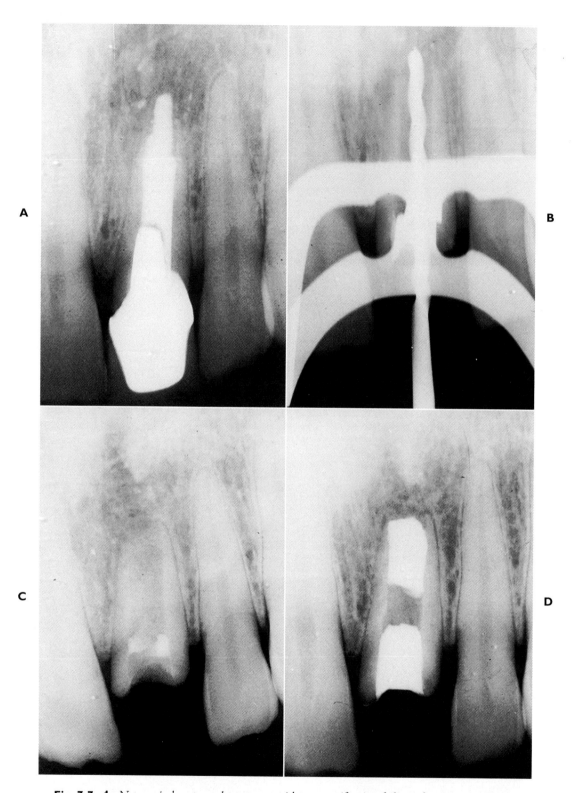

Fig. 7-7 *A, Nonsurgical root canal treatment without apexification failing after 27 years. Tooth is a central incisor restored with a cast post and a porcelain veneer crown. The patient was 34 years of age at the time of examination.* *B, Retreatment required the removal of the post and crown. Temporization during the course of treatment was provided by means of a temporary removable partial denture.* *C, Apical barrier formed after treatment with calcium hydroxide for 2 years, 8 months.* *D, Completed retreatment with post space and temporary cement restoration.*

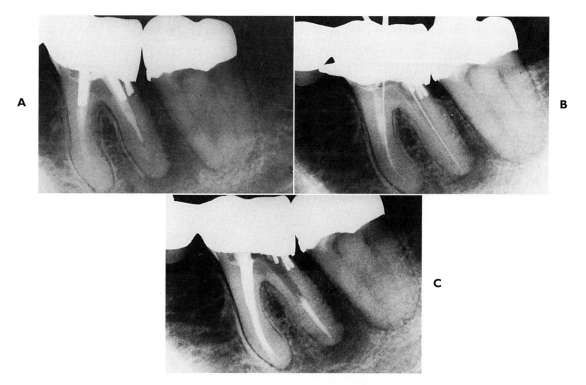

Fig. 7-8 *A, Previous root canal treatment with gutta-percha failed. Root canal fillings terminate far short of ideal location because of apparent dystrophic calcification. **B,** Radiograph obtained after removal of posts and gutta-percha. Renegotiation to the radiographic apex, though difficult, was possible in all canals. **C,** Obturation of canals; post space in distal canal.*

temporization, and function are serious considerations when one is electing to use long-term apexification techniques. In this case a temporary removable partial denture was used over a treatment span of 2 years and 8 months.

Presumably Calcified Canals

> A periradicular lesion is prima facie evidence of the presence of a canal space and necrotic tissue, even when a canal appears radiographically to be calcified.

Fig. 7-8, *A* shows a failing treatment in a mandibular molar filled short of the apical constriction in all the canals with gutta-percha. Radiographically no canal space is apparent beyond the present radicular filling material. The patient presented clinically with a long-standing gingival sinus tract. The tooth also held intraradicular posts, which should not deter the practitioner from attempting nonsurgical retreatment, since in some molars

surgery is not a viable option. Limited anatomic access, short roots, certain tooth angles, or medical contraindications frequently limit the choices to nonsurgical retreatment or extraction. From illustrations *B* and *C* of Fig. 7-8, it can be seen that the distal canal and one of two mesial canals were negotiable to the apex after post removal. Clinical examination confirmed healing of the sinus tract after the canals were débrided. The ability to negotiate one of two canals in roots such as this greatly improves the prognosis because of the frequent joining of two such canals into one at the apex.

Instrument Separation Preventing Proper Canal Cleaning and Obturation

> A separated root canal instrument is seldom, if ever, the sole cause of failure.

Since instruments are stainless steel or nickel-titanium alloy, it would be extremely rare for these materials to cause periradicular inflammation. The

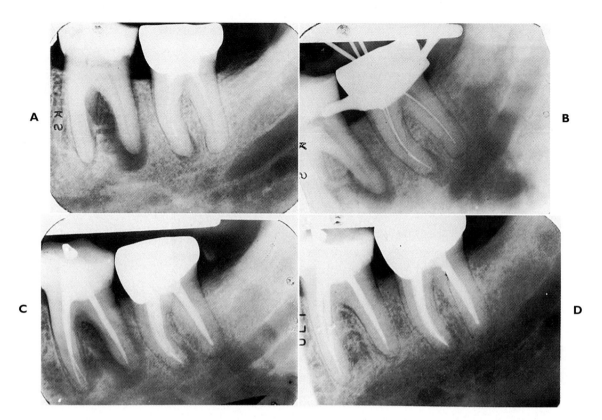

A

B

C

D

Fig. 7-9

real problem is that the separated instrument blocks proper cleaning, shaping, and canal obturation. When these instruments can be removed, successful retreatment invariably ensues. Although it is possible to remove many of these instrument fragments, the majority will not be removable because of canal curvature or total blockage of the lumen, which prevents bypassing of the segment. Occasionally it may be possible to bypass a fractured instrument segment and yet not be able to remove it. In these cases the canal is cleaned, shaped, and obturated, incorporating the fractured segment into the filling. Alternative treatment planning generally includes periradicular surgery or root or tooth resection.

CLINICAL PROBLEM: A 33-year-old female patient presented with pain of long standing in the mandibular left posterior quadrant. She was convinced that her problem was coming from the first molar, though she could not be sure. She stated that she had had root canal treatment on the second molar and was told that that tooth could not cause her any difficulty. Her pain was beginning to be

accentuated by biting. Clinical examination revealed pain to percussion and palpation on the second molar with a more subdued response on the first molar. The first molar was nonresponsive to thermal stimulation, but the second molar gave a dull ache to a cold stimulus. Periodontal probings were within normal limits. A radiograph revealed a large radiolucency on the first molar, a radiolucency on the mesial root of the second molar, and the presence of a fractured instrument in the mesial canal of the second molar. The distal canal appeared to be filled with a paste filling (Fig. 7-9, *A*). A diagnosis of pulp necrosis with subacute periradicular periodontitis was made for the first molar and incomplete root canal treatment with acute periradicular periodontitis for the second molar.

Solution: Because of the patient's symptoms and chief complaint, a decision was made to retreat the second molar first. Although needing treatment, the first molar did not give evidence of being the primary cause of the patient's discomfort. The possible explanation for the abnormal cold response with the second molar would be the

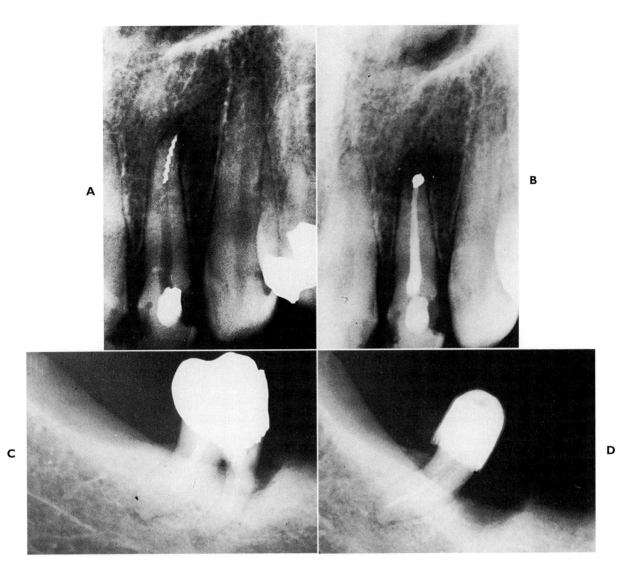

Fig. 7-10 *A,* *Fractured Hedström file protruding through the apical foramen of a maxillary lateral incisor.* ***B,*** *Appearance immediately after surgical removal of the fractured segment. The canal was cleaned, shaped, and obturated before the root-end filling was placed.* ***C,*** *Mandibular second molar presenting with severe periodontal defects around the mesial root and in the furcation. The tooth was endodontically symptomatic, and a separated file was present in the distal root.* ***D,*** *After tooth resection, which solved the periodontal problem, endodontic retreatment of the distal root was possible after removal of the instrument fragment.*

Continued.

presence of residual, degenerating pulp tissue apical to the fractured instrument in the mesial canal and apical to the paste fill in the distal canal. After significant attempts to remove the fractured instrument segment in the mesial roots, the metallic object was bypassed with a file (Fig. 7-9, *B*). Both teeth were obturated with gutta-percha and sealer, and the patient's symptoms ceased (Fig. 7-9, *C*). The fractured instrument segment was incorporated into the root canal filling. A 4-year reevalua-

tion shows excellent healing for both teeth, and the patient is symptom free (Fig. 7-9, *D*).

Fig. 7-10, *A* and *B*, shows a broken Hedström file protruding through the apical foramen of a lateral incisor in which surgery was necessary for removal and correction of the apical seal. It should be emphasized that under such conditions, the canal must still be cleaned and obturated before surgical placement of a root-end filling (Fig. 7-10, *B*). Fig. 7-10, *C* to *H*, depicts fractured instruments

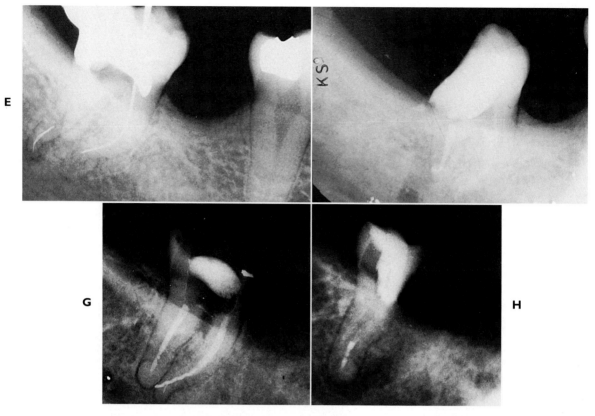

Fig. 7-10 cont'd. *E, Separated file in the distolingual canal of the mandibular third molar. F, treatment included a distolingual root resection. G, Fractured endodontic instrument in the mesiolingual canal of a mandibular second molar. H, Immediately after tooth resection.*

in the roots of mandibular molars. Since retrieval is virtually impossible around a curve in small canals and periradicular surgery in these cases was impractical, a root or tooth resection was viewed as a feasible alternative to extraction (Fig. 7-10, *D, F, H*) (see Chapter 8). In cases in which periradicular surgery or root or tooth resection cannot or should not be done, extraction or intentional replantation should be considered.[5,15]

CONSIDERATIONS IN NONSURGICAL RETREATMENT
Techniques for Removal of Gutta-Percha and Paste Fills

The simplest method of removing gutta-percha from a root canal is by softening the gutta-percha with a solvent, such as methylchloroform, rectified white turpentine, or eucalyptol[11,20,23,26,39,44] (see Chapter 6). Once the orifice of the canal has been uncovered, the access cavity is filled with solvent. The solvent must not be allowed to run onto the

rubber dam because it can denature the natural rubber and a large hole will quickly result. After 1 or 2 minutes, the solvent in the pulp chamber will dissolve the gutta-percha to the extent that a No. 15 or 20 K-file will easily negotiate the canal. Once a size 25 K-file is reached, a Hedström file or reamer can be used to engage the mass of gutta-percha laterally, often removing it in one piece (Fig. 7-11). During the penetration with the file, frequent lavage with the solvent from a 5 ml Luer-Lok syringe will both flush out softened material and provide fresh solvent for continued dissolution. The practitioner must be careful not to use any solvent at or near the apical foramen[39]: passage of these chemicals past the end of the root may result in severe postoperative discomfort.

If the solvent does not readily soften the gutta-percha, a size 20 to 30 reamer can be used to bore into the gutta-percha. This also helps to carry some of the chemical deeper into the central mass of the gutta-percha, which hastens dissolution. In larger canals, Peeso reamers can be used to remove the bulk of the gutta-percha in the coronal one half to two thirds of the canal. Subsequently, files or reamers can be used to bypass and remove the apical segment.

Many authors and clinicians recommend the use of a heated instrument to remove the coronal aspect of the gutta-percha before any of the above techniques are attempted.[16,39] The instrument can be a plugger or spreader, or a specific heat-transfer instrument (Schilder 0 or 00, produced by Caulk/Dentsply, Milford, Del., or Touch 'N Heat, by Analytical Technology, Redmond, Wash.). The instrument is heated until it is cherry red and then plunged into the coronal aspect of the gutta-percha. Do not leave the heated instrument in the gutta-percha more than 1 to 2 seconds to attain an ideal consistency for removal. Continued movement down the canal in this manner will also soften the apical mass, facilitating removal.

Many paste filling materials are largely zinc oxide and eugenol in composition and are easily soluble in solvent; however, some paste materials resist dissolution by a wide range of organic solvents. The only solution is to try to drill or bore out the set paste with rotary instruments, reamers, or ultrasonics. Fortunately, paste fills in their usual condition require no solvent. The paste looks and feels as though it had never set, or as though it had been dissolved by the action of the tissue fluid that diffused through the patent apical foramen. With the paste material already soft and mushy, a size 15 or 20 K-file can easily be passed to the apical extent of the previous preparation with the aid of copious irrigation with sodium hypochlorite (NaOCl). Ultrasonic instrumentation and flushing also works well to débride the canal of paste remnants.

Preventing the Fracture of Metallic Objects in the Root Canal

Most breakages of metallic instruments in the root canal system can be prevented by knowing how the instruments are manufactured, how they are to be used, and what limitations have been placed upon them. In general, all types of root canal instruments are too often employed beyond their usefulness, in a manner for which they were not designed, and with excessive amounts of force (see Chapter 5).

Root canal files and reamers should be inspected for irregular windings or evidence of fatigue. This is easily done by passing the instrument through a bright light and checking for irregular shiny spots, which indicate unwinding of the instrument

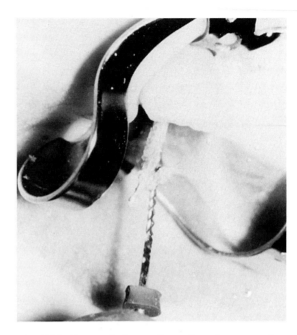

Fig. 7-11 *Removal of a poorly condensed gutta-percha filling in one piece.*

(see Fig. 4-25). Since a small file will become fatigued without visual evidence, it is wise to test each file by intentionally placing a small curve in the apical 2 to 3 mm before use and recurving it during use. It is not uncommon to have an apparently good instrument separate with only gentle curving. Smaller-sized instruments (Nos. 8 to 20) should be used minimally and replaced often.

The advent of nickel-titanium (Ni-Ti) hand instruments has had both a positive and a negative effect on the delivery of quality root canal treatment (see Chapter 5). The ability to negotiate and maintain canal curvatures has been most beneficial. However, these instruments cannot be curved before canal entry and require a different tactile sensation during working motions. Aggressive movements have led to numerous fractures of these instruments without warning (unwinding). This also occurs with the engine-driven instrument, such as the 0.04 taper Profile Ni-Ti instruments (Tulsa Dental Products, Tulsa, Okla.). These instruments do not have standard tapers found in the hand instruments and therefore often result in a locking effect against the canal wall during usage. This may easily lead to fracture. The best way to deal with the increased possibility of breakage is to practice extensively with these instruments, learning their nuances and developing an acute tactile sensation. Prevention is key to their suc-

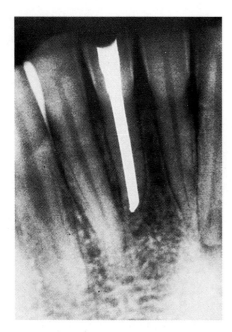

Fig. 7-12 *Radiograph of a successful silver cone root canal treatment on a mandibular incisor that required placement of an intraradicular post. Retrieval of the cone proved impossible.*

cessful usage. If they should fracture, the techniques for removal identified in this chapter will apply.

When Gates-Glidden (GG) drills and Peeso reamers are used to countersink the coronal portion of the canal, a pathway should be established with a hand instrument first. Short advances of the rotary instrument followed by complete withdrawal will allow the shavings to escape and prevent binding of the bur head in the canal orifice. Copious water irrigation is also necessary. The smaller-size burs will almost invariably bind and break if forced. When GG drills or Peeso reamers are used to flare the canal after the use of files, all cutting should be done passively as the bur is withdrawn from the canal.

Further details on the prevention of fractured instruments can be found in Chapter 5.

Although silver cones seem to be gradually losing their popularity in endodontic practice, some practitioners have achieved a high degree of long-term success with them. Careful case selection is recommended because oral conditions may change, requiring the removal of even an apparently successful silver-cone root filling. Fig. 7-12 illustrates an initially successful silver cone treatment that eventually required retreatment after more than 10 years. There were no symptoms

or evidence of pathosis. Fracture of the coronal tooth structure indicated the need for a porcelain veneer crown with an intraradicular post. The silver cone proved impossible to remove, and it would have been difficult if not impossible to drill to an adequate depth for a post. There is also the chance that the seal might be disturbed by such an attempt and that the root canal treatment might fail after restoration.

If silver cones are placed, enough length should be left in the pulp chamber for grasping should future removal be necessary. Cements should be used to cover the coronal ends of the cones in the pulp chamber. If alloy is placed in the pulp chamber, the ends of the cones will not be distinguishable from the alloy and will usually be cut off with a bur upon reentry, greatly diminishing the likelihood of successful retrieval. If a post is planned, the twist-off silver cone technique should be avoided in favor of gutta-percha. If retreatment is ever needed, it is often possible to retrieve the post, but the silver cone in the apical half of the canal may be impossible to remove nonsurgically. These same principles apply to the use of metallic core carrier techniques.

Techniques for Removing Metallic Objects from the Canal

Use of Spoon Excavators, Explorers, and Point Retrievers

A No. 31 or 33 endodontic spoon excavator with a sharp cutting edge will often lift out a silver cone if the cone is fairly loose (Fig. 7-13). If the end of the cone is bent sufficiently, it can be initially hooked with a fine No. 17 explorer or Caufield Silver Point Retriever (Moyco, Union Broach, York, Penn.) (Fig. 7-14). These instruments resemble spoon excavators with a V-shaped notch modification. Their mode of action is a prying motion, similar to that of an extraction elevator. Solvents should be used before the practitioner attempts removal of any silver cone that is firmly lodged in the canal. Some silver cones will have cement surrounding them in the orifice (Fig. 7-15) and down the canal. The solvent will help soften the cement as a small file or reamer is slowly worked beside the silver cone. Success in bypassing the silver cone will lead to the smoothest retrieval.

Use of Hedström Files

The use of solvents and fine instruments will often free up the coronal part of a silver cone. Once a pathway is negotiated, the "file-braiding" technique can be used.[14,39] One or more Hedström

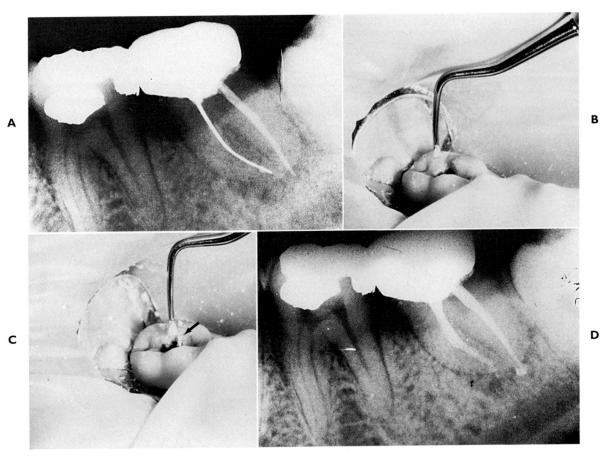

Fig. 7-13 *A, Silver cone in the mesial canal of a mandibular molar; retreatment was indicated. B, Small endodontic spoon excavator was used to engage the silver cone. C, Silver cone was lifted out of the canal (arrow). D, Retreatment with gutta-percha.*

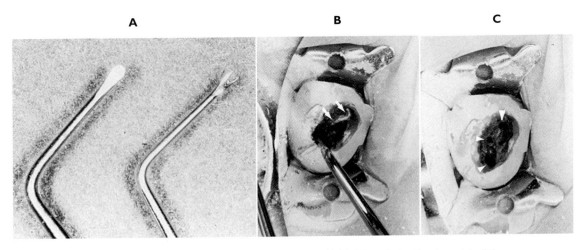

Fig. 7-14 *A, Endodontic spoon excavator (left); Caulfield Silver Point Retriever No. 35 (right). In order for the spoon excavator to engage the silver cone it must be sharp. If it was previously heated to remove gutta-percha, it will not work to remove silver cones. B, Caulfield Silver Point Retriever used to lift silver cone from the tooth (arrows). C, Silver cones removed. Notice patent orifices (arrowheads).*

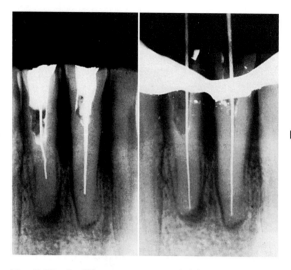

A

B

Fig. 7-15 *A, Silver cones surrounded by cement in the orifice. B, Careful excavation of the silver cones and use of solvent around cement allows removal of the silver cones and prevents particles of cement from falling into the canal orifices.*

files, usually in the No. 20 to 35 range, are placed beside the silver cone as far apically as possible and screwed into position until tight. The screwing maneuver engages the soft silver metal and yields a satisfactory purchase. If the Hedström files are twisted together, they can be simultaneously pulled out by hand (Fig. 7-16, *A* and *B*), or they can be clamped with a surgical needle holder and levered against the incisal or occlusal edge. This technique is especially useful when access is limited or the silver cone does not extend out of the orifice (Fig. 7-16, *C* to *F*). This technique may also be considered for removal of sectional or twist-off silver cones (Fig. 7-17), in addition to plastic gutta-percha core carriers. Since Hedström files will not engage stainless steel, the technique will not work on broken files, lentula spirals, or GG drills, even if they are fairly long and loose coronally.

Specialized Forceps

Several specialized forceps for the removal of metallic objects have been developed. All have narrow beaks that will extend into a reasonably conservative access opening (Fig. 7-18).[7,39,43] The Steiglitz silver point forceps (Moyco, Union Broach, York, Penn.) is a grooved needle-nosed pliers that is often too bulky to use in small access openings. The bulkier portion of the forceps can be ground away to permit better penetration into the orifice. However, the fine teeth of the instrument often

slide off the metal object to be removed rather than grasp it firmly. These detriments can be overcome by use of a Perry gold foil pliers,[14] a Peet Splinter Forceps (Silvermans, New York, N.Y.), or a Hartmen 3½ CVD Mosquito Forceps (Miltex, Lake Success, N.Y.). These forceps are generally more useful because the taper on the beaks is more gradual, allowing freedom for beak separation and engagement of the metallic object in deep access openings. The tips are not quite so delicate as the tips of the Steiglitz forceps and are less likely to bend or slip under tension. Either instrument is useful for retrieving a loosened silver cone or the shaft of a GG drill (Fig. 7-19).

If the end of a silver cone can be engaged but proves to have too much retention for unaided retrieval, a needle holder can be used to clamp the beaks of the forceps. This will increase the grip or retentive force on the silver cone. If the beaks of the needle holder are levered against a cusp, the silver cone can usually be "jacked" out of the canal (Fig. 7-20). However, this approach is seldom successful for retrieving stainless steel instruments. Although the instrument may be long enough to grasp, the serrations on the beaks will not engage the hard stainless steel shaft. Consequently the forceps will usually slip off, despite the additional force of the needle holder.

Masserann Kit

One of the most useful and versatile systems available for retrieving metallic objects from canals is the Masserann kit (MicroMega SA, Besançon, France).[4,6,24,25,28-30,47] This kit contains a series of tubular trephining drills and two sizes of tubular extractors (1.2 and 1.5 mm) (Fig. 7-21). The principle of this technique is first to create a space in the root canal around the coronal 2 mm of the metallic object so that the extractor tube will pass over it. Then the extractor plunger, a locking rod in the tube, is screwed down, locking the metallic object against a knurled ring in the tube wall. This mechanism provides adequate retention for removal of most silver cones, metallic core carriers, and some separated endodontic instruments (Fig. 7-22).

Ultrasonic Removal

Ultrasonic devices have been a part of dentistry for many years, and variations have been adapted for use in endodontics. Presently multiple devices are available with sufficient energy to loosen metallic instrument fragments lodged in the root canal. These instruments are effective in either an endodontic instrumentation mode or a scaler mode

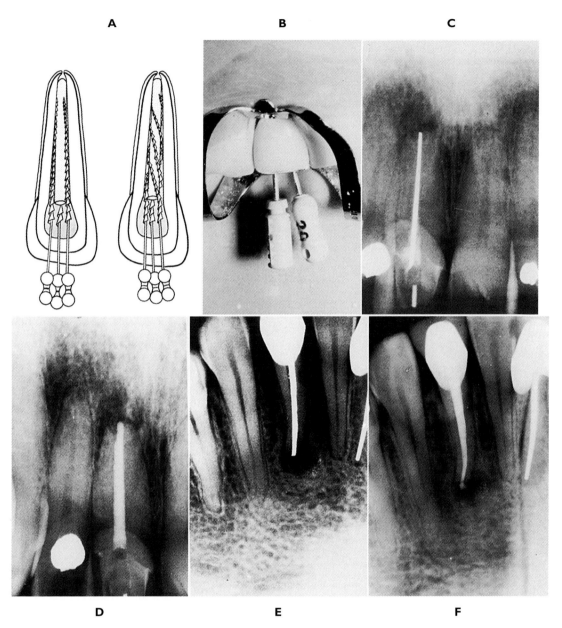

Fig. 7-16 *A, Hedström file braiding technique. B, File braiding technique requires sufficient space adjacent to the silver cone to place two or three Hedström files beside the cone in the canal. It is especially useful in canals that are wide buccolingually and contain a small, centrally located silver cone. C, Failed silver cone. The cone was removed with the file braiding technique. D, Retreatment with gutta-percha. E, Removal of silver cone with the file braiding technique in a mandibular incisor. F, Retreatment with gutta-percha.*

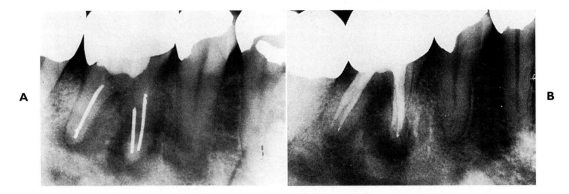

Fig. 7-17 *A,* *Radiograph showing three sectional silver cones. Cones were removed using the file braiding technique.* *B,* *Retreatment of three canals and initial treatment of the missed fourth canal.*

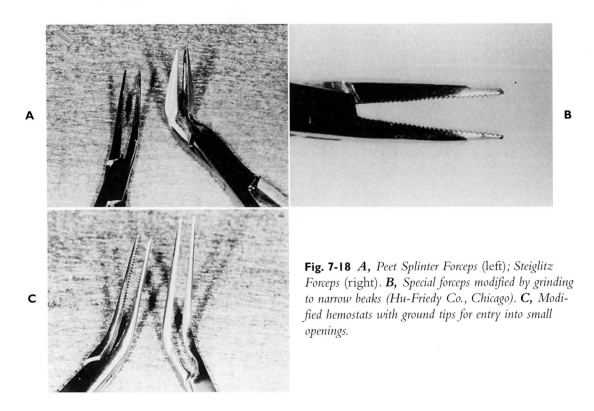

Fig. 7-18 *A,* *Peet Splinter Forceps* (left); *Steiglitz Forceps* (right). *B,* *Special forceps modified by grinding to narrow beaks (Hu-Friedy Co., Chicago). C, Modified hemostats with ground tips for entry into small openings.*

for the removal of broken endodontic instrument fragments, Gates-Glidden bur heads, posts, and other metallic objects.

Techniques for Identification, Isolation, and Removal of Silver Cones

When the tooth designated for retreatment is entered, any extension of the silver cone in the pulp chamber must be preserved. After the occlusal surface of the final restoration has been penetrated with the high-speed bur, frequent pauses for irrigation and drying will allow the earliest detection

of cement surrounding the cone in the pulp chamber. The most difficult cases are those in which an alloy has been packed to the pulp chamber floor around the silver cones. In this situation it is virtually impossible to visually identify the silver cones and dissect them out without cutting them off with the bur. In these cases, cut away the alloy from the borders of the restoration first, establishing an access opening of normal size and shape on the lingual or occlusal surface. During the cutting phase a sound finger rest must be maintained to prevent erratic movement of the hand-

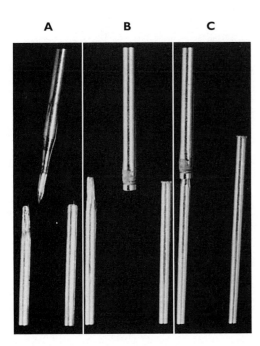

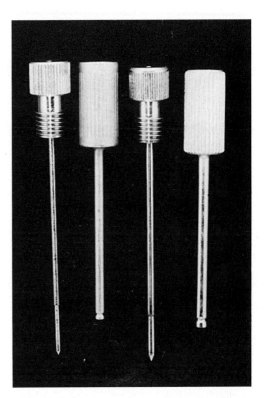

Fig. 7-26 *A, Circumferential reduction of the end of a large silver cone with a finishing bur. **B,** Reduction allows seating of the extractor on the cone. **C,** Extractor fitted on cone.*

Fig. 7-27 *Masserann extractor tubes and plungers. Uniformity of design permits the use of the small (1.2 mm) plunger in the large (1.5 mm) tube, useful for locking the extractor onto a large-diameter object.*

haps the fastest method. If there is insufficient length but the canal is negotiable around the silver cone, the Hedström braiding technique can be used.

The ultrasonic device is often useful at this point to enlarge the canal space alongside the cone. It sometimes will happen with a particularly loose silver cone that the ultrasonic energy will completely dislodge the cone. If this should occur, it may not be noticed at the time, because fragments loosened with the ultrasonic device will often be aspirated with the irrigation spray.

If these methods fail, the Masserann technique should be considered. In cases where it is possible to lock one of the two Masserann extractors directly onto the extension of the silver cone, troughing around the silver cones will not be necessary.

The extractors can be adapted and used in different ways. There are only two sizes of extractors, 1.2 and 1.5 mm; it is immediately apparent that although no object diameter is too small to be engaged, many silver cones will be too large to fit. In such cases the exposed end of the cone can usually be cut down with a fine, flame-shaped fin-

ishing bur to a diameter that will fit in the 1.5 mm extractor (Fig. 7-26). Since the screw-locking mechanism is identical on both sizes, the plunger from the 1.2 mm extractor may be used in the 1.5 mm tube, thus giving additional space in the tube for locking onto large cones (Fig. 7-27). Once the extractor has been firmly locked onto the cone, simple digital pressure will usually remove the cone. In some cases, if the silver cone does not come out with manual pressure, the ultrasonic device set on maximum power with a vibrating tip will aid in retrieval. However, it is not wise to use the needle holder in the manner shown in Fig. 7-20 with the Masserann extractor. Compression with the needle holder will collapse the tube and ruin the device. A safer approach for the most resistant cones is the impact type of crown puller, which can engage the hub of the Masserann extractor and apply sharp impact withdrawal forces. This method will loosen even the largest and tightest cones (Fig. 7-28).

If there is insufficient exposed silver cone length to engage with the extractor, it will be necessary to

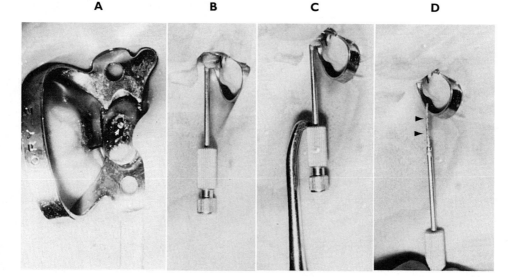

Fig. 7-28 *A, Large silver cone in a maxillary premolar* (arrowhead). *B, Attachment of extractor to silver cone. C, Impact crown remover hooked onto extractor. D, Successful silver cone removal* (arrowheads).

use the trephining drills to create a space around the cone in the canal large enough to accommodate the appropriate-sized extractor. This is a very difficult technique and must be performed with copious irrigation.

It is usually wise to begin trephining with a large drill, such as 1.6 or 1.7 mm, so that the drill will cut a wide space around the cone and avoid cutting into it. Advancing no more than 0.5 mm at a time, the drill is withdrawn. The shavings are flushed from both tooth and drill, and any solid dentin remaining around the silver cone is broken away with an explorer. Excessive pressure on the trephining drill and failure to clean the operative site frequently will cause the dentinal chips to bind inside the trephining drill, causing the cutting blades to flare and possibly break off. Flaring alone can cause perforation through the root surface. It is important to continually inspect the trephining drill for deformation and resharpen it at the earliest sign.[28-30] Chips can be removed from the inside of the drill with an endodontic file. After passing from 1 to 1.5 mm down the canal, it is wise to step down a size in drills to allow shavings to escape. Remember that the smaller extractor is 1.2 mm, which will fit into a space created by the 1.2 mm trephining drill, a fairly small drill. After the establishment of at least 2 mm of space, the extractor may be inserted and locked onto the cone as previously described, and the cone is removed (Fig. 7-29).

A trephining drill that is too close to the size of the silver cone will bind against the cone. The binding is worsened by the compaction of dentin

chips between the cone and drill. With large cones this sometimes results in the trephining drill doing double duty as an extractor (Fig. 7-30). With smaller cones, however, the binding may twist the end of the silver cone or cut into its side. In either case the silver cone will fracture on attempted retrieval and may be broken at too great a depth for a second attempt.

If the silver cone fractures or the cone is deep in the canal initially, an additional technique for exposing the coronal 2 to 3 mm involves the removal of the lateral cutting edges on a 700R tapered fissure bur.[13] This leaves a cutting edge only at the tip of the bur, which allows safe troughing around the cone without risking the cutting away of the cone. However, it must be remembered that troughing burs and trephining drills will not negotiate a curvature. Therefore care must be exercised when drilling to anticipated curvatures to prevent cutting the silver cone or perforating the root wall.

CLINICAL PROBLEM: A 27-year-old male patient presented with a history of trauma to his maxillary central incisors. The right central had been lost in the trauma, but the left central was retained after root canal treatment. Presently the patient wants to have a fixed bridge placed, but the left central incisor is tender to biting, pressure, and palpation. Clinical exam reveals that the tooth is painful to percussion and palpation. There is a small swelling around the apex of the tooth, and the tissues are inflamed. A radiograph (Fig. 7-31, *A*) shows previous root canal treatment with a split

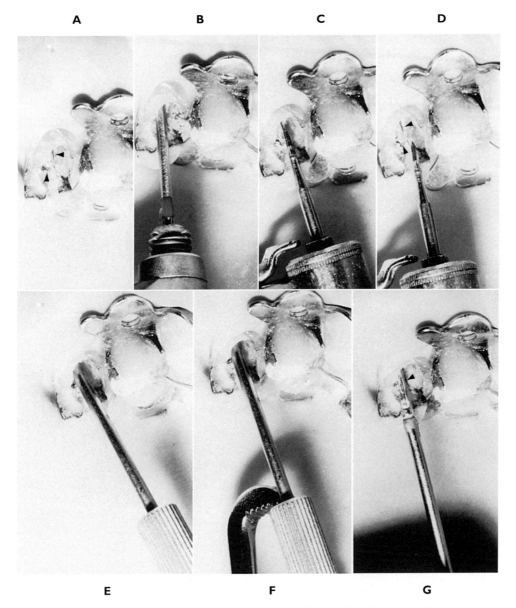

Fig. 7-29 *A, Large silver cone in palatal root* (arrowheads). *B, Troughing around silver cone with trephine. C, Bur used to reduce the top of the silver cone for extractor attachment. D, Circumferential reduction of silver cone* (arrowheads). *E, Extractor placed on silver cone. F, Crown remover hooked onto extractor. G, Successful removal of silver cone* (arrowhead).

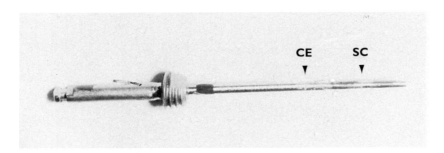

Fig. 7-30 *Silver cone (SC) unexpectedly removed when it became lodged in the cutting edge (CE) of the trephining bur.*

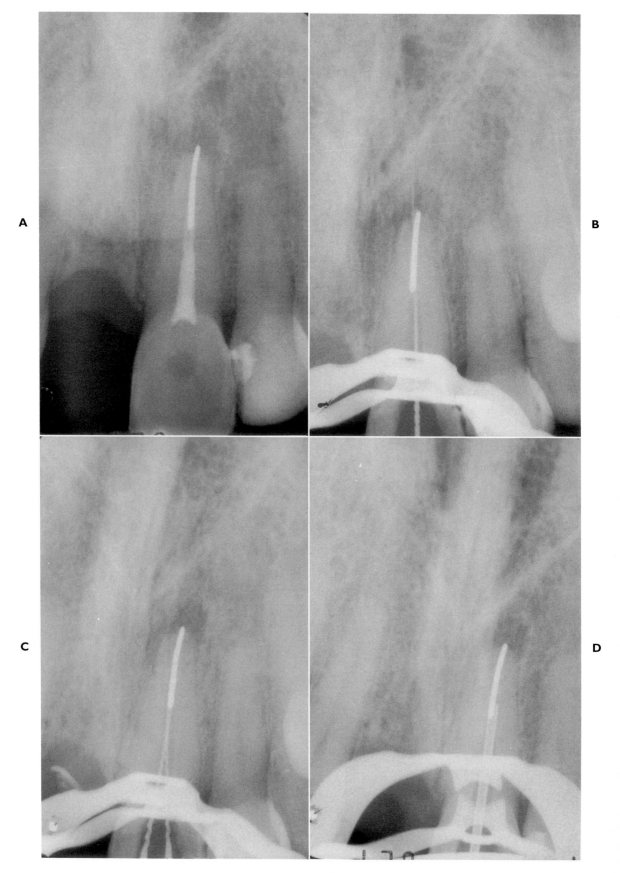

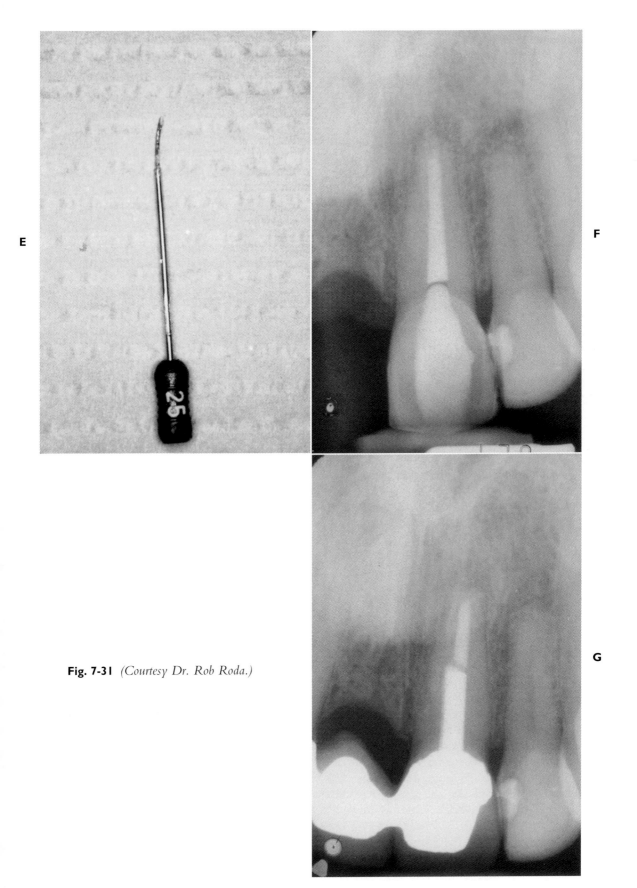

E

F

G

Fig. 7-31 *(Courtesy Dr. Rob Roda.)*

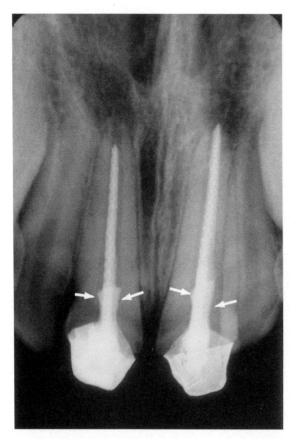

Fig. 7-32 *Two maxillary central incisors obturated with gutta-percha core carriers. Notice the amount of gutta-percha in the coronal portion (arrows) that was stripped from the carriers because the access opening was not properly prepared.*

silver cone technique. The cone protrudes beyond the end of the root, and there is apical root resorption and a periradicular radiolucency. Evidence of replacement resorption is suspected along the lateral borders of the tooth.

Solution: Based on the subjective and objective findings, a diagnosis of previous root canal treatment with acute periradicular periodontitis and apical root resorption is appropriate. Because the tooth will require extensive reconstruction for the bridge, and periradicular surgery is not the treatment of choice without attempting to replace the root canal filling, a nonsurgical approach was deemed advisable. Initially the silver cone was bypassed (Fig. 7-31, *B*) with a small file. However the cone was not loose. Second, the Hedström braiding technique was tried but without success (Fig. 7-31, *C*). Because the top of the silver cone was visible, a trephine with a small drop of cyano-

acrylate was placed around the top of the cone (Fig. 7-31, *D*). After the cement set, the trephine was teased from the tooth and the cone was removed (Fig. 7-31, *E*). The root canal was cleaned and the root filling was replaced (Fig. 7-31, *F*). A 1-year reevaluation with a fixed bridge in place is seen in Fig. 7-31, *G*. The periradicular tissues are almost healed with evidence of a new lamina dura and periodontal ligament space around the apex. Intervention nonsurgically is indicated in most cases when previous dental work requires disassembly and new restorations are to be placed.

Techniques for Identification, Isolation, and Removal of Core-Carrier Gutta-Percha Obturations

Clinical observations have identified the following indications for retreatment of core-carrier obturations: short fills, fills beyond the root apex, significant voids in the filling in the apical third of the canal, obvious stripping of gutta-percha from the carrier, or persistent symptoms after treatment, such as pain, thermal sensitivity, or discomfort to biting or pressure.

To understand the problems encountered in the retrieval of the core carriers, the major reasons for failure when using this method of obturation must be discussed.[17] It is essential that the canal preparation be a continuously tapered funnel (see Chapter 5). Failure to provide this shape will result in the lack of penetration of the carrier to the apical third of the canal and the subsequent movement of the gutta-percha to the prepared apical seat. Likewise, a shape that is too narrow at any portion of the canal will result in the stripping of the gutta-percha from the core carrier (see Fig. 6-8). This stripping will often additionally result in the cutting and binding of the core carrier into the dentin walls in the case of the metallic carrier, or the frictional binding of the plastic carriers. In either case, penetration along the walls of the carrier with a solvent or small canal may be severely hindered. If the canal is too large or too flared, gutta-percha adaptation to the walls may exhibit voids or gaps in the fill, especially in the proximal dimension.[40] This gives the clinician a false sense of the quality of the obturation.

Proper access openings are also necessary when core-carrier techniques are used. Initially, if the access is improperly shaped or insufficiently large, the softened gutta-percha will be stripped from the core carrier as it is placed into the canal (Fig. 7-32). Additionally, because both core carriers

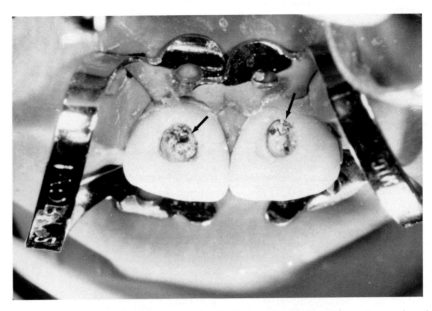

Fig. 7-33 *Two metallic core carriers* (arrows) *placed through small access openings and wedged against the unremoved lingual ledges.*

are flexible, they can lodge under unremoved lingual ledges in anterior teeth (Fig. 7-33) or pulp chamber roofs or horns in posterior teeth. This creates significant problems when attempting to reaccess the chamber during retreatment while protecting the coronal extension of the core carrier.

Carriers that are cut off at or below the canal orifice pose a different set of problems in retreatment because a purchase is restricted or impossible. Likewise it may prevent penetration of a solvent alongside the core carrier and the passage of a small instrument. Also carriers that are surrounded by composite or amalgams can be difficult to discern during reaccess and may be easily cut off (Fig. 7-34). On the other hand, core carriers, primarily metallic, which extend to the surface of the core restoration and contact the metallic crown or coronal alloy will often act as thermistors in the conduction of temperature changes. In these cases, patients report significant discomfort to thermal changes in a root canal–treated tooth. This problem is especially acute when the core carrier is beyond the root apex or has been stripped of its guttapercha in the apical third of the canal.

CLINICAL PROBLEM: A 26-year-old male patient presented as an emergency with symptoms of acute prolonged sensitivity to cold and spontaneous pain in the mandibular right quadrant. He could not bite on the first molar without excruciating pain. Root canal treatment had been completed 3 days earlier, using a metallic core-carrier obturation technique

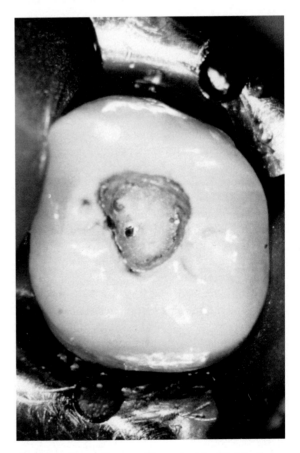

Fig. 7-34 *Protruding metallic carrier identified in the surrounding composite core during access. Care must be taken not to cut the top of the carrier (see Fig. 7-36).*

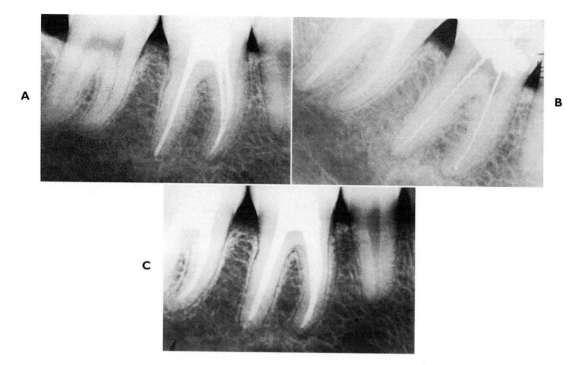

Fig. 7-35

(Fig. 7-35, *A*). When cold was applied to the teeth in question, the main source of the discomfort was the second molar. However, pain to percussion was most intense on the first molar.

Solution: A diagnosis of irreversible pulpitis and normal periradicular tissues was made for the second molar and acute apical periodontitis for the first molar. Root canal treatment was initiated on the second molar, and the occlusion was adjusted on the first molar. Percussion pain continued on the first molar for 1 week after occlusal adjustment. After completion of the root canal treatment on the second molar, using gutta-percha and sealer, the first molar was retreated (Fig. 7-35, *B* and *C*). All symptoms subsided within 2 weeks, and the first molar was obturated with gutta-percha and sealer using lateral compaction.

The retrieval of metallic core carriers has been reported more frequently in the dental literature because this was the first method introduced. Initial concerns with their removal focus on the position of the metallic carrier above the canal orifice. When their position can be identified as being surrounded by gutta-percha, composite, or amalgam, careful probing with an appropriate instrument is

indicated. For gutta-percha, an explorer, spoon, or heated instrument is sufficient. Alternatively an ultrasonic device with a scaler tip can be used. For amalgam or composite, a small bur must be carefully used to remove the surrounding material without cutting off the metallic carrier (Fig. 7-36) in a manner described for the removal of silver cones. Once removed, if sufficient coronal extension exists, the carrier can be secured with a small curved hemostat, Steiglitz silver point forceps (Moyco, Union Broach, York, Penn.), or Peet splinter forceps (Silvermans, New York, N.Y.). These forceps are quite useful because the taper on the beaks is more gradual, allowing freedom for beak separation and engagement of the metallic carrier in deep access openings or when the carrier has been cut off just above the canal orifice. Often a counterclockwise twist may be necessary to dislodge the carrier. When this fails, a heated instrument can be applied to the carrier two or three times for 5 to 10 seconds each time, or a continuously heated instrument, such as the Touch 'N Heat (Analytical Technology, Redmond, Wash.) can be applied for 20 to 30 seconds to heat the carrier (Fig. 7-37). This will soften the gutta-percha that

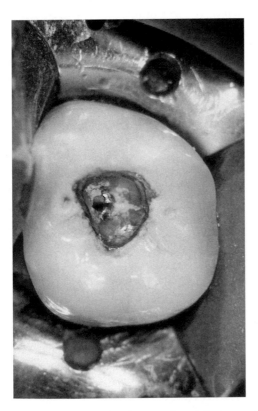

Fig. 7-36 *A small bur has been used initially to trough around the protruding core carrier. Once it is exposed and a purchase is established, removal is straightforward.*

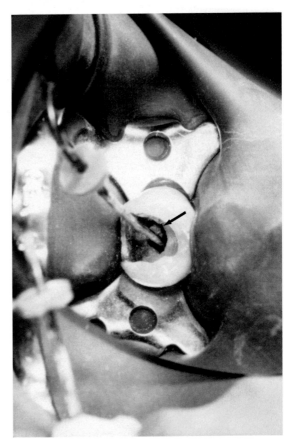

Fig. 7-37 *Use of a heat carrier to transfer heat to the metallic carrier* (arrow), *which softens the gutta-percha surrounding the core.*

surrounds the carrier, which can then be easily removed. An alternative approach would be the Masserann technique previously described.

If the heated method does not work to remove the metallic carrier, sonic or ultrasonic instruments can be used to vibrate and loosen the carrier. Coupled with heat or solvent action (methylchloroform) on the surrounding gutta-percha, easy retrieval is effected.[45,46] However, the presence of significant canal irregularities into which the gutta-percha may have flowed may lock the carrier into the canal, thereby requiring greater penetration of the solvent before the carrier can be dislodged.[45] Likewise, this creates a problem for canal cleaning and shaping after carrier removal because the position of the gutta-percha makes it relatively inaccessible to normal filing action in the canal. Removal is usually slow and multiple radiographs may be required to assess progress, especially if additional tooth structure must be

removed to gain an unimpeded access to the metallic object. Also, even after the carrier is removed, gutta-percha may be seen dispersed in the irregularities along the canal walls. Solvents alone will not remove the material, and the use of files curved or bent to contact the dentin walls in these irregularities may be indicated (Fig. 7-38).

If the metallic carrier is cut off below a pulp horn or marginal ridge because of an improper access opening, it may be difficult to grasp the object without removing excess tooth structure or risking the fracture of a crown. Attempts to bend the coronal portion of the carrier into a more favorable position for grasping are often futile and may also promote fracture of coronal structure (enamel, dentin, or porcelain). Even exposure with Masserann trephines is difficult in this situation, since the carrier may not be centered in the canal.

In cases where significant space can be created around a carrier that is bound in the canal, the

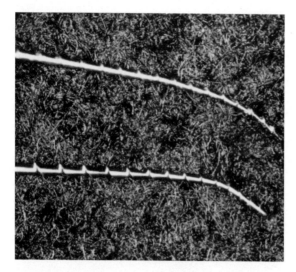

Fig. 7-38 *Apical curves in Hedström files that are necessary to assist in the removal of the carriers and associated gutta-percha.*

Hedström braiding technique, previously mentioned, can be considered. Two or three Hedström files are inserted around the core and twisted to engage the metal carrier. Even if immediate removal does not follow, loosening can occur, which facilitates removal.

Problems inherent in the retrieval of plastic core carriers include the nature of the core material, the nature of the solvent used to soften the material, the preparation shape of the root canal, the degree of extension above the canal orifice, the presence of extensive canal irregularities, and the position of the carrier at the canal terminus.

Core carriers are manufactured using two different types of plastic material. This is primarily due to the physical properties of the material required in the small sizes versus the larger sizes. In sizes through No. 40, Vectra is used, whereas for those greater than No. 40, Polysulfone is the material of choice. These materials, however, respond differently to the available solvents used to soften root canal–filling materials.[33] Ibarrola et al[21] indicated that the retrievability of the plastic core was attributed to the "adhesiveness" of the dissolve α-phase gutta-percha and the engagement of the file flutes into the softened plastic. With chloroform the plastic core carriers became softened, enabling a Hedström file to become easily engaged in its surface. Other solvents such as xylene, eucalyptol, and halothane did not soften the carrier as readily as chloroform did.

As with metallic core carriers, the shape of the prepared canal will have a significant influence on the ability to remove the plastic carrier. If insufficient taper is present in the canal shape, the carrier will be wedged between the dentin walls. This creates multiple problems in removal, such as the frictional binding and lack of space between the canal wall and carrier for penetration of solvent or a small instrument. Ibarrola et al[21] showed that the use of chloroform greatly facilitated the removal of plastic carriers in 19 out of 20 cases. However, it should be noted that this was in extracted mandibular molars where it was possible to place the solvent in a reservoir such that it was able to seep along the canal walls with the benefit of gravity. Clinically, this may not be the case when attempting to remove carriers from maxillary teeth. Likewise, the core carriers used in this study were size No. 45, which are susceptible to the action chloroform. This larger size, however, is not commonly used in smaller, more curved canals. Imura et al[22] indicated that the application of heat to the gutta-percha surrounding the coronal aspect of the plastic core carrier assisted in its removal. This was followed by xylol (xylene) to aid in the removal of the gutta-percha in the canal after the carrier was mechanically removed. Caution, however, must be exercised to prevent the cutting off or weakening of the coronal portion of the core carrier when a heated instrument is used.

If the plastic core carrier has been severed above the canal orifice, the use of grasping instruments vis à vis the metallic carriers is indicated. However, if the carrier is below the orifice, such as that found when a post space has been created, removal is limited to the use of solvents and small files. Here again, if the canal shape is narrow or constricted, penetration into the apical third of the canal may be impossible.

If extensive canal irregularities are present, such as fins, webs, and culs-de-sac, the softened gutta-percha may lock the carrier into its position. Removal with a grasping instrument may be difficult, even after softening with a solvent. Likewise if a file is being used along the length of the carrier with solvent to remove the gutta-percha, the carrier may be severed, thinned, or pushed into the canal irregularities, especially with the smaller, more flexible carriers (Fig. 7-39). If this occurs, it may give the impression that the canal is being cleaned, when in actuality the carrier is being slowly cut by the filing action. Radiographic checks during removal attempts will provide evidence that the carrier is still present, yet the canal may feel "smooth and clean" to the clinician. As with the removal of gutta-percha in the canal irregularities after metallic-carrier removal, a curved or bent Hedström file can be used to engage the adherent section of the plastic carrier for removal. Likewise this approach also favors canal cleaning and shaping.

If the core carrier is beyond the end of the root, care must be taken to avoid severance of the carrier in the apical third during removal attempts.[21] Likewise, aggressive, canal-penetrating movements may push the carrier further out of the root. This can easily occur if the plastic carrier, which is flexible, is not lying in the center of the canal or is repeatedly pushed to the side when the file penetrates the canal. If this occurs, surgical intervention may be the only choice for canal retreatment.

Techniques for Identification, Isolation, and Removal of Fractured Endodontic Instruments

If the end of a broken endodontic instrument is at the orifice of the canal, a small trephining drill may be used to create space for the extractor or choice of forceps. Since the instrument is stainless steel, there is no danger of cutting or weakening it with the trephining drill. Typically the drill will follow the instrument very easily when the techniques described in the previous section are used. Once the shaft of the instrument is exposed at least 2 mm, the extractor is used in the same manner as described in this chapter for the removal of silver cones. The 1.2 mm extractor will be adequate for instruments up to size 40. Because of the spiral

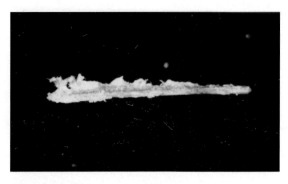

Fig. 7-39 *Thinned, plastic core carrier that was repeatedly scraped with a file during attempts at removal. Notice the grooving in the carrier. Tactile sensation could not necessarily discern that this was occurring.*

shape of endodontic instruments, a gentle counterclockwise rotational pressure is exerted during instrument withdrawal. This same technique can be used for the removal of a small metallic gutta-percha core carrier. The ultrasonic device may again be helpful if unusual resistance is encountered.

For instruments fractured at deeper levels— Gates-Glidden bur heads, Peeso reamer heads, and other metallic objects—the best approach is ultrasonic instrumentation.[24,31] The first step is to prepare the canal space coronally to the fractured segment with a series of Gates-Glidden burs or Peeso reamers in a step-back manner. The purpose of this approach is to remove any dentinal barrier to the coronal passage of the fragment after it is loosened. Next, it is absolutely essential that the fractured segment be bypassed using hand instrumentation (Fig. 7-40). This space must be carefully enlarged so

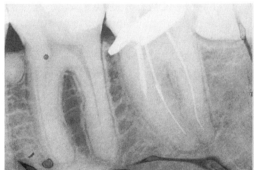
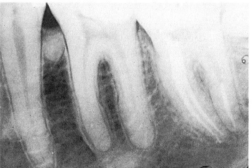

Fig. 7-40 *A, Mandibular second molar presenting with a fractured Gates-Glidden bur head in the mesiobuccal canal and a fractured Peeso reamer head in the mesiolingual canal. For removal with an ultrasonic device, it is first necessary to bypass the obstruction with small files and enlarge the space adjacent to the segment to a size 15. B, Completed case.*

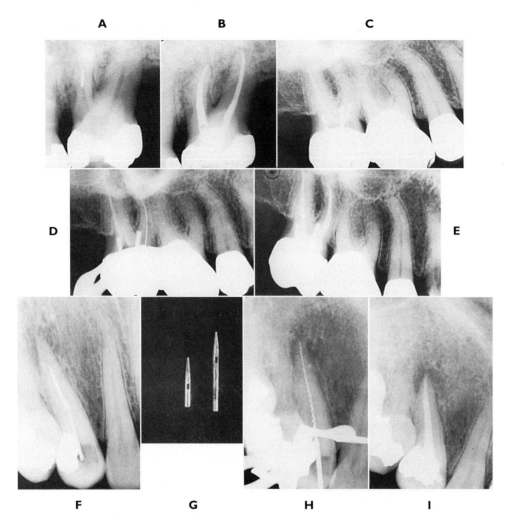

Fig. 7-41 *A, Case 1: A fractured file tip in the mesiobuccal canal on the maxillary first molar. The file tip was bypassed and removed with an ultrasonic unit at a normal endodontic instrumentation setting. B, Completed case with obturation to the apical foramen in the previously obstructed canal. C, Case 2: An endodontic explorer tip fractured in the mesiobuccal orifice of the maxillary second molar. The patient presented with symptoms of acute cold sensitivity. The endodontic treatment had been performed approximately 8 years before the onset of present symptoms. D, Immediately after ultrasonic vibration and tip removal using standard endodontic instrumentation and setting. E, Completed retreatment. F, Case 3: Maxillary canine with a history of self-treatment by the patient with sewing needles to establish drainage. The initial film showing two needle tips lodged in the canal. G, Sewing needle tips removed with an ultrasonic unit using standard instrumentation and setting. H, Measurement film after removal of the needle tips. I, Completed case.*

that a size 15 file will pass by the obstruction. At this point, a new No. 15 file in the standard ultrasonic endodontic tip is placed in the canal and energized at *normal settings for endodontic instrumentation*. File separation is a significant problem with ultrasonics, especially in the smaller sizes, and so it is vitally important to stay within the recommended settings. Usually the fragment will loosen and flow out of the access cavity undetected, along with the irrigant. This frequently occurs in the first minute of ultrasonic usage (Fig. 7-41).

When removing fractured instruments in multirooted teeth there is the potential problem of the fractured segment floating out of one canal and finding its way into one of the other orifices. To prevent this it is wise to place cotton into the other orifices or to complete the obturation on the other canals as long as there is no communication with the canal containing the obstruction (Fig. 7-42).

The removal of very deep instrument fragments is possible with the ultrasonic technique (Fig. 7-43) as long as the fragment can be bypassed.[11,31] If the instrument fractured after the tip became tightly bound in the canal (as a result of excessive rotational pressure; see Chapter 5) it will rarely be bypassed. Previous authors have diagrammatically described the retrieval of these obstructions with the Masserann technique[6,24] (Fig. 7-44). However, in clinical practice, trephining into the apical third of the root can be extremely hazardous and is not recommended even in large, straight roots with

generous use of large Gates-Glidden burs (Fig. 7-45, *A*). In most attempts the trephining drill will approach a lateral perforation as the root tapers anatomically toward the apex (Fig. 7-45, *B*). However, cleaning and shaping of the coronal portion of the canal and subsequent obturation up to the fractured object are indicated. If the fractured segment is in good contact with the surrounding dentin walls, the prognosis is more favorable, and recall observation is indicated. If the contact is obviously poor or the instrument protrudes beyond the canal system, surgical correction is indicated.

The use of small, round burs with extra-long and very thin shanks (pulp chamber bur "Müller," Hager & Meisinger, Düsseldorf, Germany), or the "Special Bur" (Maillefer, Balaigues, Switzerland) has been recommended[8] to drill around metallic objects

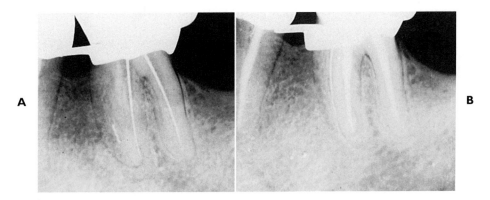

Fig. 7-42 *A, Separated metallic instrument segment in the mesiolingual canal of the mandibular first molar. B, To avoid having the fragment enter one of the other canal orifices after removal with the ultrasonic unit, it is wise to fill the other canals before the removal procedure.*

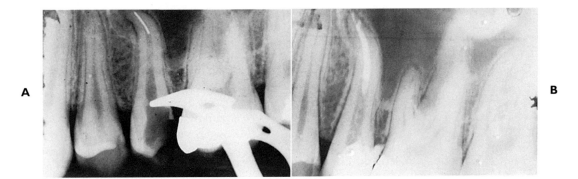

Fig. 7-43 *A, Segment of an endodontic file fractured in the apex of a maxillary premolar. Unlike the case in Fig. 7-9, this fragment was removed with the ultrasonic technique. B, Completed case.*

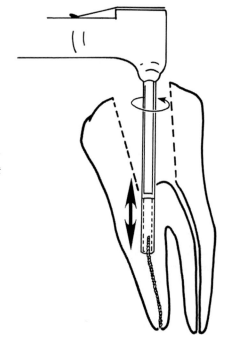

Fig. 7-44 *Method of removing a fractured instrument deep in the canal. Most attempts fail, with subsequent severe weakening of root structure or perforations.*

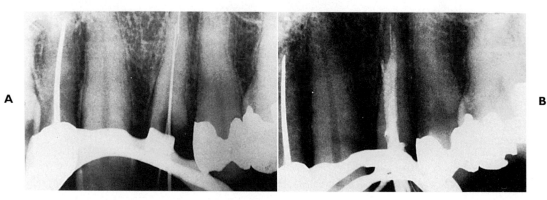

A   B

Fig. 7-45 *A, Maxillary premolar in which an attempt was made to remove a deeply fractured instrument. Notice lack of root curvature. Tooth appears to be ideal for the technique illustrated in Fig. 7-38. B, Gutta-percha obturation demonstrates a near perforation.*

when space lateral to the object exists. The small instrument shaft and head allows for good visualization of the bur as it moves apically around the object (Fig. 7-46). This approach may be useful in roots with wide buccolingual canals containing circular metallic objects. Once space is created, one of the techniques discussed can be used to grasp the object.

Techniques for Identification, Isolation, and Removal of Intraradicular Posts

With the availability of ultrasonic devices, removal of intraradicular posts has become much simpler.[4,12,14,25,37] In addition, there is minimal risk of

physical damage to the root, since no excessive forces are applied.

In recent years the use of preformed stainless steel posts has dramatically increased. The fracture of these posts from apparent metal fatigue is relatively common, typically occurring with posts of small diameter (such as the Whaledent No. 4 or 5, Parapost, produced by Whaledent International, New York, N.Y.). When fractured, the posts appear to have been used to retain buildups where very little clinical crown was remaining. As a consequence, the crown restoration is retained almost entirely by the post. The resulting post failure

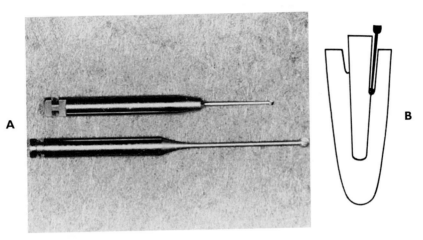

Fig. 7-46 *A, Special long shank, delicate burs for troughing around metallic objects. Top, Special Bur;* bottom, *Müller bur.* **B,** *troughing with special bur that creates space adjacent to the metallic object.*

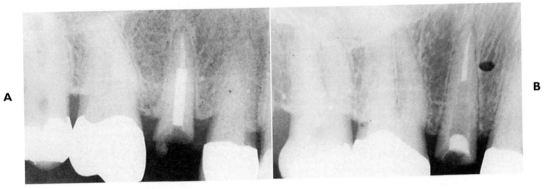

Fig. 7-47 *A, Typical example of preformed stainless steel post fracture where the crown covers minimal tooth structure at its margins.* **B,** *Post fragment removed through the combined efforts of the ultrasonic and Masserann techniques.*

occurs at or just below the occlusal surface of the remaining root surface (Fig. 7-47; see Chapter 13, Fig. 13-16). From a preventive standpoint, for any tooth with less than 2 mm of sound clinical crown circumferentially above the gingival margin, crown-lengthening procedures are indicated to increase the surface area of natural tooth structure for buildup, preparation, and retention (see Chapter 8).

The most efficient method of post removal requires the combined use of the Masserann technique[47] and an ultrasonic device. The coronal end of the post is first exposed and its margins troughed with a one-half round bur. Second, a Masserann trephining bur is selected that has a diameter slightly larger than the post. With copious irriga-

tion, frequent pauses to clean the bur, and slow penetration, a space is created around the post fragment to a depth of approximately one half the post length. During use it is important to inspect the bur for flaring and to resharpen it. Since the post is metal, there is no danger of cutting into it or of straying from it into the root. The drilling normally will take between 5 and 10 minutes.

Once the space has been created around the post, the ultrasonic device is used on the maximum setting with a vibrating tip against the exposed end of the post. Ultrasonic vibration of the post may take from 30 seconds to 10 minutes before mobility is detected. The post fragment can then be teased out of the canal (Fig. 7-48). If there is no

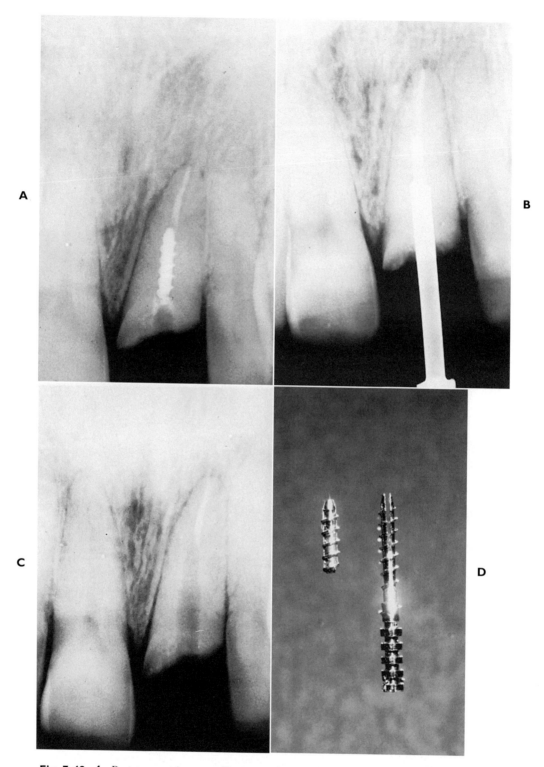

Fig. 7-48 *A,* *Post segment in a maxillary central incisor fractured 2 mm below the occlusal surface. The brand or type was unknown at the time of examination. **B,** After troughing with the one-half round bur, the Masserann extractor is used to approximately one half the length of the post fragment. **C,** The post fragment is vibrated with an ultrasonic tip and teased out of the canal. In this case, the post proved extremely difficult to tease out, although it was very loose in the canal. The reason was that it was two halves of a Flexipost (Essential Dental Systems, New York, N.Y.), which limited counter-rotation. **D,** The post fragment compared with a new Flexipost of the same size. Notice that the level of fracture is at the terminus of the slot.*

mobility after 10 minutes of continuous vibration, the Masserann bur should be used to deepen the space around the post another few millimeters, after which the ultrasonic probe is applied again in the same manner. It is highly improbable that a post fractured at the occlusal surface of the root will be loosened by ultrasonic vibration alone. It is always recommended that a space be created with the trephining bur first.

Occasionally the most difficult part of post removal is getting the loose post fragment out of the canal because of the very limited space around it and the lack of post material above the occlusal surface on which to grasp with an instrument. Aids that have worked successfully have been the ultrasonic device with an endodontic file placed in the space alongside the post, a tightly fitting Masserann extractor, and any tube that will fit over the post and that is attached with cyanoacrylate (such as Super Glue) (Post Extractor, produced by Brasseler, Savannah, Ga.) (see Fig. 7-31).

Another option that can be used with fractured threaded posts is a combination of ultrasonic vibration and the grooving of the top of the post to serve as screw. The groove can be made with a No. ½ to 1 round bur or 33½ inverted cone. A small jewelers' screwdriver is placed in the groove after the application of ultrasonic vibration. Pressure is applied in a counterclockwise fashion. The pressure can also be applied at the same time the ultrasonic is being applied. This approach is very useful when the fractured post has no place for a lateral purchase (Fig. 7-49).

The method of post removal described works reliably regardless of the type of cementing medium. Although composite resins cannot be cut with Masserann trephine burs, it is often possible to excavate enough material away from the post with a one-half round bur to enable the use of the ultrasonic unit. Fortunately, composite resin seems to be one of the easier materials to loosen because of its lack of affinity for a bond to the tooth (Fig. 7-50).

If the technique for the removal of fractured posts appears manageable, it is not hard to imagine how the same techniques can be used with full-length posts. Since ultrasonic vibration is effective only when a significant length of post is not bound in the root or restorative material, it is not necessary to use the trephining burs if there is such post length remaining after the existing core material has been cut away. It is possible to remove posts by this means from the inside of existing crowns (Figs. 7-51 and 7-52).

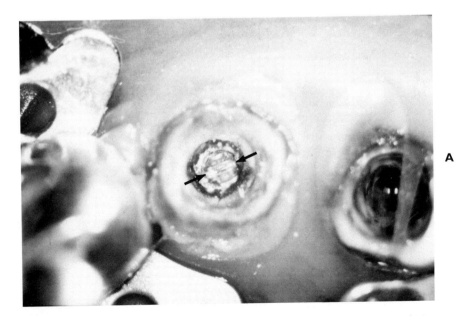

A

Fig. 7-49 *A, Fractured screw post in a maxillary central incisor viewed from the incisal. A groove has been cut with a small round bur in the top of the post to resemble the top of a screw* (arrows). *Continued.*

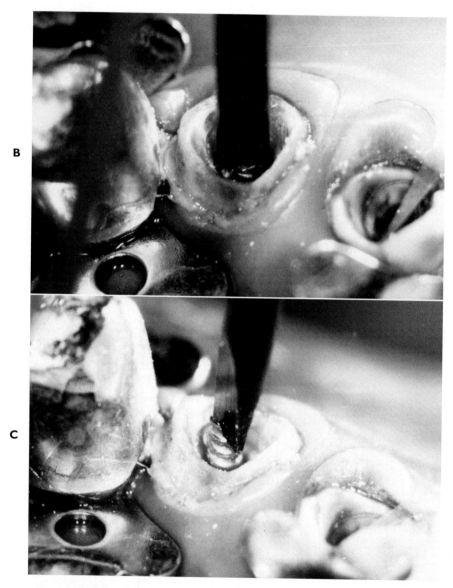

Fig. 7-49 cont'd. B, *Small screwdriver is inserted in the groove and an ultrasonic tip is applied to the screw driver while applying counterclockwise pressure on the screw driver.* **C,** *In time the seal of the cement around the post is broken and the post is unthreaded from the tooth. (Courtesy Dr. James Leonard.)*

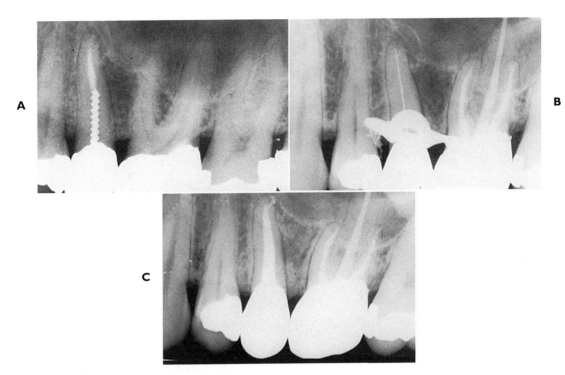

Fig. 7-50 *A,* *Previously treated maxillary premolar with a large lateral radiolucency. Patient had symptoms of irreversible pulpitis.* *B,* *After the treatment of the maxillary molar for pulpitis, retreatment was initiated on the premolar. The post in the premolar was cemented with composite resin but was not found to be difficult to vibrate loose once the portion extending into the core was reduced circumferentially with a series of one-half round burs and fine-diameter finishing burs.* *C,* *Seven-month recall showing complete regeneration of bone at the site of the lesion.*

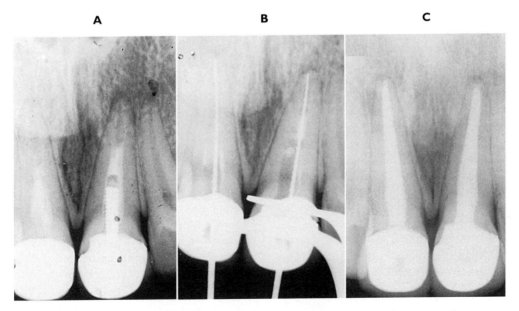

Fig. 7-51 *A,* *Case 1: Two maxillary central incisors with failing root canal treatment. Paste fills were present.* *B,* *Retrieval of the post in the tooth on the right permitted routine retreatment.* *C,* *Completed retreatment.* *Continued.*

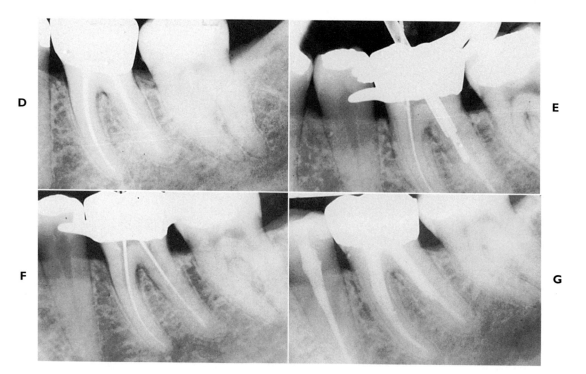

Fig. 7-51 cont'd. D, Case 2: *A mandibular molar with long-standing root canal treatment. Patient complained of acute percussion sensitivity. Symptoms did not resolve after retrieval of the silver cones in the mesial root.* **E,** *Retreatment of the distal root necessitated the removal of the post.* **F,** *Renegotiation of the distal root revealed untreated canal space. Symptoms resolved after proper canal cleaning.* **G,** *A 7-year recall film. The tooth remained symptomless. There is minimal canal enlargement from the post-removal procedure.*

Post pullers have also been available for the removal of posts since the early 1900s.[32,34] Recent versions have been modified for easier use in the oral cavity and are all used in a similar fashion (Fig. 7-53).[27,42] First, the post or post and core must be exposed and the diameter of the core or coronal aspect of the post reduced circumferentially to allow the attachment of the puller (Fig. 7-54, A). It is essential that the reduced post or core have parallel walls (Fig. 7-54, B). The occlusal root face must also be flattened, preferably with either proximal or faciolingual surfaces being parallel to each other and perpendicular to the reduced post. The post puller is slipped around the post so that the legs are in firm contact with the root face. The post must be removed in line with the long axis of the tooth to prevent torquing of the root and damage to the periodontal ligament. This is achieved by seating the legs of the post in solid contact with the prepared root face. If the proximal surfaces of the root face are not in the same parallel plane (Fig. 7-

54, C), a metal insert such as a tapered chisel can be placed between the leg and root face until the post puller is in line with the long axis of the tooth (Fig. 7-54, D). The wing nut is tightened to secure the jaws around the post. The knurled knob at the end of the puller is turned, and an apical force is directed against the root face while an opposite force draws the jaws and the post coronally, unseating the post (Fig. 7-54, E).

The use of post pullers is limited in the posterior regions of the mouth because of access difficulties and in some anterior regions when the tooth width is very small. However, post pullers have the advantage of preserving tooth structure and protecting the tooth against fracture because of the balanced force during removal. In addition, many anterior and premolar teeth can be nonsurgically retreated and retained with a minimum amount of treatment.

Often a knowledge of internal tooth anatomy will provide avenues of success (see Chapters

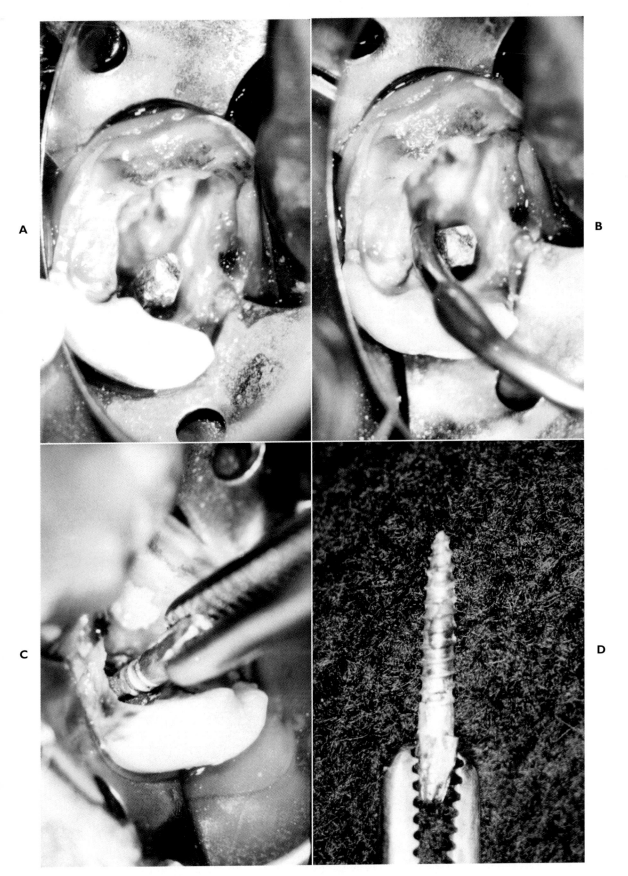

Fig. 7-52 *A, After removal of an onlay and isolation of a screw post in the palatal canal of a maxillary molar. B, Application of the ultrasonic scaler tip. C, Use of a small hemostat to purchase and unscrew the post from the canal. D, Post removed. (Courtesy Dr. James Leonard.)*

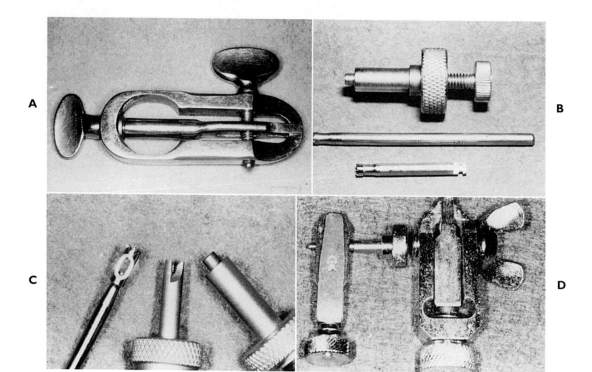

Fig. 7-53 A, *Little Giant post puller, circa 1920.* **B,** *Post-pulling device manufactured before World War II by the SS White Co.* **C,** *Present version of the SS White device.* **D,** *Various contemporary post pullers.*

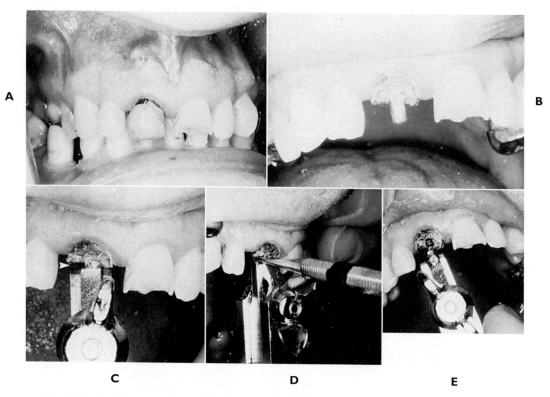

Fig. 7-54 A, *Crown requires replacement. Sinus tract is present; canal is poorly obturated.* **B,** *Crown is removed and post is reduced to have parallel walls.* **C,** *Attachment of post puller. Legs of puller are not seated on both proximal walls because of the difference in tooth structure height.* **D,** *Rather than remove tooth structure, a tapered chisel is inserted between the leg of the puller and the proximal tooth wall.* **E,** *The post is easily removed, allowing endodontic and restorative retreatment.*

1 and 7) without the necessity of post removal. Canals such as the distal canal of mandibular molars or those of the maxillary second premolar typically have a morphology that a single pre-formed stainless steel post will not completely obliterate (Fig. 7-55). This fact leads to two clinically useful approaches to retreatment. First, if the root has a second canal that has not been previously treated, the post is not likely to be in that canal and it may be possible to successfully retreat

the tooth by negotiating past the post and into the untreated canal. This assumes that the treated canal is not the source of the problem. Careful diagnostic procedures may confirm this; however, in some cases it will be apparent only when the untreated canal is cleaned and the symptoms resolve. This approach is nevertheless often easier than removing the post.

The second approach concerns the root that has only one canal. If the post is round and preformed and the canal is ovoid, it is possible to negotiate past the post and retreat the canal. In some cases this is possible without uncovering the post (Fig. 7-56).

On a final note, many endodontic specialists have chosen to use magnification in the form of operating loops or microscopes to enhance endodontic retreatment. The major assets provided by these devices are to expand the field of vision and allow the practitioner to more easily identify unwanted objects in the root canal space in most cases. These devices will not compensate for lack of knowledge or skill in the actual retreatment of cases because many practitioners who have been successfully retreating old root canal fillings or mishaps for many years without these devices will continue to do so with similar levels of success.

SUMMARY

When choosing nonsurgical endodontic retreatment, careful assessment and treatment planning with each case is the cornerstone to success.

With a keen awareness of and skill in the techniques advocated for retreatment, with an appreciation for the support provided by adjunctive tech-

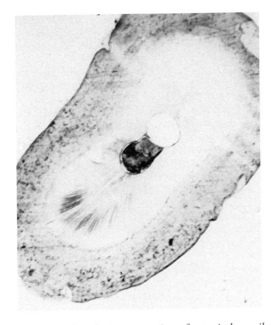

Fig. 7-55 *A histologic cross-section of a typical maxillary premolar showing an ovoid canal only partially cleaned and shaped. If this canal were obturated and a post were placed, contaminated, unfilled canal space would remain as a potential source of failure.*

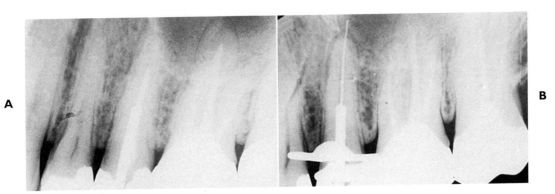

Fig. 7-56 *A, Maxillary premolar with post and canal voids in a symptomatic patient. B, Without removing the post, it was possible to bypass the post and retreat the canal.*

nologies, and with an understanding of the potential hazards encountered in retreatment, the astute practitioner will enjoy a significant level of success in this approach to the prevention, identification, and management of these endodontic challenges.

References

1. Abou-Rass M: Evaluation and clinical management of previous endodontic therapy, *J Prosthet Dent* 47:528-534, 1982.

2. Allen RK, Newton CW, Brown CE: Statistical analysis of surgical and nonsurgical endodontic retreatment cases, *J Endod* 15:261-266, 1989.

3. Brady JM, del Rio CE: Corrosion of endodontic silver cones: A scanning electron microscope and X-ray microprobe study, *J Endod* 1:205-210, 1975.

4. Chalfin H, Weseley P, Solomon C: Removal of restorative posts for the purpose of nonsurgical endodontic retreatment: report of cases, *J Am Dent Assoc* 120:169-172, 1990.

5. Dumsha TC, Gutmann JL: Clinical guidelines for intentional replantation, *Compend Cont Dent Educ* 6:604-609, 1985.

6. Feldman G, Solomon C, Notaro P, et al: Retrieving broken endodontic instruments, *J Am Dent Assoc* 88:588-591, 1974.

7. Fors UGH, Berg J-O: A method for the removal of broken endodontic instruments from root canals, *J Endod* 9:156-159, 1983.

8. Fors UGH, Berg J-O: Endodontic treatment of root canals obstructed by foreign objects, *Int Endod J* 19:2-10, 1986.

9. Frank AL: Therapy for the divergent pulpless tooth by continued apical formation, *J Am Dent Assoc* 72:87-93, 1966.

10. Friedman S, Stabholz A: Endodontic retreatment—case selection and technique. Part 1: Criteria for case selection, *J Endod* 12:28-33, 1986.

11. Friedman S, Stabholz A, Tamse A: Endodontic retreatment—case selection and technique. Part 3: Retreatment techniques, *J Endod* 16:543-549, 1990.

12. Gaffney JL, Lehman JW, Miles MJ: Expanded use of the ultrasonic scaler, *J Endod* 7:228-229, 1981.

13. Gerstein H, Weine FS: Specially prepared burs to remove silver cones and fractured dowels, *J Endod* 3:408-410, 1977.

14. Glick DH, Frank AL: Removal of silver points and fractured posts by ultrasonics, *J Prosthet Dent* 55:212-215, 1986.

15. Grossman LI: Intentional replantation of teeth: A clinical evaluation, *J Am Dent Assoc* 104:633-639, 1982.

16. Grudin L: Softened gutta-percha technique. In Gerstein H, editor: *Techniques in clinical endodontics,* Philadelphia, 1983, Saunders, pp 121-132.

17. Gutmann JL, Battrum DE: Challenges in retreatment of Thermafil obturated root canals, *Lebanese Dent J* 33(2):57-66, 1994.

18. Gutmann JL, Dumsha TC: Cleaning and shaping of the root canal system. In Cohen S, Burns R, editors: *Pathways of the pulp,* ed 4, St Louis, 1987, Mosby, pp 156-182.

19. Hession RW: Long-term evaluation of endodontic treatment: anatomy, instrumentation, obturation—the endodontic practice triad, *Int Endod J* 14:179-184, 1981.

20. Hunter KR, Doblecki W, Pelleu GB: Halothane and eucalyptol as alternatives to chloroform for softening gutta-percha, *J Endod* 17:310-312, 1991.

21. Ibarrola JL, Knowles KI, Ludlow MO: Retrievability of Thermafil plastic cores using organic solvents, *J Endod* 19:417-418, 1993.

22. Imura I, Zuolo ML, Kherlakian D: Comparison of endodontic retreatment of laterally condensed gutta-percha and Thermafil with plastic carriers, *J Endod* 19:609-612, 1993.

23. Kaplowitz, GJ: Evaluation of the ability of essential oil to dissolve gutta-percha, *J Endod* 17:448-449, 1991.

24. Krell KV, Fuller MW, Scott GL: The conservative retrieval of silver cones in difficult cases, *J Endod* 10:269-273, 1984.

25. Krell KV, Jordan RD, Madison S et al: Using ultrasonic scalers to remove fractured root posts, *J Prosthet Dent* 55:46-49, 1986.

26. Ladley RW, Campbell AD, Hicks ML, Li S-H: Effectiveness of halothane used with ultrasonic or hand instrumentation to remove gutta-percha from the root canal, *J Endod* 17:221-224, 1991.

27. Machtou P, Sarfati P, Cohen AG: Post removal prior to retreatment, *J Endod* 15:552-554, 1989.

28. Masserann J: L'extraction des instruments cassés dans les canaux radiculaires: technique nouvelle, *Actual Odontostomatol* 47:265-274, 1959.

29. Masserann J: Entfernen metallischer Fragmente aus Würzelkanalen, *J Br Endod Soc* 5:55-59, 1971.

30. Masserann J: L'extraction des fragments de tenons intra-radiculaires, *Actual Odontostomatol* 75:329-342, 1976.

31. Nagai O, Tani N, Kayaba Y et al: Ultrasonic removal of broken instruments in root canals, *Int Endod J* 19:298-304, 1986.

32. Neaverth EJ, Kahn H: Re-treatment of dowel-obturated root canals, *J Am Dent Assoc* 76:325-328, 1968.

33. Parker H, Glickman GN: Solubility of plastic Thermafil carriers, *J Dent Res* 72:188, 1993.

34. Prothero JH: *Prosthetic Dentistry,* Chicago, 1923, Medico-Dental Publishing Co, p 844.

35. Seltzer S, Green DB, Weiner N et al: A scanning electron microscopic examination of silver cones removed from endodontically treated teeth, *Oral Surg Oral Med Oral Pathol* 33:589-605, 1972.

36. Stabholz A, Friedman S: Endodontic retreatment—case selection and technique. Part 2: Treatment planning for retreatment, *J Endod* 14:607-614, 1988.

37. Stamos DG, Haasch GC, Chenail B et al: Endosonics: clinical impressions, *J Endod* 11:181-187, 1985.

38. Stamos DE, Stamos DG, Perkins SK: Retreatodontics and ultrasonics, *J Endod* 14:39-42, 1988.

39. Taintor JF, Ingle JI, Fahid A: Retreatment versus further treatment, *Clin Prev Dent* 5(5):8-14, 1983.

40. Taylor J, Baumgardner K, Walton R: Coronal leakage: comparison of lateral condensation vs Thermafil obturation, *J Dent Res* 71:123, 1992.

41. Trope M: Flare-up rate of single-visit endodontics, *Int Endod J* 24:24-27, 1991.

42. Warren SR, Gutmann JL: Simplified method for removing intraradicular posts, *J Prosthet Dent* 42:353-356, 1979.
43. Weisman MI: The removal of difficult silver cones, *J Endod* 9:210-211, 1983.
44. Wennberg A, Orstavik D: Evaluation of alternatives to chloroform in endodontic practice, *Endod Dent Traumatol* 5:234-237, 1989.
45. Wilcox LR: Thermafil retreatment with and without chloroform solvent, *J Endod* 19:563-566, 1993.
46. Wilcox, L R, Juhlin, JJ Endodontic retreatment of Thermafil vs. laterally condensed gutta-percha, *J Endod* 20:115-7, 1994.
47. Williams VD, Bjorndal AM: The Masserann technique for the removal of fractured posts in endodontically treated teeth, *J Prosthet Dent* 49:46-48, 1983.

▼

Chapter 8

Problems in Tooth Isolation and Periodontal Support for the Endodontically Compromised Tooth

Paul E. Lovdahl

Curtis K. Wade

"Probably the first requisite for a successful operation is that the operator should be thoroughly familiar with the anatomy of the region."*

Endodontic problem solving often addresses the questions of tooth isolation, periodontal integrity, and restorability. A common example is a carious tooth margin below the free gingival margin. When such a lesion is excavated, the traditional approach favors a restorative orientation; that is, buildup with temporary or permanent materials. More recently, interest has turned to the application of periodontal and orthodontic techniques to resolve these problems.[1,3,4,11,20] This chapter is a discussion of the diagnosis, treatment planning, and appropriate periodontal, orthodontic, and surgical procedures in the integrated treatment of endodontically compromised teeth with deep carious or fractured tooth margins. The advantages of these approaches over a purely restorative approach are emphasized.

Endodontic treatment is enhanced by reliable isolation and minimal operational and visual restraints.

Restoration is also improved by maintaining supragingival margins and avoiding a structurally weakened buildup with an access opening. Within

these principles, three classes of cases are described in which the level of tooth structure is below the free gingival margin: first, cases in which only local periodontal surgical techniques are indicated; second, cases in which a combination of orthodontic and periodontal techniques are required; and third, cases in which some form of root removal is appropriate, in combination with periodontal procedures.

CASES REQUIRING LOCALIZED PERIODONTAL SURGERY

These cases are distinguished by caries or fracture below the free gingival margin but above crestal bone. Several variations are commonly encountered clinically, such as interproximal caries, caries below an existing crown, cusp fractures, and so forth. Various techniques of gingivectomy using a scalpel or electrosurgical units have been recommended.[14] Frequently these techniques are contraindicated because of an inadequate zone of attached gingiva, the presence of osseous defects, or an anatomic form that precludes an optimal periodontal result. In these cases an apically repositioned flap in combination with a reverse bevel incision is the technique of choice. The advantages include preservation of maximum attached gingiva, correction of minor osseous defects, and creation of optimal tissue contours postoperatively. Potential disadvantages are more complicated

---

* From Blayney JR: *Dent Cosmos* 74:635-653, 1932.

instrumentation and increased procedure time, though the time spent in this phase of treatment is easily made up during the endodontic and restorative phases.

Diagnosis and Treatment Planning

1. Ensure that there is no contraindication to minor oral surgery under local anesthesia.
2. The dentin margin should be below the free gingival margin.
3. The periodontal status should ideally be within normal limits (Fig. 8-1), though sulcus depths of 4 to 5 mm around the involved

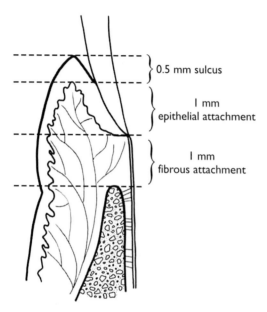

Fig. 8-1 *Normal periodontium in the region of the dentinoenamel junction.*

tooth can be treated. It is important to assess the overall periodontal condition of the patient and to distinguish the indication for a localized procedure as described herein from the indication for complete periodontal therapy.

Equipment Needed

1. Scalpel: Bard Parker No. 15 or 15C
2. Periosteal elevator
3. Retractor
4. Periodontal curettes
5. Surgical-length high-speed bur No. 2, 4, 6, and 8
6. Needle holder and suture: 3-0 gut
7. Periodontal pack or cold-cure temporary crown and bridge acrylic
8. Wiedelstadt chisel

Surgical Procedures

The objective of the surgical procedure is to place a sound dentin margin approximately 1+ mm above the free gingival margin. Since the optimal sulcus depth of the normal periodontium is 1 to 2 mm, the dentin margin will necessarily have to be 3 mm above the crestal bone (Fig. 8-2). With consideration for the anatomic and histologic differences between the buccal or labial aspect of a tooth and the palatal or lingual aspect, one surgical technique with two minor variations will be considered. For purposes of discussion, the labial or buccal approach will be described first in a step-by-step manner.

1. With adequate local anesthesia, a reverse bevel incision (Fig. 8-3, *A* and *B*) is made at the crest of the free gingiva to the gingival

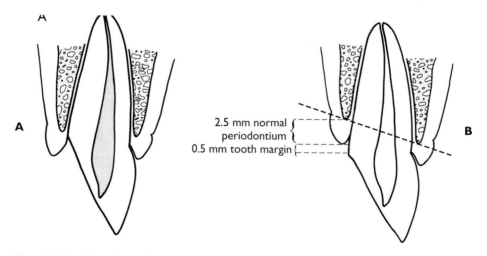

Fig. 8-2 *A, Normal periodontium immediately after a subgingival cuspal fracture. B, Healing after crown-lengthening procedure. There is a 1.5 to 1 mm dentin margin above the gingival crest.*

attachment beginning in the midlabial aspect of the tooth immediately anterior to the tooth requiring crown lengthening, continuing through the mesial and distal papillae, and ending midlabial to the tooth immediately posterior. Scalloping is important in the horizontal incision. If the zone of attached gingiva is more than 4 mm wide, a more apical level of incision can be used over the fractured tooth structure to enhance the result. A zone of at least 4 mm of attached gingiva should be preserved. If, when the envelope flap is reflected, insufficient relaxation is obtained, a vertical relaxing incision may be considered. This should be located anterior to the tooth being treated and should include the papilla (Fig. 8-3, C).

2. Curette the resected tissue lining the sulcus and all interproximal tissue.
3. Using the scalpel, make a second incision to the bone parallel to the surface of the gingival tissue through the papillae and any thick areas

of tissue to produce a uniform flap thickness of approximately 2 mm (Fig. 8-4, A)
4. Use the curette to remove the second wedge of tissue under the flap (Fig. 8-4, B).
5. Elevate as an envelope flap and retract it. In most cases where 2 to 3 mm of crown lengthening is required, it will not be necessary to make a vertical incision.
6. Assess the distance between crestal bone and the tooth margin. Three millimeters of exposed tooth is required; therefore if the bone is thin, the Wiedelstadt chisel may be used to pry the bone away from the tooth. If the bone is thick, use the No. 6 or 8 round bur to thin the overlying bone so that the chisel may be used. The bony contours should favor ramping into interproximal areas and

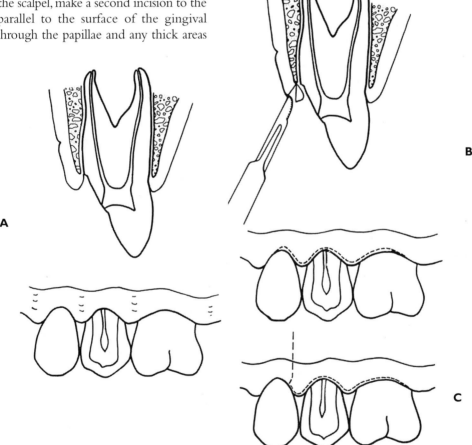

Fig. 8-3 *A, Maxillary premolar with a subgingival fracture of the buccal cusp. B, Incision for full mucoperiosteal envelope flap (broken line). Incision extends from the gingival crest to the crestal bone. C, If insufficient relaxation is anticipated with the envelope flap, a vertical relaxing incision is made to include the gingival papilla on the mesial aspect.*

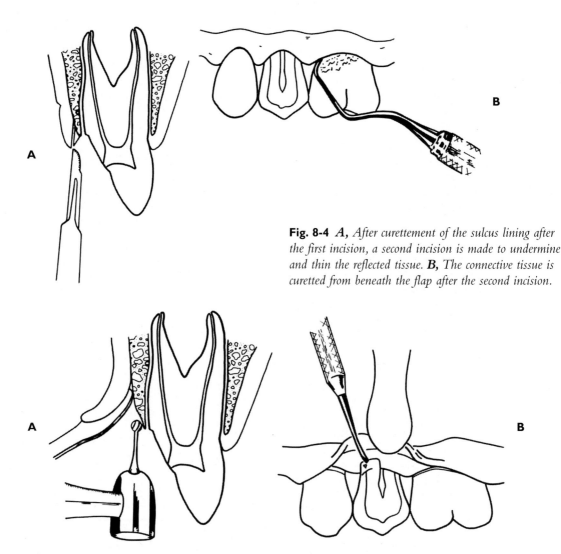

Fig. 8-4 *A, After curettement of the sulcus lining after the first incision, a second incision is made to undermine and thin the reflected tissue. B, The connective tissue is curetted from beneath the flap after the second incision.*

Fig. 8-5 *A, Osseous recontouring performed using a No. 8 round bur on a high-speed hand-piece with copious irrigation. If the bony crest is to be apically repositioned, thin this area as much as possible, avoiding contact with the root. B, Wiedelstadt chisel is used to remove and recontour the thinned bone to apically reposition the bony crest.*

should not leave sharp ridges or grooves (Fig. 8-5). The smaller No. 2 and 4 round burs may be necessary to reshape bone in narrow inter-proximal areas. Burs are used only to remove the surface layers of bone, avoiding contact with tooth structure. Subsequently the Wiedelstadt chisel is used to remove bone up to the dentinal surface at right angles.

7. Use the curette again to remove the small, jagged irregularities at the crest of the bone as it attaches to the tooth.
8. Apically position (Fig. 8-6) and suture the flap in place with simple sutures or a sling suture from the mesial papilla to the distal papilla.
9. Place a periodontal dressing.

CLINICAL PROBLEM: A 36-year-old male patient was referred for tooth extraction of the mandibular second premolar before the construction of a fixed partial denture from the first premolar to the first molar. The second premolar had carious margins below the free gingival margin (Fig. 8-7, *A*). The patient wished to retain the tooth if possible, as opposed to extraction and bridge construction.

Solution: Crown lengthening was deemed a reasonable alternative, depending on the depth of carious tooth structure and the ability to establish healthy soft- and hard-tissue contours without compromising the supporting periodontium. A reverse-bevel, mucoperiosteal tissue flap with an

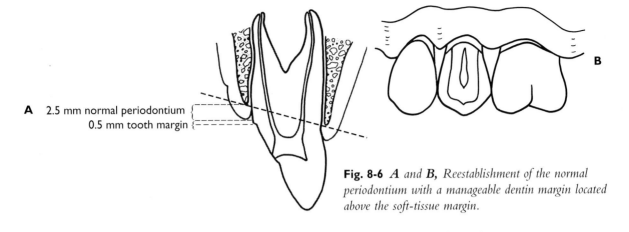

Fig. 8-6 *A* and *B,* *Reestablishment of the normal periodontium with a manageable dentin margin located above the soft-tissue margin.*

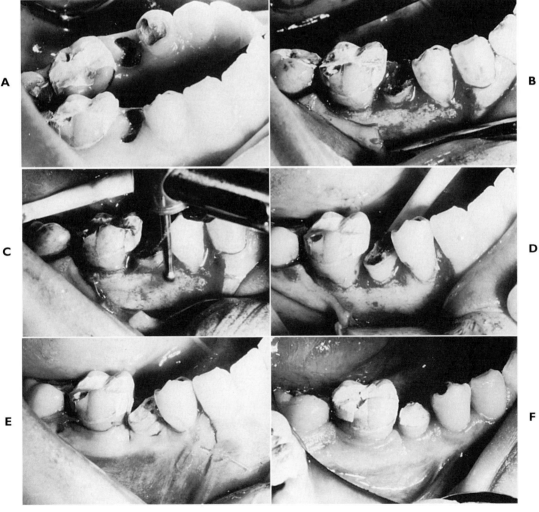

Fig. 8-7

207

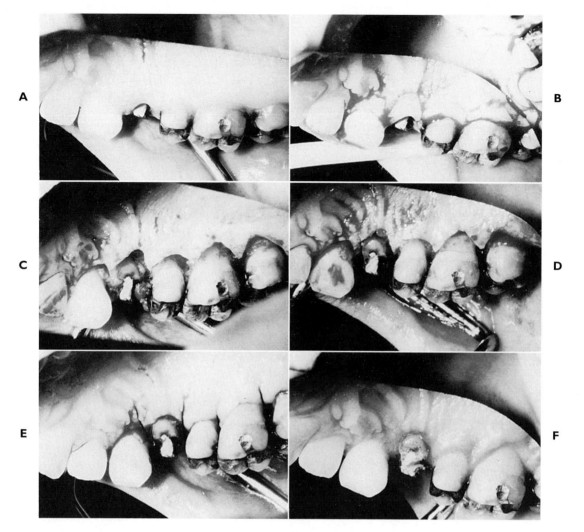

Fig. 8-8

anterior releasing incision was reflected from the distal of the canine to the distal of the first molar (Fig. 8-7, *B*) on the buccal with an envelope flap on the lingual. Notice that there is minimal tooth destruction, and the integrity of the supporting bone is quite good. Using a high-speed No. 6 round bur, the bone was carefully removed and contoured to expose sufficient tooth structure both buccally and lingually, while at the same time blending the removal with the adjacent teeth (Figs. 8-7, *C* and *D*). Fig. 8-7, *E,* shows the tissue repositioned and sutured. Four weeks later there is excellent postoperative healing, and the tooth is ready for the completion of root canal treatment along with a post or post and core buildup and crown (Fig. 8-7, *F*) (see Chapter 13).

The palatal gingiva differs from the buccal gingiva in the width of the zone of keratinized tissue and in thickness to the extent that even after the first and second incisions and curettages are performed the flap will not be sufficiently mobile for apical positioning. It will therefore be necessary to make the first incision exactly at the osseous level and in the form desired for the final repositioned flap margin. This will take careful preoperative measuring. It is better to be conservative, since more tissue can always be removed if needed.

CLINICAL PROBLEM: A 52-year-old male patient presented with a coronally fractured maxillary lateral incisor (Fig. 8-8, *A*—palatal view). Previously there had been a crown on this tooth. The fracture occurred while the patient was eating corn on the

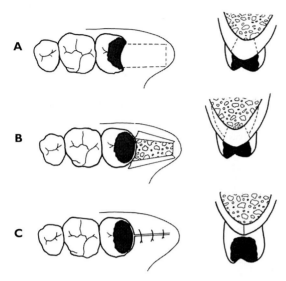

Fig. 8-9 A, *Distal carious lesion on a maxillary second molar that extends below the gingiva of the tuberosity. Broken lines indicate initial incision.* **B,** *Incision margins are undermined and connective tissue wedge is removed.* **C,** *Closure of tissue flaps results in supragingival dentin margin.*

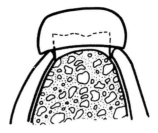

Fig. 8-10 *Directly fabricated temporary crown with intentionally bulky margins allows the flaps to be tucked under during suturing and to serve as a stint.*

cob. Retention of the tooth was critical for this patient. Probings were deep on the palatal aspect of the lateral incisor. No other periodontal defects were noted.

Solution: Often palatal defects pose significant problems when considering crown lengthening. Careful probing is essential to determine the extent of the fracture, that is, the level of remaining tooth structure. Treatment planning resulted in the choice of crown lengthening, with the knowledge that other adjunctive procedures may have to be considered depending of the depth of the fracture. A scalloped reverse-beveled incision was made along the palatal tissues (Fig. 8-8, *B*) and on the facial tissues. The tissue was reflected, exposing the fractured margin (Fig. 8-8, *C*), and the resected connective tissue was removed from the surgical site with periodontal curettes (Fig. 8-8, *D*). The reflected tissues were repositioned at an apical level (Fig. 8-8, *E*). Subsequent healing with sufficient tooth margins for proper tooth restoration is seen in Fig. 8-8, *F*.

Special Considerations for Periodontal Surgical Techniques

Distal Tooth in the Arch
Frequently the tooth requiring crown lengthening is the distal tooth in the arch. In the maxilla,

this is commonly the tuberosity area, which is often little more than a mass of fibrous connective tissue. A distal-wedge procedure may easily be incorporated into a crown-lengthening procedure.

1. Two parallel incisions approximately 4 or 5 mm apart are made in the tuberosity to the underlying bone. The width and depth will depend on the thickness of fibrous connective tissue on the tuberosity. A conservative initial width will allow future trimming of the flaps to achieve good approximation. A third incision in the mucosa connects the two parallel incisions distal to the tuberosity (Fig. 8-9, *A*).
2. The rectangle of tissue between the parallel incisions is removed.
3. The flaps are reflected as previously described. The undermining incisions are made around the tooth and extended distally to include the buccal and lingual flaps. The buccal undermining incision penetrates to or slightly beyond the mucogingival line to enhance flap mobility (Fig. 8-9, *B*).
4. After osseous recontouring, the two flaps of the distal wedge are approximated with sutures (Fig. 8-9, *C*).

Freestanding Tooth
A tooth without an immediate proximal neighbor may be treated in the same manner as any other tooth. Since there is frequently little clinical crown, the major problem arises in trying to suture the flap securely. It will frequently fail to stay well adapted to the bone and tooth. An excellent solution to this problem is to festoon an oversized, temporary aluminum-shell crown well short of crestal bone. Fill the crown with a periodontal dressing and seat it while the material is soft. This will maintain the position of the gingival tissues during initial healing. It is usually sufficient to leave this in place for 3 to 4 days (Fig. 8-10).

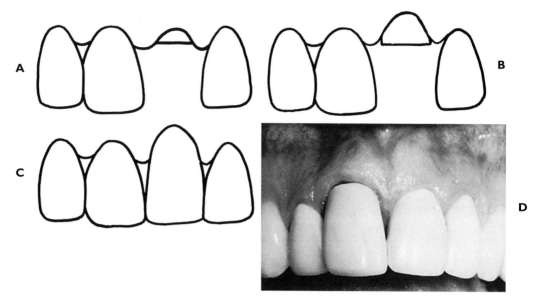

Fig. 8-11 *A, Maxillary central incisor immediately after traumatic fracture. Fractures of incisors are usually oblique and extend much farther subgingivally on the palatal or lingual aspect. **B,** If crown lengthening alone is chosen, the gingival crest of the fractured tooth will be significantly higher than that of the adjacent teeth. **C,** A porcelain veneer crown in this case would be excessively long and unesthetic. **D,** Aesthetically unacceptable restoration following crown lengthening alone on a fractured tooth.*

CASES REQUIRING ORTHODONTIC EXTRUSION AND PERIODONTAL SURGERY

The most common indication for orthodontic extrusion is a fractured tooth margin below the crestal bone.[8,10,20,23] Other indications are caries[3,11,18] or perforations from resorption,[7,20] post-space preparation,[20] and aberrant access openings[20] (see Chapter 3). Extrusion is also useful in the management of some infraosseous periodontal defects.[9,19] At the outset it must be emphasized that since bone and soft-tissue attachments usually follow the tooth during extrusion,[9,10] crown-lengthening procedures after extrusion are necessary to achieve the desired clinical crown length and to restore biologic and aesthetic tissue relationships.[3,21] Therefore the following diagnostic considerations must be evaluated before a course of treatment is chosen in a given clinical situation.

Diagnostic and Treatment Planning Considerations

Extraction and Prosthesis

Cases of subosseous tooth fracture require full-coverage restorations. If the fracture is a result of trauma, many adjacent teeth are also injured and will require similar restorations. In other situations, the adjacent teeth may already require full coverage. In these specific cases, serious consideration must be given to extraction of the deeply fractured tooth and placement of a fixed prosthesis or implant-supported prosthesis. It is important to consider the cost-benefit ratio in the selection of the ultimate treatment plan.

Crown Lengthening Only

If crown lengthening is necessary, it must be decided at the outset whether root extrusion is indicated. It is important to consider the potential esthetic problem of an exceptionally long clinical crown and the periodontal maintenance problems of uneven gingival contours (Fig. 8-11).

Extrusion Only

As previously described, extrusion alone will seldom produce the desired clinical length because the gingival attachment and alveolar bone will "follow" the tooth as it is erupted. In addition, the result will usually be unacceptable esthetically because of coronal movement of the marginal gingiva (Fig. 8-12).[2]

Tooth Type

Although it is possible to extrude nearly any tooth, the simplest cases are those that have single

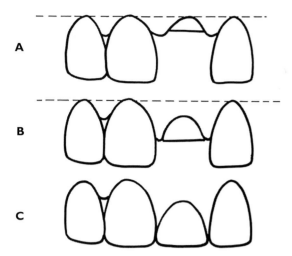

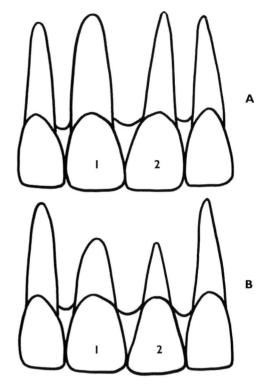

Fig. 8-12 *A, Diagram of a fractured tooth corresponding to that shown in Fig. 8-11, A. B, Appearance after extrusion alone. The gingival crest has migrated coronally with the tooth. C, A porcelain veneer crown made for this tooth would be excessively short and unaesthetic.*

Fig. 8-13 *A, Two maxillary central incisors with different root morphologies. Tooth 1 has a root of fairly uniform diameter, wheras tooth 2 tapers considerably from the cervical line to the apex. B, After extrusion of both teeth, a porcelain veneer crown on tooth 1 would appear aesthetically normal in size and contour. Because of a smaller cervical diameter, a crown on tooth 2 would appear distinctly narrow cervically, with unaesthetically wide embrasures.*

roots and an immediate proximal tooth on either side for appliance anchorage. Molars are generally difficult to treat, as are terminal teeth in the arch or freestanding piers. An orthodontic consultation may be necessary in these cases.

Crown-Root Ratio

In determining the suitability of a root for extrusion, the final crown-root ratio must be estimated. If a root is fractured completely below the crestal bone, the postoperative root length will be at least 3 mm less than the overall root length because of the allowance for 1 mm of clinical crown and 2 mm of gingival sulcus. Since most fractures tend to be oblique rather than horizontal, the fracture should be measured with a periodontal probe to determine the deepest extension. Effective root length will begin below this level. Orthodontic extrusion and crown lengthening may result in an unacceptably short root. Short root length may also be the result of advanced periodontal bone loss or may be normal for the patient. Such teeth will, at the very least, require splinting to adjacent teeth in the final restoration. Serious consideration must be given to possible extraction in preference to extrusion.

Aesthetics of Root Width

The esthetic appearance of the gingival contours and crown width is important in the maxillary anterior region. An evaluation of anterior

tooth morphology reveals a variation in root taper from the cervix to the apex. In the case of an extruded root with a relatively uniform width, the cervical diameter does not change as eruption continues. Therefore the width of the crown restoration will be similar to that of the natural crown. In the case of the steeply tapering root, the cervical diameter diminishes as the root is extruded, and the crown restoration will have a distinctly narrow dimension at the cervix, leaving excessively wide and unaesthetic embrasures[10] (Fig. 8-13).

Treatment Planning for Endodontic Procedures

In most severe root fractures or extensive cervical decay, little if any sound clinical crown remains. Consequently there is limited tooth structure for engaging and isolating the tooth intended for eruption. Furthermore, the pulp is invariably

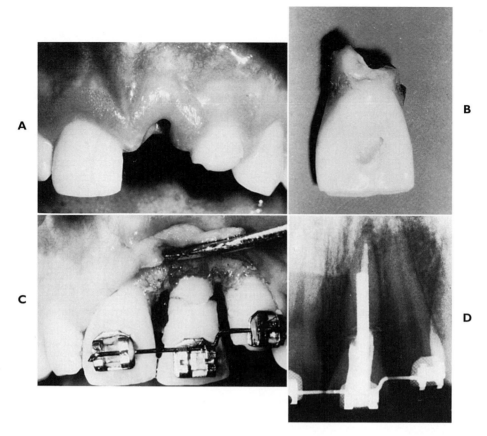

Fig. 8-14

exposed and requires immediate attention. Two
alternatives for the clinical management of this situation are described below.

Completion of Endodontic Treatment after Extrusion

1. The fractured root is visualized and hemostasis is established chemically (CUT-TROL,
   Ichthys Enterprises, Mobile, Ala.). Avoid the
   use of electrosurgery because it can have
   serious destructive effects on the bone.
2. A rubber dam is stretched across the two
   adjacent teeth. The pulp is extirpated and the
   canal is temporarily sealed.
3. A temporary buildup is completed using two
   or three TMS Minim (0.21 mm) pins (Whaledent International, New York, N.Y.) and composite resin or dentin-bonded composite.

4. A bracket is bonded to the resin and the
   tooth is extruded.
5. After extrusion, crown lengthening, and stabilization, the root canal treatment is completed in the routine manner by removing the
   buildup.
6. A post core and a crown are fabricated and
   cemented.

The advantages to this approach are, first, that the
treatment rendered is suitable for all preoperative
conditions of the pulp (vital, necrotic, and suppurative); second, that the root canal treatment is ultimately performed under routine conditions of
asepsis; and third, that a multitude of restorative
options are available, such as a cast post and core, a
prefabricated post and buildup, and so forth. The
disadvantage is that an endodontic flare-up can

occur during extrusion. In addition, pin buildups are sometimes difficult to place and can fracture or loosen under orthodontic traction.

Completion of Endodontic Treatment before Extrusion

1. The fractured surface is exposed and hemostasis is established chemically (CUT-TROL, Ichthys Enterprises, Mobile, Ala.). Avoid the use of electrosurgery because it can have a serious destructive effect on the bone.

2. Place a rubber dam across the two adjacent teeth.

3. Extirpate the pulp and perform complete root canal treatment.

4. A preformed stainless steel post of appropriate size for the final restoration is permanently cemented with zinc phosphate cement. Temporary cementation will invariably fail under orthodontic traction.

5. The bracket can be attached in one of several ways, depending on aesthetic needs:

   a. Bond the bracket directly to the post with composite resin.

   b. Fabricate an acrylic crown over the post by the direct technique and cement it with zinc phosphate cement. Exact marginal fit is not possible but also is not necessary because the extrusion will be completed quickly. Bond the bracket to the crown. Grind the acrylic crown as extrusion proceeds to relieve occlusal interferences.

   c. If available, the natural crown may be adapted to the post by drilling out the canal from the fractured surface into the crown and cementing the crown to the post with zinc phosphate or glass ionomer cement and adjusting occlusion as extrusion proceeds (Fig. 8-14).

   d. Or consider more elaborate orthodontic techniques such as a fixed or removable double-arch wire appliance with attached crown.[5,18]

6. After extrusion, the acrylic crown, natural crown, or arch wire appliance is removed, leaving the post as permanent retention for a buildup of composite resin or alloy.

7. After suitable stabilization and crown lengthening, the permanent crown is fabricated and cemented.

The advantages to this approach are that the best possible anchorage for eruption is available and that the treatment is more aesthetically pleasing. The disadvantages include the possibility of moisture contamination during the endodontic procedure or cementation of the post.

CLINICAL PROBLEM: A 27-year-old male patient was referred from a hospital emergency room shortly after receiving a blow to the mouth. The left central incisor had been fractured below the gingival margin in an irregular manner (Fig. 8-14, *A* and *B*). Because of the nature of the fracture, he had been told that the tooth would probably have to be extracted. Emotionally he was not prepared to deal with this eventuality, nor was he prepared to leave the office without a tooth or a replacement in his mouth. The patient was given a thorough examination, and radiographically the remaining root appeared to have sufficient length, width, and taper to consider extrusion.

Solution: The facial tissue was reflected sufficiently to examine the fractured root surface. There was no evidence of fracture in the retained segment. The root segment was endodontically treated and a post was cemented into the root. A palatal opening was created in the crown portion and this was fit over the post and cemented to the fractured root face (Fig. 8-14, *C* and *D*). An orthodontic appliance, as previously discussed, was applied to the crown to begin active extrusion. Once brought into position, crown lengthening can be performed to ensure proper tissue margins and contours.

Treatment Planning for Orthodontic Extrusion

The objective of orthodontic extrusion is to erupt the tooth sufficiently to provide 2 to 3 mm of tooth length above the crestal bone for a biologic attachment after crown lengthening. The basic equipment for this procedure includes a bird-beak pliers, wire cutters, straight nitinol wire, 0.022 × 0.025 inch seat direct-bond brackets, elastics, acid-etch bonding resin, and, for some applications, round (0.016 or 0.018 inch) or rectangular (0.019 inch) wire for shoe-loop appliances.

Bracket Placement

Ideally, brackets should be placed on the teeth immediately adjacent to the tooth to be erupted. These should be placed as close to the occlusal or incisal surfaces as possible without interfering with the occlusion. On the tooth intended for eruption, the bracket is placed as close to the gingival margin as possible.

Mechanics of Extrusion

Although several mechanical applications can be used to extrude teeth, the procedure can be accomplished for most teeth in the shortest time

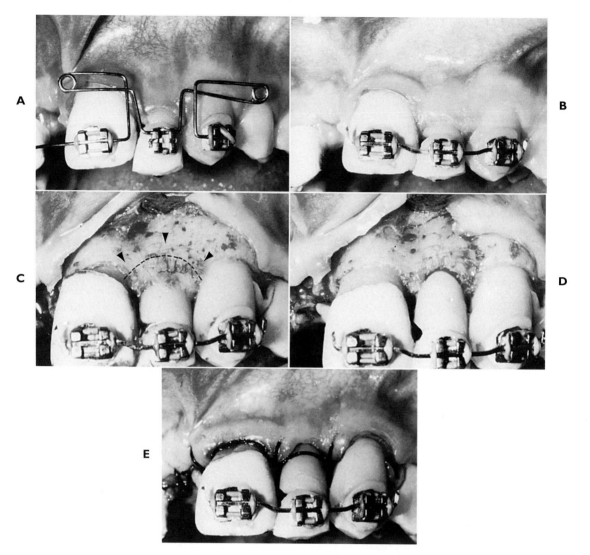

Fig. 8-15 *A,* *Post extrusion of maxillary lateral incisor. Notice the considerable difference in gingival marginal heights of extruded and adjacent teeth. The shoe-loop appliance is inactive.* *B,* *Rigid segmented arch wire placed for retention before crown lengthening. Notice reduction of incisal edge to compensate for extrusion.* *C,* *Reflection of full mucoperiosteal envelope flap reveals fibrous jellylike osteoid material on root surface (arrowheads).* *D,* *Curettage of the newly formed bony matrix and recontour of the crestal bone resulted in a level bony crest across the arch.* *E,* *Flaps repositioned and sutured. Notice level gingival margins across the arch and longer clinical crown on the fractured tooth.*

and with the fewest appointments by placing more loops and bends in the wire, which effectively lengthens the wire and its period of activity. On the other hand, a straight wire displaced into the brackets will not have a long period of activity but exerts a great deal of force and increases the need for frequent adjustments.

The shoe-loop,[3] or T-loop,[22] is an appliance that includes a sufficient number of loops and bends to sustain an eruptive force on a tooth for up to 2 weeks. Most single-root applications will require a 0.016 inch wire. The shoe loop is bent so that the horizontal bar is above the bracket of the tooth to be erupted before activation. The wire is then secured to the adjacent teeth by elastic bracket ligatures, and the shoe loop is depressed and secured into the bracket on the tooth to be erupted by the same means.

During the course of eruption it may be necessary to relieve the occlusion as the tooth erupts above the occlusal plane. Failure to provide space for eruption will result in extreme occlusal trauma on the erupting tooth. The usual length of time for eruption of single-rooted teeth is 2 to 4 weeks; molars may require up to 8 weeks. Factors affecting the length of time for eruption include age of the patient, surface area of the root, relative bone density, and achievement of optimal force. A molar may require a heavier wire if there is no evidence of movement within 7 to 10 days. Once the tooth has erupted to the desired level, it should be splinted with a heavy, rigid wire bonded into the brackets. Without stabilization the tooth may relapse and intrude. To prevent a relapse, a resection of the coronal periodontal fibers during extrusion has been recommended, although it has not been shown to be effective in every case.[15] It is reasonable to schedule the crown lengthening in 2 to 3 weeks; however, retention should continue for an additional 3 weeks after the crown lengthening.

Crown Lengthening Considerations Unique to Extrusion

After 2 to 3 weeks, the new bone forming around the erupted tooth will be approximately 70% mineralized and will appear as a fibrous, jellylike substance that is soft and easy to curette off the root during the crown-lengthening procedure. Preoperatively the attachment should be probed to clarify the exact width of osseous tissue to be removed. Care must be taken to avoid overzealous curettage because the new bone will also be found at the level of desired osseous contour and, as healing progresses, will become supporting bone after 2 to 3 months. Bone should be contoured to establish a positive or convex architecture with the adjacent teeth. If aesthetics is a concern in the anterior region, and there are wide embrasures, it may be better to leave as much osteoid as possible in the interproximal areas to support the gingival papilla and fill the embrasure (Fig. 8-15).

The method of suturing is not important as long as primary closure is achieved. Secondary healing may result in soft-tissue cratering interproximally.

Rapid and uncomplicated healing will be compromised by occlusal trauma and inflammation.

Therefore it is essential that the tooth not be in occlusion, that hygiene be strictly maintained, and that the surgical site be carefully evaluated during the healing period. After 1 week, sutures are removed and hygiene reinforced. Prophylaxis and hygiene monitoring should continue at 2-week intervals for three additional visits. In most cases, complete healing should occur within 6 to 8 weeks. The posteruption stabilizing splint can be removed at this time. If there is considerable mobility, it is reasonable to delay restorative procedures for another 4 weeks. If the degree of mobility is still unacceptable, it is best to splint the erupted tooth to an adjacent tooth during the restorative phase of treatment. Ultimately the objective of combined therapy for the severe subosseous fractured tooth is a restorable aesthetic tooth, with a normal biologic soft-tissue attachment. Figs. 8-16 to 8-18 are clinical cases illustrating the principles of orthodontic extrusion and crown lengthening discussed in this section.

CLINICAL PROBLEM: A 41-year-old male patient presented with a chief complaint that his crown will not stay on his tooth. Examination shows decayed tooth structure and food debris inside the crown, with deep carious margins on the remaining root (Fig. 8-17, *A*). Remaining root length of the second premolar was sufficient to consider root extrusion after root canal treatment.

Solution: A shoe-loop appliance was attached to the adjacent molar and to the canine because there was a porcelain crown on the first premolar. A bracket was attached to the horizontal component of the appliance above the second premolar and secured to this tooth by using a post and composite for anchorage (Fig. 8-17, *C* and *D*). Notice in *C* the space that is developing apically to the root because of extrusion over a 2-week period (Fig. 8-17, *D*). This area will be repaired with new bone. Fig. 8-17, *E*, shows the premolar in the extruded position with a new core buildup immediately after crown lengthening. Notice the quality of soft-tissue adaptation and available tooth margins for restoration. Fig. 8-17, *F* and *G,* show the tooth with a new crown and osseous repair at the 6-month recall evaluation.

CLINICAL PROBLEM: A 58-year-old male patient presents with a fractured lingual wall of the mandibular left second molar. He has a history of bruxism. The third molar is impacted, and there is no history of pain or evidence of pathosis with this tooth (Fig. 8-18, *A*). The patient wishes to retain the tooth; however, crown lengthening alone would not be indicated because of the position of the furcation of the adjacent tooth and the need to remove excessive amounts of soft tissue and bone.

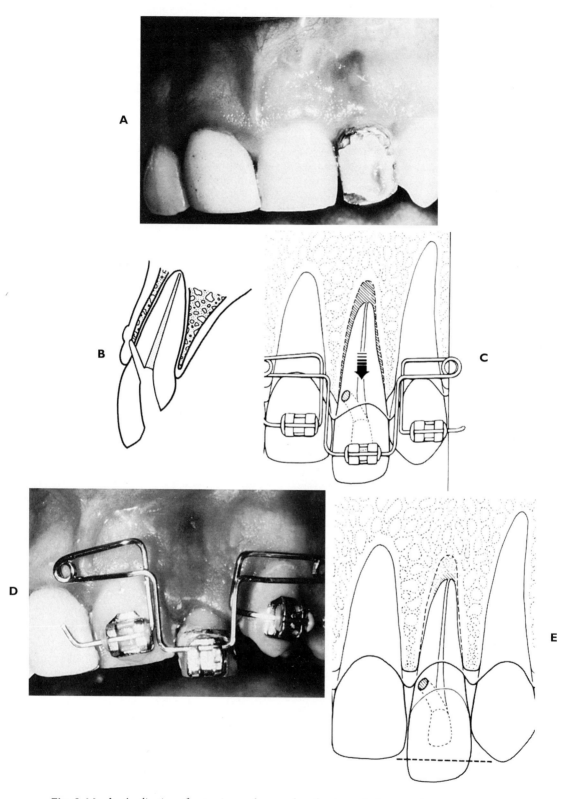

Fig. 8-16 *A, Application of extrusion and crown-lengthening techniques to correct a severe localized periodontal defect that resulted from perforation of the root during post-space preparation. B, Proximal diagram of the perforation to be managed. C, Diagram of root extrusion with coronal movement of bone and gingival attachment. D, Tooth extruded before periodontal management. E, Diagram of perforation above the gingival margin after crown lengthening and incisal reduction.* Continued.

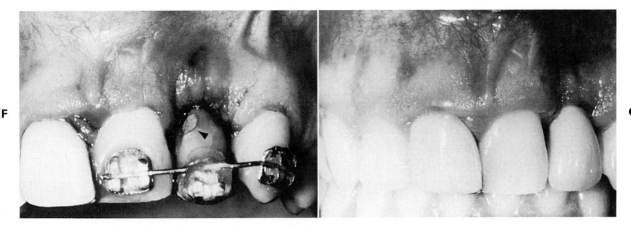

Fig. 8-16, cont'd. *F, Clinical representation of procedures accomplished in* **D**. *Perforation has been sealed with amalgam* (arrowhead). **G,** *Recall appearance; new crown has been placed encompassing the repaired perforation. (**C** and **E** from Gutmann JL, Harrison JW:* Surgical endodontics, *Boston, 1991, Blackwell Publications.)*

SOLUTION: Treatment planning of this case indicated the need to consider both extrusion and crown lengthening. The position of the furcation of the second molar would allow occlusal movement without exposure. After root canal treatment, a shoe-loop appliance was attached from the second premolar and first molar, with a horizontal bar extending to a bracket placed on the buccal of the second molar (Fig. 8-18, *B* to *D*). The tooth was extruded, during which time occlusal adjustments were necessary. Fig. 8-18, *E*, shows the radiographic appearance of the extruded tooth, and Fig. 8-18, *F* and *G*, show the lingual and buccal aspect of the tooth after crown lengthening. The tooth was restored with a crown (Fig. 8-18, *H*). The entire case took 6 weeks to complete.

Rapid orthodontic extrusion with a fiber resection has been suggested as an alternative to incorporating crown lengthening with the extrusion procedure.[15-17] With this technique, coronal migration of the attachment and bone are prevented during extrusion by repeated resection of the crestal periodontal fibers in the sulcus. The procedure is repeated several times during the extrusion period. The potential for adverse sequelae, such as resorption or relapse, is minimal, though patients will most likely require gingival recontouring to create an optimal relationship between the gingiva and the margin of the restoration. In this respect, then, crown lengthening may still be the treatment of choice after extrusion.

Surgical Repositioning

With increased understanding of the parameters of success for intentional replantation has come the suggestion of coronal surgical repositioning to expose restorable tooth margins. Although this approach is experimental, success has been reported with marginal luxation, followed by interdental sutures and surgical dressings for stabilization.[12]

CLINICAL PROBLEM: A 17-year-old male patient presented as an emergency after a blow to his mandible during football practice. The patient was sore but did not have acute pain. Fig. 8-19, *A,* shows a noncarious, unrestored maxillary premolar with a palatal cusp fracture 3 mm below the crestal bone. Since the relationship between the level of the fracture and the level of the furcation was not known, it was questionable whether to commit the tooth to orthodontic extrusion and crown lengthening. Because of the cause of the fracture—facial trauma—it was important to rule out additional fractures not apparent radiographically or clinically. Even with the removal of the fractured segment (Fig. 8-19, *B*), the integrity of the remaining root-tooth segment could not be adequately ascertained.

Solution: Surgical eruption and repositioning (Fig. 8-19, *C*) allowed immediate inspection and determination of suitability for retention. No additional fractures were noted. The tooth was repositioned coronally and splinted to produce and stabilize restorable margins. After a 6-month retention

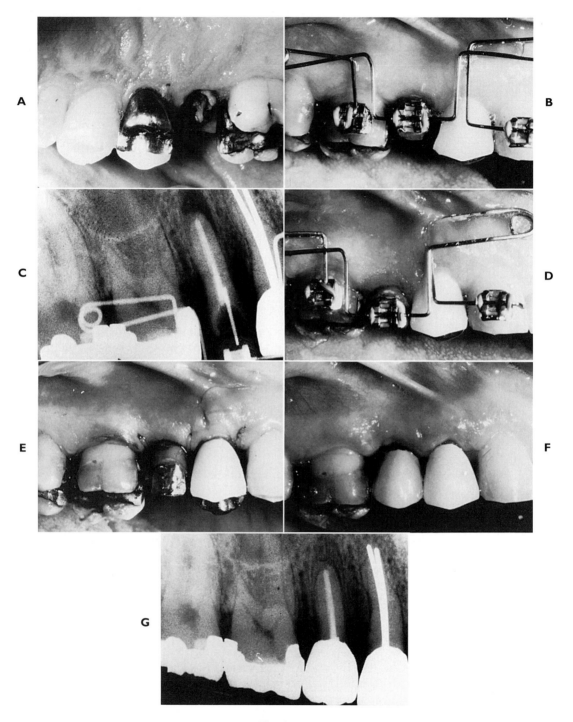

Fig. 8-17

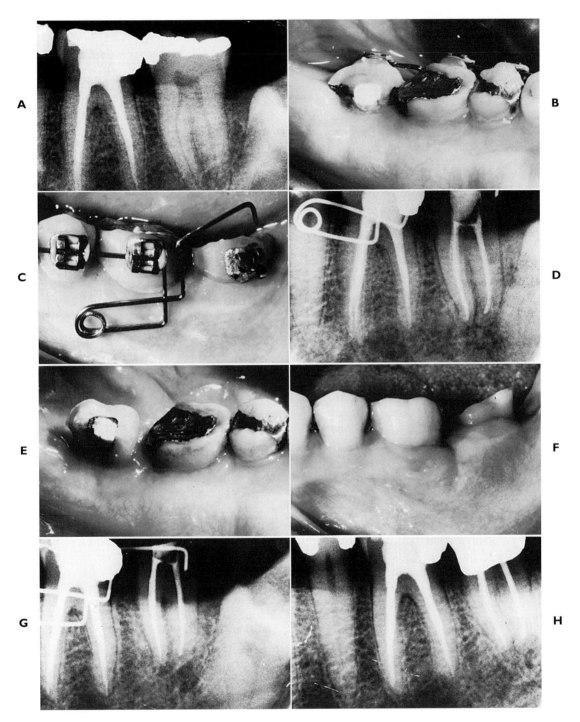

Fig. 8-18

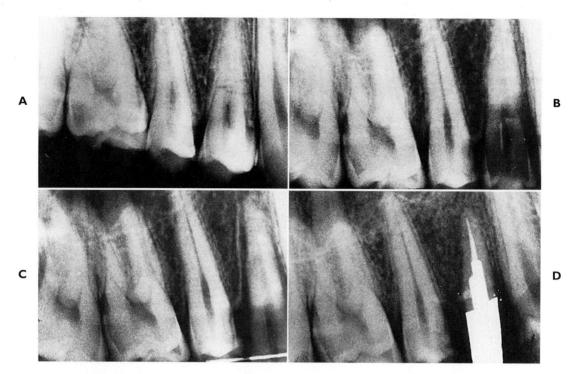

Fig. 8-19 *A, Surgical coronal repositioning in lieu of orthodontic extrusion. Notice fracture in coronal third of root. **B**, Fractured segment removed. **C**, Apical segment surgically extruded and repositioned; 6-week retention period. **D**, Subsequent post and amalgam core buildup. Notice regeneration of periradicular tissues.*

period, root canal treatment was completed and a post-core and crown were placed (Fig. 8-19, *D*).

CASES REQUIRING ROOT OR TOOTH RESECTION (AMPUTATION AND HEMISECTION)

A third option in the treatment of the deep subgingival margin applies only to multirooted teeth. Although any multirooted tooth is theoretically eligible for this approach, in clinical practice premolars have rarely been found suitable, and so only molars are discussed here. Root resection (amputation) and tooth resection (hemisection or bicuspidization) procedures are useful for a variety of clinical problems. Periodontally involved furcations can be eliminated or opened for maintenance. Teeth with severe problems confined to one root may be retained by elimination of a particular root. In considering the deep subgingival margin, these techniques are useful for teeth in which deep caries or a fracture has occurred in a limited area. Perhaps the ideal case is that in which the deep margin is localized over a single root.

Clarification of terminology and technique is important at this point. *Tooth resection* is the division of a molar into multiple single-rooted teeth.[6] It may include the extraction of a segment or the retention of all segments. For example, in a mandibular molar, tooth resection and retention of both segments have historically been referred to as *bicuspidization*. By its very nature, the crown and root portion of the tooth are resected. *Root resection* refers to the removal of a root from any molar without sectioning through the crown.[6] In this discussion, root resection would by necessity include the removal of that portion of the crown, if any remains, that contains the deep subgingival margin.

Endodontic Considerations before Root Resection

If the tooth to be treated has not previously been submitted to root canal treatment, it is usually best to do the root canal treatment before root resection, for two important reasons. First, it is exceedingly difficult to complete root canal treatment on the retained root. Postsurgically, rubber dam placement, leakage control, and canal management are more difficult. Second, the difficulty of root canal treatment cannot be determined preoperatively. If the canals prove to be difficult to penetrate or if a

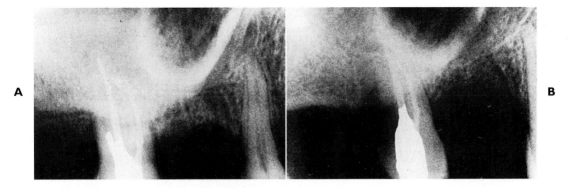

Fig. 8-20 *A, Radiograph of a tooth for which distobuccal root resection is indicated. After root canal treatment an amalgam was condensed into the distobuccal orifice. **B,** After root resection the orifice is permanently sealed.*

procedural accident compromises the anticipated result, the tooth can be extracted, thus limiting the patient to one surgical procedure instead of two (root resection plus extraction).

If the tooth has previously been treated endodontically, it is essential that the success of the treatment be confirmed and the integrity of the root filling preserved in the retained root. Although it is not the purpose of this section to delineate the parameters of endodontic success, the most important diagnostic factors would be the lack of periradicular radiolucency, lack of sensitivity to percussion, absence of vertical fracture, and an adequately dense gutta-percha root canal filling in all canals to the apical constriction. Although in some cases there may be apparently successful silver cone fillings, retreatment with gutta-percha is still indicated because of the likely need for post space (see Chapters 6 and 7).

If the tooth has not had root canal treatment, it is necessary only to complete it in the retained root or roots. In the case of root amputation it is additionally helpful to condense alloy into the orifice of the canal in the root to be extracted, so that the canal openings on the cut surfaces of the crown are completely sealed internally (Fig. 8-20).

Periodontal Considerations before Root Resection

The level of supporting bone is of primary importance in assessing the periodontal condition of the root to be retained. Even with splinting, a root with only 2 to 3 mm of supporting bone must be considered unsuitable. A safe minimum would be 50% bone loss; that is, a crestal bone height no lower than half the distance from the cemento-enamel junction to the apex. There must also be a

relatively uniform crestal bone height around the root, that is, no localized deep periodontal defects.

Of equal significance is the level of the furcation relative to the level of crestal bone on both the mesial and distal aspects of the tooth. The ideal relationship would be a furcation height above interproximal bone height as might be found in a tooth with generalized periodontal disease. These cases are suitable for tooth or root resection and result in an acceptable postoperative periodontium (Fig. 8-21, *A* to *C*). The cases unsuitable for resection alone are those in which the furcation level is 2 mm or more below the crestal bone. Simple tooth resection and extraction in these cases will heal with a bone level on the furcation side of the root no higher than the furcation itself (Fig. 8-21, *D*).

For example, if the furcation level is 3 mm below crestal bone and the postoperative healing is ideal, the sulcus depth on the nonoperatively treated surface of the retained root would be 2 mm whereas on the furcation surface it would be 5 mm, clearly undesirable and difficult to maintain. Some cases may be treated by osteotomy on the interproximal crestal bone to make it level with the furcation. However, the routine removal of large amounts of healthy bone from the adjacent tooth is seldom indicated and technically difficult. Extrusion is another alternative suitable if the root is long enough. Teeth with fused roots or the C-shaped mandibular molar are not suitable for resection.

Restorative Considerations before Root Resection

Before a resection procedure is begun, the practitioner must determine whether adjacent teeth should also be treated for full restorative coverage. It must be decided at the outset whether or not

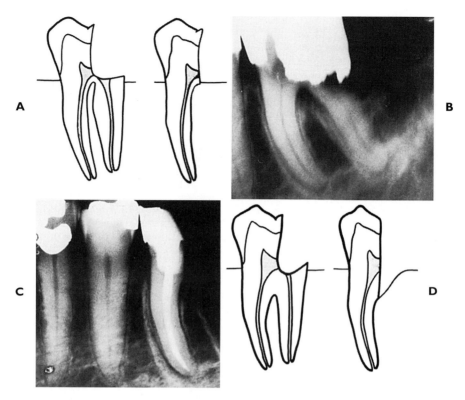

Fig. 8-21 *A, Diagram showing a favorable furcation level relative to the adjacent crestal bone necessary for tooth resection. B, Preoperative radiograph of a case in which tooth resection was indicated because of severe caries distally and in the furcation. C, Appearance after root canal treatment and tooth resection, retaining the mesial root. D, Diagram of a furcation level not suitable for tooth resection.*

tooth resection and full crown coverage would be superior to extraction of the involved tooth and placement of a fixed prosthesis (Fig. 8-22). Although the remaining root may be splinted to an adjacent tooth, the problems of hygiene, cost, and difficulty of restoration must be weighed. A second consideration is the restorability of the remaining root segment. Even with crown lengthening incorporated into the tooth-resection procedure, can the root be restored with a full crown, is it capable of bearing an occlusal load, and is it periodontally sound?

Surgical Techniques for Root Resection

A complete treatise on resection procedures is provided in other texts.[6,13] However, for simplicity in a straightforward case the after guidelines will apply.

1. The surgical equipment is the same as for the crown-lengthening procedure.
2. A horizontal sulcar incision is made both buccally and lingually (or palatally) at least one complete tooth width mesial and distal to the tooth to be resected.

3. Curette the interproximal tissue and any connective tissue tags and identify the precise location of the furcation.
4. Using a No. 557 crosscut fissure bur or a No. 170L or XL straight-cutting, tapered bur, divide the crown from the occlusal surface to the furcation with a cut parallel to the long axis of the tooth and centered over the root intended for extraction. This will prevent cutting into the part of the crown and root to be retained. If there is a through-and-through furcation defect, a periodontal probe may be placed through the defect buccolingually to act as a visual guide for accurate resection. Silver cones can also be used in this manner (Fig. 8-23).
5. Once the root has been completely severed from the retained tooth structure (verified either radiographically or clinically), the segment to be removed is carefully extracted.
6. Use a tapered diamond bur designed for full-crown preparations to shape the surface of the

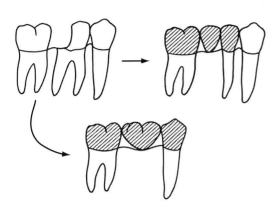

Fig. 8-22 *Restorative options that depend on the suitability of retaining root segments after resection.*

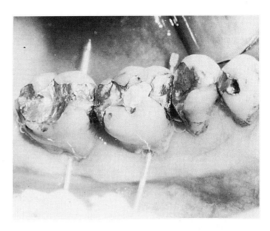

Fig. 8-23 *Silver cones can be placed through the furcations of molars to serve as a visual guide for accurate bur placement during resection.*

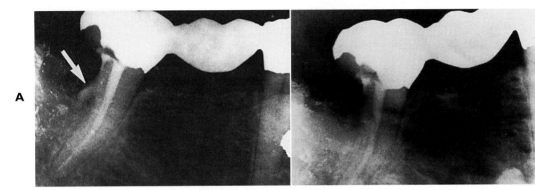

Fig. 8-24 ***A,*** *Radiograph obtained during root resection procedure to check for dentin overhangs (arrow) in the furcation. Further reduction and contouring is required.* ***B,*** *Reduction of overhang in the furcation.*

cut crown so that a smooth transition exists from the crown surface to the root surface.

7. Obtain a radiograph to verify that no fluting or overhanging spurs of tooth structure are left protruding into the furcation (Fig. 8-24).

8. Compare the level of bone on the furcation side with the level of bone on the opposite side of the root. If there is a discrepancy in height, a combination of round burs and the Wiedelstadt chisel may be used to level the bone height, as in the crown-lengthening technique.

9. Wound closure and dressing are the same as described for the crown-lengthening procedure.

Tooth Stabilization after Resection

Although splinting may be a direct result of placing a fixed prosthesis on some resected teeth, other cases require specific splinting procedures to enhance arch stability and to support the teeth during function as healing progresses. Frequently such teeth already have a full crown that is to be retained. Because unfavorable occlusal forces may result in fracture of the supporting root, the crown should be splinted to the tooth adjacent to the extracted root. One method is to cut a 2 × 2 mm Class II cavity preparation in both teeth and place a flexible stainless steel wire covered by a light-cured composite resin to allow some movement between the two crowns (Fig. 8-25). Dentin-bonded techniques are also effective when natural tooth structure is available. Attempts to create a rigid splint with heavy wire and alloy will usually fail because the alloy fractures. Temporary bridges may also be used to stabilize the retained segment or segments, retain interproximal space, and protect the remaining tooth structure and soft tissue during healing (Fig. 8-26).

CLINICAL PROBLEM: A symptom-free 53-year-old male patient presented with decay in the roots of the mandibular second molar at the furcation level. The decay had proceeded into the furcation region, making it difficult for the patient to clean the tooth and prevent further breakdown of the furcation bone. Radiographically this is visible in

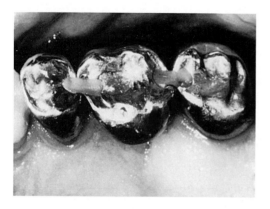

Fig. 8-25 *Molar splinted to adjacent teeth by means of an interproximal wire and composite splint.*

Fig. 8-27, *A,* and clinically in Fig. 8-27, *B.* This tooth was the distal abutment for a fixed partial denture, and its maintenance was crucial to future restoration of the dental arch.

Solution: A combination of issues entered into the treatment planning for this case, including the need for root canal treatment, tooth resection, orthodontic segment repositioning and stabilization, periodontal management, and prosthetic restoration. The fixed partial denture was resected (Fig. 8-27, *C*) and root canal treatment was completed (Fig. 8-27, *D*). The tooth was resected using the crown-contouring method. Initially a silver cone was threaded through the furcation as a guide (Fig. 8-27, *E*). This was followed by cutting into the furcation from the buccal and lingual until resection was complete (Fig. 8-27, *F* to *H*). Subsequently, posts and cores were placed, and the segments were orthodontically bracketed. Separation occurred over a 2-month period (Fig. 8-27, *I* to *J*). Ultimately the segments were crowned and stabilized by a new fixed partial denture. A 2-year reevaluation, with buccal, lingual, and radiographic views respectively, indicates a stable oral environment (Fig. 8-27, *K* to *M*). The patient is symptom free

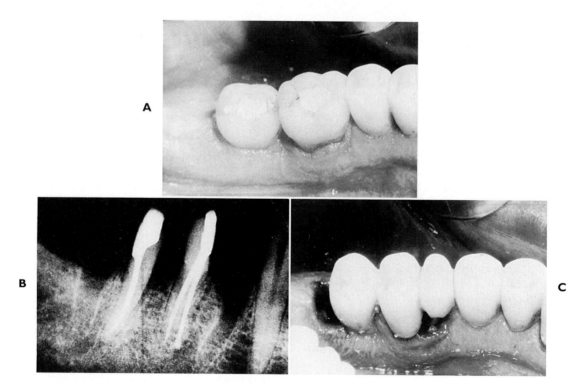

Fig. 8-26 *A, Two mandibular molars suitable for tooth resection and select segment retention. Root canal treatment is performed before resection. B, Resected teeth retaining key, sound abutments. C, Temporary acrylic bridge acts as a splint during the healing process after tooth resection.*

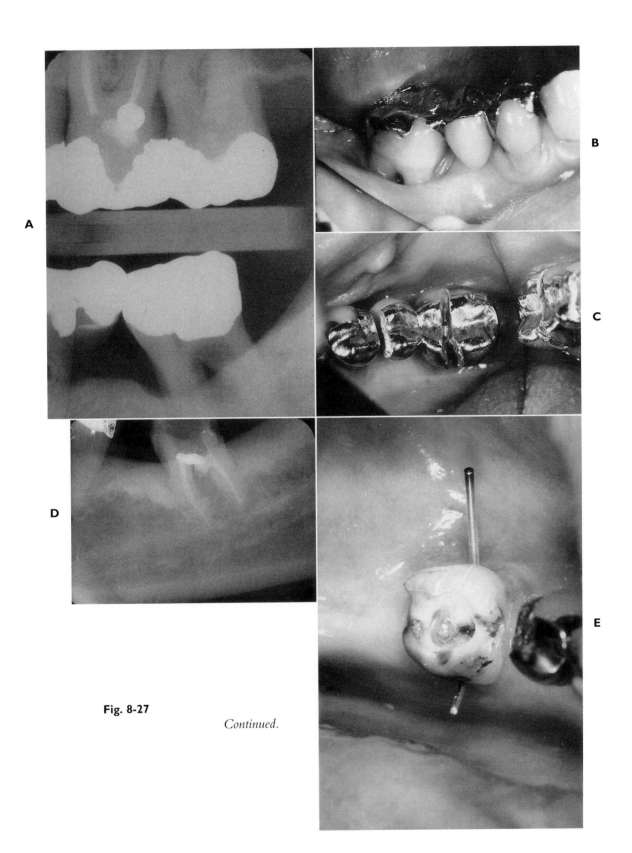

Fig. 8-27

Continued.

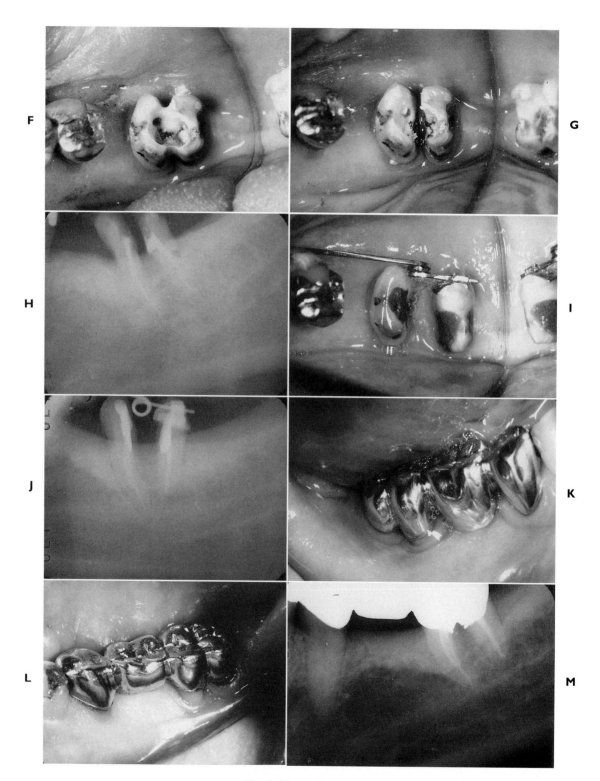

Fig. 8-27 cont'd.

and able to maintain his appliance. This case stresses the importance of creativity and integration of all dental disciplines in a problem-solving manner.

SUMMARY

This chapter has focused on problem-solving techniques in the management of the subgingival tooth margin in conjunction with endodontic procedures. Crown-lengthening techniques can be used to expose margins that are subgingival but above the osseous crest. Orthodontic extrusion will result in exposure of subosseous margins when followed by crown lengthening. Specific restorative procedures to enhance the management of these cases have also been highlighted. Finally, resection procedures may be considered appropriate for retaining periodontally sound, restorable roots of multirooted teeth unrestorable because of caries, fractures, perforations, and unanticipated endodontic misfortunes during treatment.

References

1. Assif D, Pilo R, Marshak B: Restoring teeth after crown lengthening procedures, *J Prosthet Dent* 65:62-64, 1991.
2. Batenhorst KF, Bowers GM, Williams JE: Tissue changes resulting from facial tipping and extrusion of incisors in monkeys, *J Periodontol* 45:660-668, 1974.
3. Biggerstaff RH, Sinks JH, Carazola JL: Orthodontic extrusion and biologic width realignment procedures: methods for reclaiming nonrestorable teeth, *J Am Dent Assoc* 112:345-348, 1986.
4. Davis JW, Fry HR, Krill DB, Rostock M: Periodontal surgery as an adjunct to endodontics, orthodontics, and restorative dentistry, *J Am Dent Assoc* 115:271-275, 1987.
5. Delivanis PD, Delivanis HP: Esthetic solutions in orthodontic extrusion of compromised teeth, *J Endod* 10:221-226, 1984.
6. Gutmann JL, Harrison JW: *Surgical endodontics,* St. Louis, 1994, IEA [Ishiyaku EuroAmerica] Publishers Inc, pp 409-448.
7. Hartwell GR, Cecic PA: An esthetic restorative technique for use during the stabilization period after vertical root extrusion, *J Am Dent Assoc* 107:59-60, 1983.
8. Heithersay GS: Combined endodontic-orthodontic treatment of transverse root fractures in the region of the alveolar crest, *Oral Surg Oral Med Oral Pathol,* 36:404-415, 1973.
9. Ingber JS: Forced eruption: Part I. A method of treating isolated one or two wall infrabony osseous defects—rationale and case report, *J Periodontol* 45:199-206, 1974.
10. Ingber JS: Forced eruption: Part II. A method of treating nonrestorable teeth—periodontal and restorative considerations, *J Periodontol* 47:203-216, 1976.
11. Ivey DW, Calhoun RL, Kemp WB et al: Orthodontic extrusion: its use in restorative dentistry, *J Prosthet Dent* 43:401-407, 1980.
12. Kahnberg K-E: Surgical extrusion of root-fractured teeth—a follow-up study of two surgical methods, *Endod Dent Traumatol* 4:85-89, 1988.
13. Lost C: *Hemisektion und Würzelamputation,* Munich, 1985, Carl Hanser Verlag.
14. Lovdahl PE, Gutmann JL: Periodontal and restorative considerations before endodontic therapy, *J Acad Gen Dent* 28:38-45, 1980.
15. Malmgren O, Malmgren B, Frykholm A: Rapid orthodontic extrusion of crown root and cervical root fractured teeth, *Endod Dent Traumatol* 7:49-54, 1991.
16. Pontoriero R, Celenza F, Ricci G, Carnevale G: Rapid extrusion with fiber resection: a combined orthodontic-periodontic treatment modality, *Int J Periodontol Rest Dent* 5:30-43, 1987.
17. Reitan K: Clinical and histological observations on tooth movements during and after orthodontic treatment, *Am J Orthodont* 53:721-745, 1967.
18. Ries BJ, Johnson GK, Nieberg LG: Vertical extrusion using a removable orthodontic appliance, *J Am Dent Assoc* 116:52-523, 1988.
19. Ross S, Dorfman HS, Palcanis KG: Orthodontic extrusion: a multidisciplinary treatment approach, *J Am Dent Assoc* 102:189-191, 1981.
20. Simon JHS, Kelly WJ, Gordon DG et al: Extrusion of endodontically treated teeth, *J Am Dent Assoc* 97:17-23, 1978.
21. Stern N, Becker A: Forced eruption: biologic and clinical considerations, *J Oral Rehabil* 7:395-402, 1980.
22. Tuncay OC, Cunningham CJ: T-loop appliance in endodontic-orthodontic interactions, *J Endod* 8:367-369, 1982.
23. Wolfson EM, Seiden L: Combined endodontic-orthodontic treatment of subgingivally fractured teeth, *J Can Dent Assoc* 41:621-624, 1975.

Chapter *9*

▼

Problems in Managing Endodontic Emergencies

Thom C. Dumsha
James L. Gutmann

"To cure the Tooth-ach, Take a new Nail, and make the Gum bleed with it, then drive it into an Oak. This did Cure William Neal, Sir William Neal's Son, a very stout Gentleman. When he was almost Mad with the Pain, and had a mind to have Pistoll'd himself."*

The alleviation of dental pain is one of the prime objectives of the dental profession. The key to the successful management of dental pain is to establish a diagnosis and treat the condition efficiently and effectively. This chapter outlines some problems that may be encountered in the management of both acute and chronic pain arising from diseases of the pulp and periradicular sequelae.

Although numerous classifications of pulpal and periradicular disease states have been proposed in endodontic texts,[44,46-48,52] only a limited number of clinical diagnostic situations require identification before effective treatment can be rendered.

SYMPTOMS AND CHRONOLOGY OF PAIN

Often a diagnostic decision concerning the pulpal status of a particular tooth with respect to endodontic treatment can be made before any clinical tests are performed. An immediate working diagnosis of either an irreversible disease state requiring emergency treatment or a reversible disease state requiring palliative treatment or observation can often be made based on symptoms alone. For example, if the patient reports a history of severe,

spontaneous pain in a tooth for several days, there is an irreversible pulpitis that requires root canal treatment. However, if the patient has had a recent restoration in the sensitive tooth or complains of a recent sensitivity to thermal changes, a more conservative approach is recommended. These are not hard-and-fast rules in the total management of pulpal problems, since the most probable diagnosis is determined by integrating a complete subjective and objective evaluation in some situations.

However, attention to the key subjective symptoms noted by the patient or elicited by the practitioner will very often uncover the most probable status of the pulp or periradicular conditions.

In general, a watch-and-wait approach is adopted or minimal treatment is rendered when the following conditions are present:
1. Short-term sensitivity or discomfort (several days or weeks)
2. A history of recent dental treatment, gingival recession, loss of restoration, or possible fractured cusp

On the other hand, definitive pulpal treatment is more often indicated when these conditions are present:
1. A history of moderate to severe pain, with frequently recurring episodes of spontaneous pain, over long periods of time
2. Painful symptoms produced by specific stimuli, such as biting, touching, and hot or cold

---

*From Aubrey J, as cited in Foley GH: *Foley's footnotes,* Wallingford, Penn., 1972, Washington Square East.

229

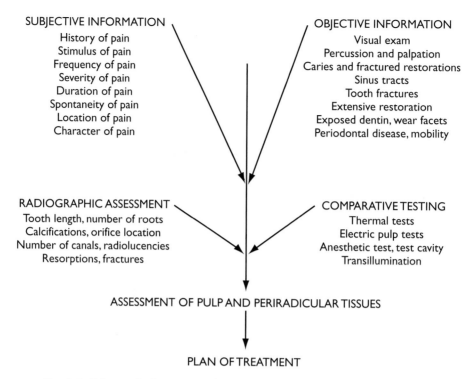

SUBJECTIVE INFORMATION
History of pain
Stimulus of pain
Frequency of pain
Severity of pain
Duration of pain
Spontaneity of pain
Location of pain
Character of pain

OBJECTIVE INFORMATION
Visual exam
Percussion and palpation
Caries and fractured restorations
Sinus tracts
Tooth fractures
Extensive restoration
Exposed dentin, wear facets
Periodontal disease, mobility

RADIOGRAPHIC ASSESSMENT
Tooth length, number of roots
Calcifications, orifice location
Number of canals, radiolucencies
Resorptions, fractures

COMPARATIVE TESTING
Thermal tests
Electric pulp tests
Anesthetic test, test cavity
Transillumination

ASSESSMENT OF PULP AND PERIRADICULAR TISSUES

PLAN OF TREATMENT

Fig. 9-1 *Scheme of information gathering for pulpal and periradicular diagnosis.*

DIAGNOSIS AND TREATMENT: PULPAL AND PERIRADICULAR

Diagnostic categories should correspond to treatment-oriented categories. That is, the diagnosis should indicate the pulpal and periradicular status and the kind of treatment needed to eliminate the problem. Therefore the diagnosis should be clinically based and must represent both a pulpal and a periradicular analysis, which includes the integration of all diagnostic information (Fig. 9-1). Clinical characteristics of pulpal inflammation and its spread to the periradicular tissues are presented in Tables 9-1 and 9-2 and are integrated into the problem-solving discussions in the subsequent sections.

Vital Pulps

Reversible Pulpitis: Treatment

In the case of reversible pulpitis, the pulp is inflamed, and removal of the causative factors, such as a high restoration, incipient caries, a fractured restoration, a fractured cusp, or exposed cervical dentinal tubules, will usually alleviate the patient's discomfort. However, observation and evaluation are warranted in each case to ensure that the problem resolves and a chronic degenerative pulpitis does not develop.

Pulpal pain can occur after restorative procedures. In some cases the pain resolves within a few hours or days. In other cases it may linger for weeks or months, with varying levels of discomfort. Even when the restoration is removed and a sedative dressing is placed, the patient may experience continued low-grade pain. In these cases the pulp is probably undergoing chronic degeneration because of the cumulative effect of the restorative procedures, coupled with previous episodes of pulpal inflammation and irritation. If pain does not resolve within a few weeks and the patient wishes to be pain free, it is probably wise to consider rediagnosing the condition as irreversible pulpitis.

CLINICAL PROBLEM: A 29-year-old female patient is referred for root canal treatment on her mandibular left second molar. She has no chief complaint. In fact she cannot understand why she needs root canal treatment. Subjectively she knows there may be decay in the tooth. She lost a restoration approximately 3 months earlier. Food gets caught in the tooth, but she cannot remember having any discomfort. The reason she went to her general dentist was to replace the filling because her tongue was being irritated by the edge of the tooth where the filling was lost. Clinically there is evi-

▼ **Table 9-1** Clinical characteristics of pulpitis

REVERSIBLE PULPITIS	IRREVERSIBLE PULPITIS
Sensitivity to mild discomfort	Pain may be absent or present
Short duration or shooting sensation	History of pain is usually given
Not severe	Pain is often moderate to severe
Infrequent episodes of discomfort	Pain is often spontaneous
Seldom hurts to bite unless tooth also fractured or restoration is loose and occlusion is affected	Pain is increasing in frequency, often to the point of being continuous
Could result in irreversible pulpitis if cause not removed	Pain usually lingers, especially with increasing episodes
Symptoms usually subside immediately or shortly after removal of cause	Patient often requires some type of analgesic
Common causes include exposed dentin, cracked restorations, recently placed restorations, initial carious attack or rapidly advancing caries, altered occlusion	Thermal stimulation often elicits severe lingering pain
	May be able to identify specific or multiple stimuli
	Pain radiates or is diffuse or may be localized
	History of trauma, extensive restorations, periodontal disease, or extensive recurrent caries is present
	Radiographic changes may be absent or include calcifications, resorptions, or radiolucencies

▼ **Table 9-2** Clinical characteristics of periradicular periodontitis

CHRONIC	SUBACUTE	ACUTE	ALVEOLAR ABSCESS
Radiolucent lesion	Slight tenderness to biting or percussion	Pain to biting or percussion	Severe pain with biting, percussion, and palpation
Patient asymptomatic	No lesion present on radiographs	No thickened ligament space or lesion present	Tooth elevated in socket
If sinus tract present, referred to as "suppurative"		Tooth may be mobile	Tooth very mobile
Percussion produces little or no discomfort		Often tender to palpation	Swelling may be present
Variation includes condensing osteitis, which is represented by a diffuse radiopacity indicative of low-grade pulpal degeneration			Often radiolucency present
			Often systemic symptoms

dence of a fractured restoration, of which the distal portion is missing. There is surface decay in the area where the restoration was lost. Compared to the adjacent and contralateral teeth, the second molar responds normally to palpation, percussion, and sensibility testing (thermal and electric pulp tests). Radiographically, other than the obvious lost restoration, all findings are normal (Fig. 9-2, *A*).

Solution: Based on the subjective and objective findings, a diagnosis of reversible pulpitis with normal periradicular tissues is indicated. Also there is no evidence of calcifications or resorptions in the pulp chamber or canal system that might indicate an adverse pulpal response to irritation. Likewise, radiographically the lamina dura and periodontal ligament space are intact. Unless a direct pulp exposure

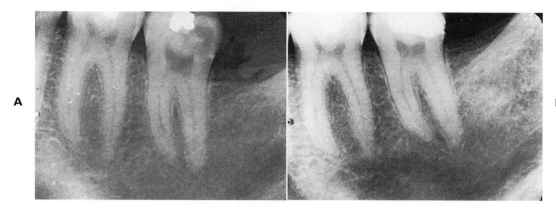

Fig. 9-2

occurs during caries excavation, *root canal treatment is not indicated*. The decay was removed and sound dentin was identified. The tooth was restored with an IRM (Fig. 9-2, *B*) and the patient was informed that unless symptoms developed, the tooth should receive a restoration in within a few weeks.

Irreversible Pulpitis with Localized Symptoms

In an emergency, the most obvious way to determine the cause of discomfort is to ask the patient if the pain is localized to a particular tooth or to a point on the gingiva or mucosa.

If the patient can isolate the tooth, then the diagnostic process is partially complete. If the patient is not sure which tooth is sensitive or is causing pain, the next procedure is to duplicate the painful response. Therefore, if a patient complains of cold sensitivity, an ice stick or other source of cold stimulus is applied to each tooth in the area of concern. Begin with presumably normal teeth and test several teeth individually in the quadrant. In addition, test contralateral teeth and teeth that have already had root canal treatment, to serve as controls. Depending on the duration of pain, that is, whether short (immediate remission within 10 seconds) or long (remission within 15 to 60 or more seconds); the intensity of pain (slight pain to some sensitivity with relief shortly after removal of stimulus versus severe throbbing pain after removal of the stimulus); and the reproducibility of the pain, one can usually determine if the pulp is irreversibly inflamed.

Patients often complain of sensitivity to heat and cold, but in the vast majority of cases cold is the primary stimulus causing pain. Sensitivity to

hot foods or liquids can also occur but this finding is not correlated to any specific histopathologic state of the dental pulp. Some think it may relate to the presence of an intrapulpal abscess, while others feel it relates to more of a degenerative pulpal state.

Another patient complaint is the inability to chew or tap on a particular tooth. This factor does not relate to or indicate pulpal vitality.

When coupled with other pulpal symptoms, pain when chewing implies the presence of inflammation in the periradicular tissues resulting from an inflamed, degenerating, or necrotic pulp.

The replication of the response to this stimulus (percussion) is not an aid in diagnosing the status of the pulp. However, if sensitivity to percussion is an isolated symptom, occlusal adjustment and observation may be the only treatment indicated. More often than not, however, if a tooth is sensitive to percussion, along with other symptoms of irreversible pulpitis, the pulp or tooth must be removed to eliminate the patient's problem.

CLINICAL PROBLEM: A 31-year-old male patient presents with severe toothache that is accentuated by biting. He also indicates that he cannot stand to have something cold on his tooth. He claims to have had a temporary filling placed in the tooth 8 months earlier but has not sought treatment because there was no pain. He can point to the mandibular left second molar as the source of the pain. Clinical examination reveals a temporary restoration of the distoocclusal portion of the tooth. The third molar has already begun shifting into the defect. Compared with the adjacent and

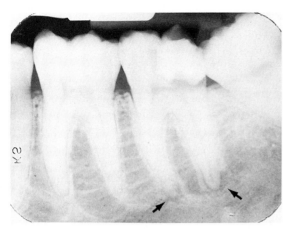

Fig. 9-3

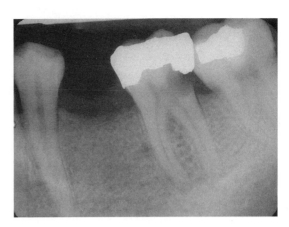

Fig. 9-4

contralateral teeth, the second molar is exquisitely painful to percussion. Sensibility tests are not indicated to locate the source of the patient's problem, and the use of ice might only cause the patient further discomfort. A radiograph shows a diminished pulp chamber and canals, a potentially leaking temporary restoration, and significant changes in the lamina dura and periodontal ligament space on all the roots (Fig. 9-3, *arrows*).

Solution: Based on the subjective and objective findings, a diagnosis of irreversible pulpitis with acute periradicular periodontitis is indicated. Emergency treatment should be complete removal of the pulp to the desired apical termination in the roots. The symptoms and signs indicate that inflammation is into the periradicular tissues and removal of the cause (pulp tissue) is necessary. Generally a pulpotomy alone will not relieve the patient's symptoms.

A diagnostic problem arises when multiple teeth in a quadrant are sensitive to cold. In this case, it is difficult to isolate the tooth that is causing the symptoms. A good method to determine the offending tooth is to individually isolate each tooth in the quadrant with a rubber dam. Often the pulpally involved tooth will ache for several minutes after exposure to a cold stimulus. Therefore the practitioner must wait several minutes between testing each tooth to decide if the stimulus has elicited this pain. If the tests are performed too rapidly, several teeth will have been cold tested by the time the patient reports the aching sensation, and the test results will be inconclusive. Another approach is to alternate between a hot and a cold stimulus, allowing ample time before advancing to the next

tooth. This is necessary because the pain associated with the chief complaint is often slow in onset.

CLINICAL PROBLEM: A 52-year-old female patient presents with a throbbing toothache that is accentuated by thermal changes. She can point directly to the mandibular left first molar. She indicates that she always gets food caught behind that tooth. Clinically there is a large amalgam restoration in this tooth. Also evident is a deep carious lesion on the distobuccal margin below the tissue line. Placement of an explorer into this area causes severe pain for the patient. Percussion and palpation do not accentuate the patient's discomfort and are considered as normal. Radiographically the extent of the carious lesion is obvious (Fig. 9-4). There is a large pulp chamber, and slight periradicular changes are noted at the root apices.

Solution: Based on the subjective and objective findings a diagnosis of irreversible pulpitis with normal periradicular tissues is indicated. Root canal treatment is necessary. However, before beginning the definitive treatment, the restoration should be removed, the caries excavated, and the restorability of the tooth assessed. Crown lengthening may also be necessary. Failure to address these concerns may lead to problems with coronal leakage during appointments, or poor treatment planning that will result in the loss of the tooth for reasons other than endodontic ones.

Irreversible Pulpitis with Symptoms Not Localized

Nonlocalized pulpitis poses the most difficult and challenging diagnostic problem for the practitioner, since neither the patient nor the practitioner can readily identify the tooth in question. (In rare cases a radiograph may provide the answer.) In this situa-

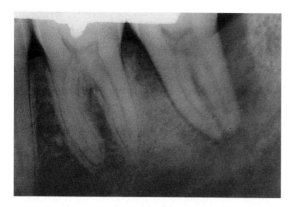

Fig. 9-5

tion the patient complains only of vague pain, usually chronic in nature and sometimes severe but without any known stimulus to evoke the discomfort. More often than not, the symptoms cannot be reproduced by heat, cold, or mastication, but nonetheless chronic pain is still present. This commonly occurs under full-coverage restorations. If the radiographic picture is unclear, the astute practitioner will do nothing for this patient but wait until the symptoms localize to a specific tooth. Inevitably the symptoms do localize, though it may take several weeks or longer for the process to occur.

The removal of a deep restoration and replacement with a sedative dressing (zinc oxide–eugenol) may initially alleviate the symptoms. However, long-standing chronic pulpal inflammation will not resolve with this procedure and root canal treatment is indicated once the tooth or cause is determined.

The final treatment alternative for nonlocalized pulpitis is to alert the patient to the lack of diagnostic conclusions. If the pain is severe enough, the patient may opt for a speculative diagnosis. However, if there is less than a 70% to 80% assurance of determining the offending tooth, it is recommended to watch and wait until localization occurs.

Resist the temptation to open the tooth to see if it will help the patient in pain.

Too often multiple teeth are opened with this intent and without a relatively conclusive diagnosis. In many cases this approach does not eliminate the patient's symptoms, and vague, nonlocalized pain continues.

CLINICAL PROBLEM: A 39-year-old male patient presents with vague discomfort in the mandibular left posterior region. His discomfort is difficult to describe, and he cannot localize the origin. At times he says he has sensitivity to thermal changes, at times discomfort to biting. The discomfort was infrequent until recently when it began to appear more often without warning. He points to the last two teeth in this quadrant. Clinical examination reveals an occlusal restoration is present in the first molar. The second molar is intact except for the presence of fracture lines on the proximal marginal ridges. Percussion is normal on the second molar. The patient is more aware of tapping on the first molar and says it feels different from the contralateral tooth. Palpation is noncontributory. Sensibility testing indicates that the second molar is nonresponsive, whereas the first molar is abnormally sensitive to thermal testing. Probing indicates deep pocket formation on the distal with an incipient pocket on the mesial of the second molar. Radiographically a large enveloping radiolucency is obvious around the distal of the second molar with loss of bone mesiocervically (Fig. 9-5). The pulp canal system is patent on the second molar; however, the first molar exhibits extensive pulp stone formation in the chamber and in the distal pulpal space. The first molar also has a thickened lamina dura typical of a localized sclerosis.

Solution: Based on the subjective and objective findings, a multiple diagnosis is indicated. First, the second molar has a necrotic pulp with a chronic periradicular periodontitis subsequent to tooth fracture (see Chapter 11). Retention of this tooth is poor, and extraction is indicated. The first molar was diagnosed with irreversible pulpitis with chronic to subacute periradicular periodontitis and is probably responsible for the patient's present symptoms. Root canal treatment is indicated, and because of the potential predisposition to tooth fractures, the tooth should receive a full coronal restoration (see Chapter 13).

Irreversible Pulpitis: Treatment

Rapid and effective management of irreversible pulpitis requires removal of the bulk of the inflamed tissue, especially when there is pain on percussion. This is often accomplished by a pulpotomy, which removes the bulk of the vital, inflamed tissue from the pulp chamber and reduces the pressure in the soft tissue. However, in multirooted teeth, a partial pulpectomy can also be performed, since the palatal or distal roots of molars are usually quite large and most of the pulp tissue in these canals can be removed. Since the mesial canals of mandibular molars and the buccal canals of maxillary molars are usually quite small, adequate

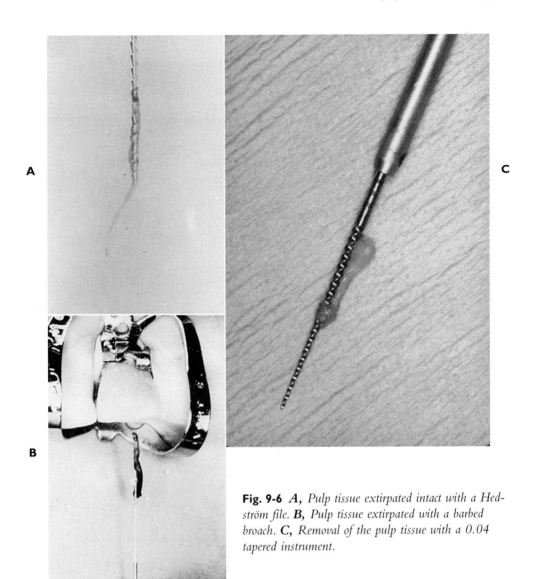

Fig. 9-6 *A, Pulp tissue extirpated intact with a Hedström file. B, Pulp tissue extirpated with a barbed broach. C, Removal of the pulp tissue with a 0.04 tapered instrument.*

removal of the pulp tissue in these canals is difficult without total instrumentation. Therefore it is prudent to leave these canals untouched in vital cases rather than clean them inadequately, which might cause hemorrhage and inflammation, along with the potential for further discomfort. If there is acute tenderness to percussion, however, it may be wise to determine the accurate working length of each canal and clean and shape the canals to a minimum size of a No. 20 to 25 K-file. This will usually ensure tissue removal in the apical third of these small canals, thereby minimizing or negating continued inflammation in the periradicular tissues from pulpal sources.

Hedström files are convenient for removing intact soft tissue from the root canal system. The largest Hedström file that will fit in the canal without binding is carefully twisted clockwise into the canal completely to the apex, penetrating the pulp tissue in the canal. Once the file is at the most apical portion of the canal it is removed with light pressure applied against the circumference of the canal, bringing with it the pulp tissue in toto (Fig. 9-6, *A*). Another method is to use barbed broaches to grasp the tissue (Fig. 9-6, *B*). However, if these instruments are forced into the canal or bind against the wall in the canal, they can easily break, or shred the tissue on removal; therefore their use is generally recommended only in moderate- to large-sized canals. The recent introduction of the 0.04 tapered Ni-Ti instruments (Tulsa Dental Products, Tulsa, Okla.) has provided an additional method

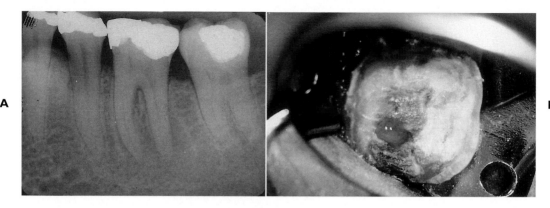

A

B

Fig. 9-7

for pulp tissue removal. Pulps can be routinely removed intact with these instruments (Fig. 9-6, *C*).

To expedite the management of irreversible pulpitis, the following guidelines are recommended. If the tooth is not painful to percussion, a minimum of a pulpotomy is indicated. If the tooth is painful to percussion, a pulpectomy will be necessary along with occlusal adjustment.

Necrotic Pulps

The diagnosis and management of an advanced degenerative or necrotic pulp are often straightforward, since both diagnostic aids and radiographs are quite useful. If the pain can be localized to a particular tooth, the diagnosis is almost complete. However, if the pain is not localized, comparative tests such as thermal tests or the electric pulp test are required, along with radiographic findings that support the diagnosis (see Fig. 9-1). Likewise, the situation becomes more confusing when the pain cannot be localized and multirooted teeth are suspect. In these situations comparative tests are of limited value, since in some cases the pulp may be partially vital and these tests may elicit positive or weakly positive responses. The practitioner must rely heavily on radiographic signs of early periradicular changes (loss of lamina dura, thickening of the periodontal ligament space), size and extent of caries (if radiographically visible), sensitivity to mastication, and previous extensive restorations in the tooth.

Necrotic tissue must always be removed from the pulp chamber. Unlike cases with vital pulp, however, the tissue in the root canals must also be removed—if not totally, then as much as can be removed at the emergency visit. Total pulp space débridement is the ideal treatment for symptomatic teeth with necrotic pulps and can be easily accomplished in anterior teeth and single-rooted posterior teeth with patent canals. In multirooted teeth, total débridement may be more complicated because of root canal anatomy and limitations of canal working length. Also, full instrumentation may be warranted. However, the risk of pushing some necrotic debris past the apical constriction during débridement must be considered. Many authors and practitioners believe that if no necrotic debris is pushed beyond the apex the patient will have less postoperative discomfort.[35] Since the patient is already in pain, it is incumbent on the practitioner to prevent additional pain by maintaining the files 2 to 3 mm from the apex of the roots. Likewise, if the necrotic tissue is considered the major irritant and the source of the patient's discomfort, thorough removal by means of careful cleaning and shaping within the confines of the root along with copious irrigation with sodium hypochlorite (NaOCl) is indicated. Therefore, there are two treatment modalities for the necrotic pulp. Either protocol may be selected; the choice will depend on the practitioner's expertise, the diagnosis, the patient's symptoms, anatomic constraints, and the time available for treatment.

Treatment Plan A

1. Establish proper access to all canals.
2. Irrigate thoroughly with NaOCl.
3. Débride pulp chamber.
4. Débride the coronal and middle portions of the root canal with K-files, Hedström files, or broaches, and use copious NaOCl irrigation, making sure not to penetrate the apical 2 to 3 mm of the canal.

5. Temporarily seal the access opening.

6. Use analgesics as necessary (see discussion of analgesics, p. 250-251).

Treatment Plan B

1. Establish proper access to all canals.

2. Irrigate thoroughly with NaOCl.

3. Débride pulp chamber.

4. Débride the coronal and middle portions of the root canal with K-files, Hedström files, or broaches, and use copious NaOCl irrigation.

5. Carefully place a small file (No. 15 K) 1 mm short of the anticipated working length as determined from a good radiograph.

6. Correct the length as necessary, using radiographs for verification. Be sure not to penetrate the apical constriction.

7. Complete canal cleaning and shaping, taking care not to push apically but applying force to the file on the outstroke to remove debris coronally.

8. Temporarily seal the access opening.

9. Use analgesics as necessary.

CLINICAL PROBLEM: A 44-year-old female patient presents with constant pain in the mandibular left jaw. She cannot isolate the source of the pain that has already begun to radiate to her ear and the back of her neck. Although she had previously had some discomfort in this area, it always went away. Now it is constant and she cannot function with pain medication. Clinical examination reveals restorations in all the posterior teeth. The largest restoration is in the first molar. There are multiple defects in the margins that would indicate some degree of long-term coronal leakage. Percussion and palpation are abnormal on the first molar, with the adjacent teeth also exhibiting some soreness. Sensibility tests are normal for all teeth except the first molar, which does not respond. Radiographically there is a deep restoration in the first molar, and a large radiolucency is evident around the roots (Fig. 9-7, *A*).

Solution: Based on the subjective and objective findings, a diagnosis of pulp necrosis with acute periradicular periodontitis is indicated. Although some might believe that an acute alveolar abscess is present, the pathognomonic signs of such are absent, that is, excessive tooth mobility and elevation of the tooth in its socket. After the coronal restoration was removed because of poor margins and the potential for recurrent decay under the restoration, root canal treatment was initiated. Upon exposure of the pulp chamber, a purulent exudate was evident (Fig. 9-7, *B*). Thorough canal cleaning and shaping was accomplished on this visit. Likewise the restorability of the tooth had been determined along with the elimination of potential avenues of leakage during treatment.

Acute Alveolar Abscess

The acute alveolar abscess poses a particularly difficult problem in treatment and postoperative patient management because of the potential for severe discomfort and swelling after treatment. The diagnosis of an abscessed tooth is probably the least difficult to make, since a radiolucent area is often present on the radiograph. The tooth is mobile or extruded from its socket, the patient cannot touch or chew on the tooth, and swelling is often present intraorally or extraorally, or both. Sinus tracts are not usual with an acute alveolar abscess, since once a sinus tract opens to the oral cavity, the intracortical pressure and swelling decrease and the pain is relieved.[10] However, sinus tracts can periodically open and close, and in the interim periods the patient may be in acute pain.

Treatment of the acute alveolar abscess is essentially no different from treatment of the necrotic pulp, except for managment of the swelling that may be present. Depending on the type of swelling (fluctuant or nonfluctuant, localized or diffuse) and the presence or absence of drainage, the practitioner can decide on the most appropriate treatment. However, since most abscessed teeth have concomitant intraoral or extraoral swellings or both, an understanding of the different types of swellings is necessary before proper treatment can be rendered.

Localized Swelling

Localized swellings associated with abscessed teeth may take a variety of forms (Fig. 9-8). Small loculations of pus can form directly adjacent to the abscessed tooth. In these situations the tooth must be opened and an attempt should be made to establish drainage through the tooth (apical trephination; see also p. 240). Drainage is achieved by placing a No. 15 to 25 K-file 1 to 3 mm through the apex of the tooth. In many instances drainage will begin through one or more canals, and some of the purulence will be eliminated. If the intraoral swelling is small, this treatment will often suffice to alleviate the patient's discomfort. However, if the area adjacent to the tooth is moderately large and fluctuant, incision and drainage should be performed (see p. 238-241). There is no need for antibiotic coverage since the swelling is localized and con-

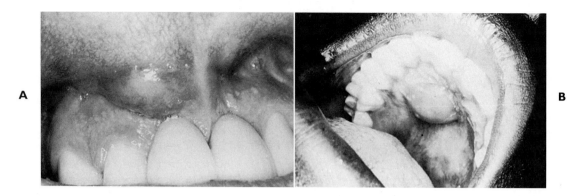

Fig. 9-8 *A, Moderately large-sized purulent loculation adjacent to the central incisor. **B,** Large palatal swelling required immediate drainage.*

fined within the oral cavity. Likewise, if incision and drainage are anticipated, it may behoove the practitioner to fully clean the canal system and seal the tooth before the procedure. This removes all the irritating tissue from the canal and creates a clean environment that can be obturated as soon as the patient is symptom free. This cleaning will not create postoperative problems for the patient because the incision and drainage will relieve any potential inflammatory responses in the periradicular tissues resulting from canal instrumentation. If the canal is not cleaned, it must still be addressed at a future date, with the possibility of pushing debris past the root apex and causing additional pain for the patient.

Diffuse Swelling

Diffuse swelling must be managed aggressively to avoid major complications. Diffuse swelling is defined as generalized tissue edema or cellulitis (Fig. 9-9). Because the swelling is diffuse, there is no indication for incision and drainage, since the purulence is not localized to any one specific area. These patients are in need of both immediate antibiotic coverage (see p. 251) and aggressive removal of any necrotic tissue in the pulp canal system. Often drainage cannot be established through the canals of these teeth, and treatment plan A or B for necrotic pulps is indicated.

Following are guidelines for assessing proper treatment for a localized or diffuse swelling:

1. Tissue swelling fluctuant—drainage through tooth
   a. Open tooth and establish drainage (Fig. 9-10); clean tooth (treatment plan A or B); close tooth.
   b. Incise and drain (see next section).

c. Use hot saline rinses.
2. Tissue swelling fluctuant—no drainage through tooth
   a. Open tooth, no drainage obtained; clean tooth (treatment plan A or B); close tooth.
   b. Incise and drain.
   c. Use hot saline rinses, to be held in the mouth as long as possible.
3. Tissue swelling nonfluctuant—drainage through tooth
   a. Open tooth and establish drainage; clean tooth (treatment plan A or B); close tooth.
   b. Consider antibiotics (see p. 251).
   c. Do not incise and drain.
4. Tissue swelling nonfluctuant—no drainage through tooth
   a. Open tooth, no drainage obtained; clean tooth (treatment plan A or B); close tooth.
   b. Use hot intraoral saline rinse.
   c. Use antibiotic coverage.
   d. Do not incise and drain.

Incision and Drainage

Incision is performed with a No. 11 or 15 scalpel blade and a pair of hemostats. After the appropriate nerve block and local circumferential infiltration of anesthetic solution, a horizontal incision is made in the center of the swelling along its dependent base, to the depth of the bone (Fig. 9-11, *A* and *B*). The maximum amount of purulent debris will be removed if the incision is placed immediately below the crest of the purulence and the incision depth is to bone. In some cases, depending on the anatomy of the swelling, an elliptical or even vertical incision may be indicated to achieve maximum access to the most dependent portion of the swelling (Fig. 9-12).

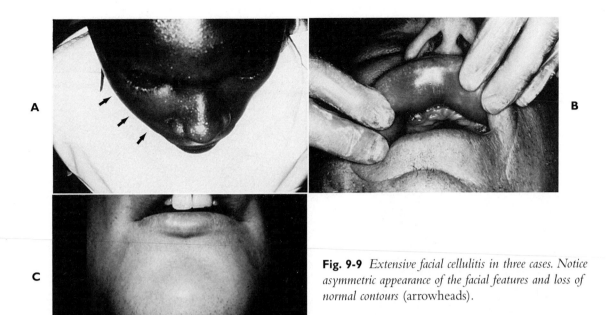

Fig. 9-9 *Extensive facial cellulitis in three cases. Notice asymmetric appearance of the facial features and loss of normal contours (arrowheads).*

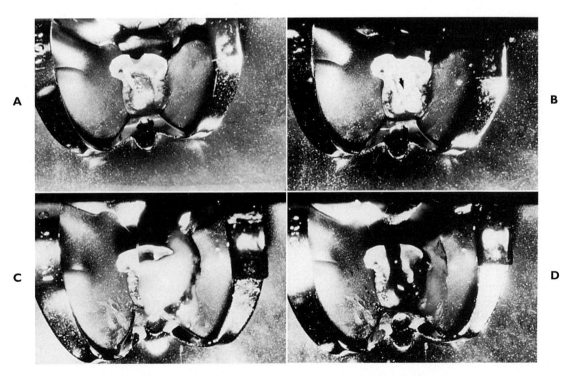

Fig. 9-10 *A, Tooth with severe decay; the patient was symptomatic. B, Initial drainage was purulent (arrowhead). C, Within a short time the rate of drainage increased, and some hemorrhage was noted. D, Eventually the purulence ceased and only hemorrhagic exudate was visible.*

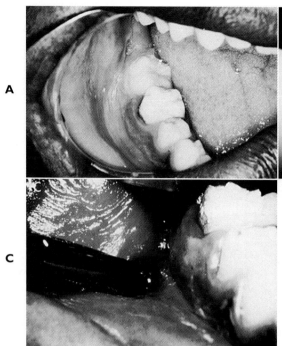

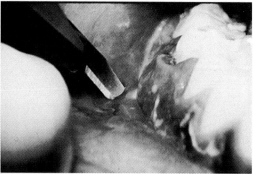

Fig. 9-11 *A, Preoperative view of area to be incised. B, No. 15 scalpel blade is used to make an incision to the depth of bone. C, Closed hemostats are placed into the incision and opened, releasing purulence and hemorrhagic exudate.*

Next, closed hemostats are placed into the incision and opened, thus dislodging loculated areas of purulence (Fig. 9-11, *C*).

In most instances a drain is not necessary, since the incision will remain open for 12 to 24 hours. However, in cases with moderate to severe cellulitis, a drain may be indicated.[21] If placed, it should be secured to prevent it from being either enclosed in the wound or loosened by normal oral forces and dislodged completely from the incision. Sutures may be used if a rubber drain is chosen. If a gauze drain is preferred, the blood clot that forms around the margins of the incision will usually stabilize the drain. Drains should remain in place no longer than 2 to 3 days, after which time the swelling should have abated.

In an attempt to prevent bacteremia, which may occur during the incision and drainage procedure, it has been recommended that the contents of the swelling be removed by needle aspiration before the incision procedure.[16] In many cases this may be appropriate if drainage could not be obtained through the tooth before the surgical procedure, and the swelling has a high degree of fluctuancy.

Trephination: Apical and Surgical

As previously discussed, apical trephination is accomplished by aggressively placing a No. 15 to 25 K-file beyond the confines of the apex. In most cases this will establish drainage. Each case should have radiographic verification of the file position beyond the apex. This procedure can introduce some treatment problems, such as destruction of the natural apical constriction or zipping of the canal at the apex in curved canals (see Chapter 5). However, the benefits of the procedure far outweigh the potential problems. Surgical trephination is rarely needed to manage pain if good principles of diagnosis and treatment are followed. However, it is a reliable procedure to manage intractable pain when all other methods have failed. In all likelihood, the severe pain is caused by an increase in intracortical pressure in the periradicular tissues, which can only be relieved through a surgical opening when apical trephination has failed or cannot be performed.

Surgical trephination involves a soft-tissue incision, cortical penetration with a rotary instrument, and the creation of a pathway for drainage from the periradicular tissues.[21] Three approaches may be considered.

Treatment Option 1
1. Proper anesthesia is obtained.
2. A No. 15 scalpel blade is used to make a small (5 mm) horizontal or vertical incision in the mucosa apical and proximal to the root apex.

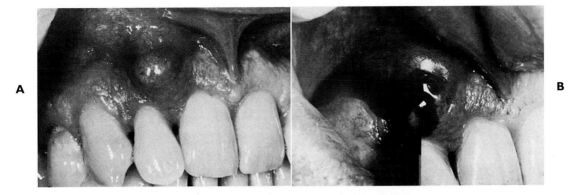

Fig. 9-12 *A, Circumscribed swelling between the lateral and central incisors. **B**, Vertical to curved incision made in the most dependent portion of the swelling. Notice extensive drainage.*

This positioning is critical to avoid penetration into tooth structures.

3. Retract the mucosa with a tissue retractor, periosteal elevator, or the wide end of a sterile No. 7 wax spatula.
4. A No. 6 or 8 round bur is used to penetrate the cortical plate at an angle designed to reach the periradicular tissues or lesion; avoid contact with the root. This approach works well when a large periradicular lesion is present.
5. Immediate drainage for relief of intracortical pressure is usually obtained.
6. The patient is treated with hot saline rinses.

Treatment Option 2

1. Proper anesthesia is obtained.
2. A No. 15 scalpel is used to make a small (5 mm) incision vertically adjacent to the root of the tooth in question (Fig. 9-13, *A* and *B*).
3. Retract the mucosa with a tissue retractor or wide end of a sterile No. 7 wax spatula (Fig. 9-13, *C*).
4. A No. 6 or 8 round bur is used to penetrate the cortical plate only (Fig. 9-13, *D*).
5. A large K-file (No. 40 minimum) is used to bore a path through the cancellous bone to the periradicular tissues or lesion, avoiding contact with the root apex (Fig. 9-13, *E* and *F*).
6. Immediate drainage or relief of intracortical pressure is usually obtained.
7. The patient is treated with hot saline rinses.

More often option 2 is a safer approach, especially if vital structures are adjacent to the tooth in question, if roots are closely approximated, or if the vestibule is shallow. Failure to adhere to these principles can result in destruction of the root structure

and periodontal ligament, with the potential for subsequent external root resorption (see Chapter 10).

Treatment Option 3

An alternative to either of the previous options is to use a large endodontic spreader to penetrate the cortical plate.[14] After the penetration site has been anesthetized, a No. 3 spreader is placed parallel to the root surface with a silicon stop as a reference point. The spreader is then rotated to a point nearly perpendicular to the root apex. Apical pressure is applied as the spreader pierces the alveolar mucosa, periosteum, and cortical bone into the periradicular lesion. The value in this approach is that no incision or surgical flap is necessary, and the chance of damage to the root structure is minimized. However, entry to the lesion may be very difficult in the presence of thick cortical bone.

ANESTHESIA IN THE MANAGEMENT OF TOOTH PAIN

One of the greatest problems in managing pain of tooth origin is inability to provide adequate anesthesia for the patient in distress. With the advent of newer anesthetic devices, much if not all of the discomfort can be eliminated.

Once a diagnosis, in particular of acute pulpal pain, acute periradicular pain, acute alveolar abscess, or cellulitis is made, one of the greatest problems in managing the patient's discomfort is the inability to provide adequate anesthesia. With an understanding of the inflammatory processes involved, a knowledge of the osseous and neural variations of the area to be anesthetized, knowledge of the action of anesthetic solutions, skill in the administration of solution to the target area, and an appreciation for the psychologic make up of the patient,

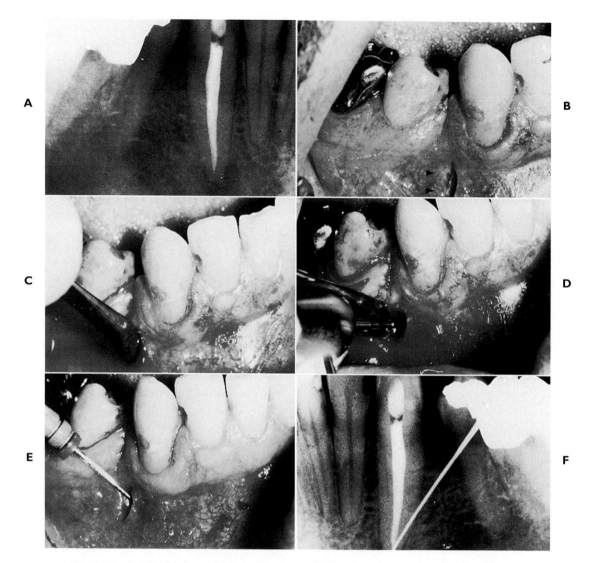

Fig. 9-13 A, *Mandibular canine recently obturated. The patient reported severe pain. No swelling is present but a large radiolucency is visible.* **B,** *Small vertical incision (arrowheads) is made distal to the canine eminence in the midroot portion.* **C,** *Mucosa is retracted with a small tissue retractor.* **D,** *No. 6 round bur is used for initial penetration of the heavy mandibular cortical plate.* **E,** *No. 40 K-file is used to penetrate the cancellous bone to the periradicular lesion.* **F,** *Radiographic verification of the position of the file.*

endodontic emergencies can be efficiently and effectively managed in a problem-solving, painless manner.

Impact of Tissue Inflammation/Infection on Achieving Anesthesia

Pulpal and Periradicular Changes

The normal pulp has a relatively high blood flow that is minimally influenced by vasodilator substances (irritational products). This results in only minor increases in localized blood flow during irritation and inflammation.[25] In this inflamed environment, capillary permeability appears then to be more significant than blood flow, with regard to the inflammatory response of the pulp. This rules out the concept of generalized pulpal edema, despite the low-compliance environment within the tooth. The localized inflamed tissues experience an increase in tissue pressure that results in a focal vascular stasis, ischemia, and tissue necrosis. These focal areas of necrosis serve as additional insults within the pulp, and the subsequent cyclic episodes of inflammation and cellular death result in the incremental, circumferential spread of tissue destruction.[50]

The periodic irregular inflammation and destruction of localized tissue components coupled with bacterial invasion can partially explain the clinical experience of episodic pain. Further explanation for this episodic phenomenon may include neural fluctuations, with cycles of increased nerve fibers and peptide cytochemical alteration followed by decreases, perhaps associated with cycles of intrapulpal abscess expansion and pulpal attempts at repair.[6] Interestingly in this respect, the sprouting of new nerve fibers and alterations in neuropeptides associated with a painful carious attack has been identified.[56] Likewise, sustained, severe pain might be interpreted as multiple areas of tissue simultaneously undergoing demise. In many patients, episodes of severe pain are often followed by the absence of symptoms, indicating pulpal necrosis, or an effective avenue of drainage from the inflammatory process has been obtained.

The inflammatory process of pulpal disease and degeneration is basically the same as elsewhere in the body's connective tissue.[46] When coupled with endodontic procedures, coronal leakage of bacteria and their products from inferior dental restorations, or toxic root canal filling materials, the periradicular tissues will appear variable with regard to inflammation and repair. Histologically the lesion consists predominantly of granulation tissue, exhibiting significant angioblastic activity, many fibroblasts, connective tissue fibers, an inflammatory infiltrate, and often a connective tissue encapsulation.[54] The inflammatory infiltrate consists of plasma cells, lymphocytes, mononuclear phagocytes, and neutrophils. Occasionally cholesterol clefting is seen along with foreign-body giant cells. If, in addition, adjacent strands of epithelium or rests of Malassez have been stimulated by the inflammatory response to form a stratified squamous epithelium–lined cavity filled with fluid or semisolid material, a cyst will be present.

As long as there is an egress of tissue irritants and bacteria from the root canal system, or there is a failure of the phagocytic macrophage system to control this irritation, the histologic pattern of the periradicular lesion will be one of concomitant repair and destruction.[49] Often this variable tissue response is subjected to superimposed inflammatory, infective, or immunologic processes, and patient signs and symptoms will reflect these changes, moving from a chronic clinical state of minimal to no symptoms to an acute state with the complete litany of painful characteristics (see Tables 9-1 and 9-2). It is this environment that the astute practitioner must control with properly chosen and administered anesthetic solutions.

CLINICAL PROBLEM: The presence of old paste fillings in root canals poses a significant problem from the preventive standpoint. The root canals in these teeth have had an interchange of tissue fluids and paste materials for long periods during which the immunologic and inflammatory responses have often struck a balance and the patient is reasonably comfortable. If bacteria are superimposed through coronal leakage or a hematogenous route, or if the contaminated paste materials are suddenly thrust beyond the root apex into the periradicular tissues during retreatment, acute problems often result. Notice that both cases in Fig. 9-14 represent similar situations where this potential is real.

Solution: Management of these cases in the quiescent stage requires a careful coronal removal of the canal contents, without pushing any contaminated material beyond the apex. The crown-down approach or coronal preflaring techniques work quite well in these cases (see Chapter 5). Copious irrigation is essential, along with the cleaning and shaping of the canal within the confines of the root space. Although some clinicians choose to place the patient on nonsteroidal antiinflammatory agents before treatment, others routinely advocate antibiotic coverage. Although the former is reasonable, the latter lacks substantive scientific support and is usually done for the sake of the treating dentist. If the teeth are already in an acute stage, drainage must be obtained if possible along with complete canal space débridement. In these cases, depending on signs and symptoms, antibiotics may be warranted (see discussions on p. 251).

Inflammation and Neural Considerations

The inflammation that accompanies pulpal and periradicular degenerative-infective changes results in a reduced tissue pH over variable areas depending on the extent and acuteness of the process. This has been suggested as the explanation for the difficulty in achieving quality anesthesia because the ability of the weak anesthetic base (pK_a 7.5 to 9) to dissociate is significantly affected.[12] Others have suggested that the inflammation present alters peripheral sensory nerve activity,[43] possibly because of neurodegenerative changes along the inflamed neural element distal from the inflammatory site.[37] Wallace and coworkers[51] have

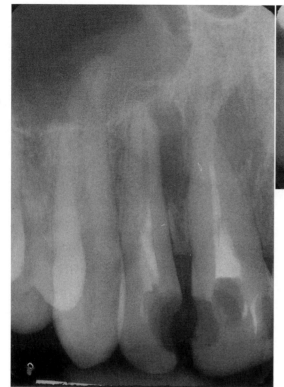

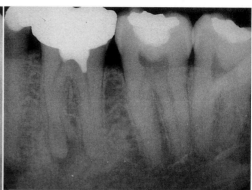

Fig. 9-14

hypothesized that "nerves arising in inflamed tissue have altered resting potentials and excitability thresholds and that these changes are not restricted to the inflamed pulp itself but affect the entire neuron cell membrane in every involved fiber. The nature of these changes is such that the reduction in ion flow and in action potential created by local anesthetic agents is not sufficient to prevent impulse transmission for the reason that the lowered excitability threshold allows transmission even under conditions of 'anesthesia'." As suggested by Wong and Jacobsen,[55] an increase in anesthetic concentration (not necessarily volume) is required to lower the neural action potential when attempting to achieve complete anesthesia in the presence of inflamed tissues. An alternative approach would be to administer the local anesthetic remote from the area of inflammation, such as the use of a regional nerve block whenever possible,[15,39] especially in the case of extensive cellulitis.

Osseous Variations and Aberrant Neural Structures

Variations in the osseous anatomy surrounding tooth roots and aberrant neural structures have received renewed attention as potential impediments to the administration of successful anesthesia. The common variations encountered are discussed relative to the maxilla and mandible, along with the suggested sequence for achieving profound anesthesia in each jaw.

Maxilla

Generally the outer cortical plate of the maxillary bone is thin and sufficiently porous in the adult to make infiltration anesthesia effective. However, in facial or buccal areas of the zygomaticoalveolar crest (Fig. 9-15, *A*) penetration of the anesthetic solution to the middle superior alveolar nerve may be restricted,[38] especially in children.[39] Likewise, the absence of this neural branch has been reported, requiring more extensive placement of the anesthetic solution to manage the first molar and premolars.[23,28]

Anteriorly the prominence of the anterior nasal spine and prominent floor of the piriform aperture (Fig. 9-15, *B*) may preclude approximation of the root apices of the incisor teeth. In the premolar and molar region, the position of the palatal roots relative to the buccal cortical plate may by necessity require the placement of palatal infiltration anesthesia.

Anesthesia for Maxillary Teeth. Providing adequate anesthesia in the maxillary arch is not difficult, and a suggested sequence is found in Table 9-3. Most often the inability to do so cannot

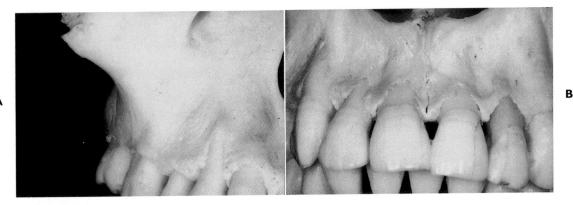

Fig. 9-15 *A,* Anatomic osseous section demonstrating the position of the zygomaticoalveolar crest over the maxillary first molar. *B,* Thickness of bone in the anterior nasal spine and piriform aperture, along with root position may prevent immediate and profound anesthesia in the maxilla.

be attributed to the presence of infection but rather to error in technique and placement of the anesthetic solution. For the patient in pain, maxillary infiltration in the buccal or labial vestibule of one carpule (1.8 cc) is usually sufficient for anterior teeth; however, some maxillary anterior teeth are palatally inclined (lateral incisors, some central incisors, canines), whereas others have palatal roots that must also be anesthetized). These roots are often overlooked after the buccal infiltration, and the patient experiences needless discomfort.

Infiltration on the facial or buccal side *should vary* from the standard approach of depositing the solution near the apex with the needle parallel to the long axis of the root (Fig. 9-16, *A*). Rather an angulated approach directed at the root apex will usually provide a more rapid and accurate diffusion through the bone (Fig. 9-16, *B* and *C*).

Palatal infiltration should be used routinely, especially when the patient is already somewhat hypersensitive.[32] Knowledge of the exact location of the palatal apex with respect to the palatal vault is critical for proper placement of the anesthetic solution and elimination of any painful response. Block anesthesia, such as an infraorbital block, posterior superior alveolar block,[27] or injection into the greater palatine foramen, is considered very good for achieving maximum anesthesia, especially in cases where the patient has minimal discomfort. For additional techniques or variations of those suggested, refer to other expert sources.[32,33]

Mandible

The mandibular foramen is the primary target for the deposition of anesthetic solution for pro-

found anesthesia of the mandibular teeth. Although the position of the foramen is variable, it is usually found anterior to the midpoint of the ramus of the mandible when the anterior border of the mandible is defined as the internal oblique ridge.[36] Studies have identified this position as slightly above the occlusal level of the molar teeth,[5] though Nicholson[36] indicated that it was below the occlusal surface in 75% of the mandibles studied (Fig. 9-17). The importance in this variability cannot be overemphasized for the clinician because the angle and level of needle penetration will have to be reassessed and altered accordingly in many cases in which profound anesthesia is not readily achieved with a standard approach.

Although rare, the potential for extreme variability in the coursing of the mandibular canal has been identified, even to the extent of bifidity.[7,22,24] Conventional attempts at mandibular blocks in these cases may lead to failure. Examination of panoramic views of the mandible are extremely helpful to anticipate variations of this nature, at least two-dimensionally.

Of all the variables that create controversy in achieving profound anesthesia in the mandible, the presence of accessory innervation has received the most attention. These range from the presence of well-defined foramina in the retromolar fossa[7,8,22,26,29] (Fig. 9-18), to the extension to and innervation of both posterior and anterior teeth by branches of the mylohyoid nerve,[17,22,30] to the presence of median symphyseal crossover from branches of the incisive nerve,[18,42,43] to finally the existence of a transverse cervical cutaneous nerve

▼ **Table 9-3** Suggested sequence for maxillary anesthesia

- *Supraperosteal injection:* Infiltration from the facial side with the needle tip in the immediate area of the root apex at an angle of 45 to 90 degrees (Fig. 9-16, *B* and *C*)
- *Palatal injection:* To supplement the facial infiltration when necessary
- *Regional injection or block:* When infiltration fails or extensive infection or swelling is present
- *Periodontal ligament injection:* Often requiring multiple injection sites and may be limited in scope when extensive discomfort is present
- *Intraseptal injection:* Useful when bone is less dense
- *Intraosseous injection:* Requiring osseous penetration with rotary instrument and caution with amount of solution injected; used as adjunct with intrapulpal injection

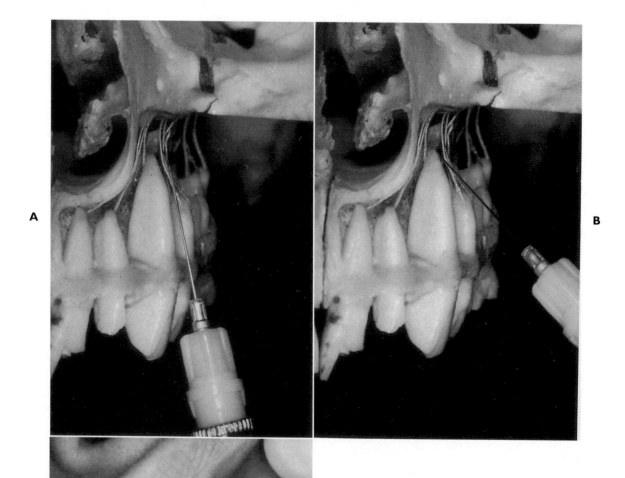

A

B

C

Fig. 9-16 *A, Normal angle and position for the delivery of anesthetic solution to the maxillary teeth. B, Altered approach to enhance the rapid movement of the anesthetic solution to the root apex. C, Clinical demonstration of the altered technique.*

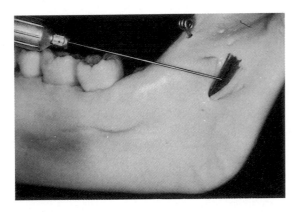

Fig. 9-17 *Angle and position of needle entry for the inferior alveolar block injection.*

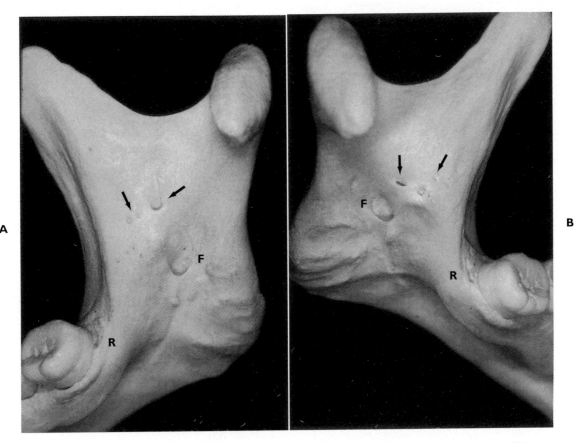

Fig. 9-18 *A and B, Right and left views of the internal surface of the ramus of the mandible. Notice the major foramina (F) for the entry of the inferior alveolar nerve and vessels. The minor foramina (arrows) also can carry branches of the nerve and provide innervation to the mandibular teeth. Likewise small openings in the retromolar region (R) can also carry small innervative branches. All possibilities must be considered when obtaining profound mandibular anesthesia.*

247

▼ **Table 9-4** Suggested sequence for mandibular anesthesia

- *Inferior alveolar injection:* Administered by the traditional method, with the potential variables indicated being taken into account
  - *Gow-Gates injection:* Requires practice to achieve proficiency
  - *Akinosi closed-mouth injection:* Used with limited mandibular opening
- *Buccal infiltration:* For soft-tissue anesthesia
- *Mylohyoid infiltration:* If teeth continue to be inaccessible endodontically
- *Mental foramen infiltration:* If teeth continue to be inaccessible endodontically
- *Periodontal ligament injection:* Often requires multiple injection sites and may be limited in scope when extensive discomfort is present
- *Intraseptal injection:* Useful when bone is less dense
- *Intraosseous injection:* Requires osseous penetration with rotary instrument and caution with amount of solution injected; used as adjunct with intrapulpal injection
- *Intrapulpal injection:* Efficient; administer rapidly

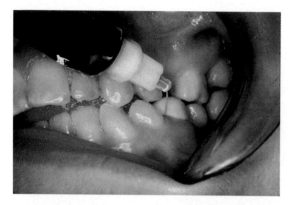

Fig. 9-19 *Placement of a needle for the periodontal ligament injection. The solution is delivered with significant pressure.*

that may intermingle with fibers of the mental nerve or has been suggested actually to enter the mental foramen and course posteriorly, innervating the premolars or molar teeth.[11,38,41,55] Support for this speculated phenomenon is primarily empirical.[9,32,40] A further in-depth discussion of the complexities of mandibular innervation can be found in other treatises.[34,40]

Anesthesia for Mandibular Teeth. The mandibular posterior teeth are perhaps the most difficult to anesthetize adequately. The reasons are multiple and include accessory nerve innervation, inadequately administered mandibular blocks, and lower pain thresholds for inflamed teeth. However, a few basic principles can aid in achieving profound anesthesia. A suggested sequence for administration is found in Table 9-4.

1. Do not infiltrate for the purpose of anesthetizing accessory innervation until the mandibular block has been given and lip signs indicate profound anesthesia.
2. Infiltrate one-third carpule of anesthetic solution around the affected tooth.
3. Use a mental block and/or mylohyoid infiltration with mandibular molars.[32]
4. Do not attempt endodontic treatment until the tooth can undergo percussion (if originally sensitive) or until the stimulus of pain (cold, heat) can be placed on the tooth without discomfort.

> Too often the practitioner fails to wait an adequate amount of time before initiating emergency treatment, and the cold water or air from the turbine causes severe pain for the patient. This lessens the patient's confidence in the practitioner and decreases the patient's pain threshold.

If after these basic principles have been followed adequate anesthesia still has not been achieved, intraligamental injection may be considered[31] (Fig. 9-19). However, with multirooted teeth, intraligamental injections should be placed beside each root for complete anesthesia. This is especially true in molar teeth, where in some cases the distal root is separated from the mesial root by a considerable distance.

If all other techniques fail to provide proper anesthesia, intrapulpal anesthesia can be used. This technique may initially evoke pain until the pulp has been penetrated. Therefore, attention to proper technique is mandatory. To gain entrance to the pulp chamber with the least amount of patient discomfort, a No. 1 or 2 round bur is used in short incremental strokes. The bur is used to cut into the

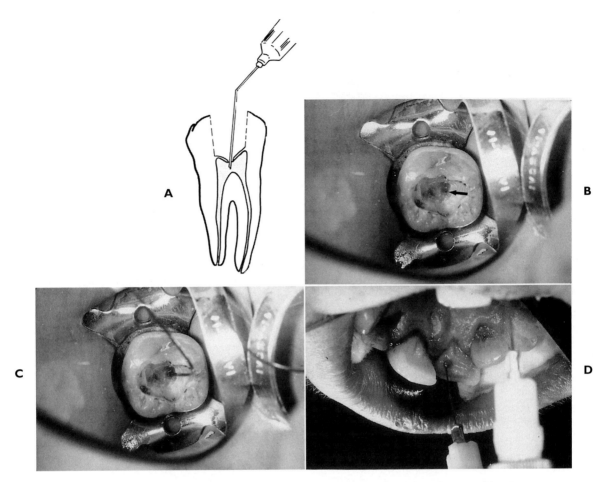

Fig. 9-20 *A, Intrapulpal injection technique. A small opening is made with a round bur into the pulp chamber; then a 30-gauge needle is passed into the pulp chamber as the anesthetic solution is slowly injected. If resistance is met, more pressure is placed on the syringe plunger to force the solution into the pulp chamber.* **B,** *Mandibular molar with small pulp exposure (arrow).* **C,** *Placement of a 30-gauge needle for intrapulpal anesthesia.* **D,** *Use of a needle directly into a pulp exposure immediately after a complicated coronal trauma fracture.*

center of what would normally be the outline of the access-opening preparation, or it is directed to the highest pulp horn. If the bur penetrates only a few tenths of a millimeter at a time into the tooth, severe discomfort is minimized, and access to the pulp is achieved. A 30-gauge needle is passed into the small opening in the roof of the pulp chamber, with the anesthetic agent injected during penetration (Fig. 9-20, *A* to *C*). Often only a few drops of solution are necessary to anesthetize the pulp tissue. It should be noted, however, that the intrapulpal technique may anesthetize only the coronal pulpal tissue. Often the vital tissue in the canals has not been properly anesthetized, and a pulpectomy should not be attempted. In some cases total pulpal

anesthesia can be achieved and the pulp can be removed in its entirety. After complicated crown fractures (see Chapter 11) especially in the presence of soft-tissue swelling, injections can be given directly into the site of the pulp exposure (Fig. 9-20, *D*). Rapid anesthesia is achieved with minimal patient discomfort.

CONSIDERATIONS IN LEAVING TEETH OPEN FOR DRAINAGE

One of the greatest misconceptions in the management of endodontic emergencies is that teeth must be left open for drainage between appointments.

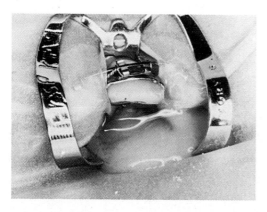

Fig. 9-21 *Maxillary central incisor with extensive drainage upon opening. Even with this amount of drainage, the tooth should be allowed to drain; it should then be measured (if possible), cleaned, and closed.*

In almost every case, regardless of how much purulent material is obtained from the opened tooth, it can usually be dried and safely closed if the etiologic factors have been alleviated (Fig. 9-21).[35] If left open, the tooth will eventually have to be closed, and so there is little if any rationale for leaving the tooth open.[1,2,13] In fact, there are several reasons why the tooth should not be left open for drainage,[45] such as:

1. Additional bacterial contamination
2. Contamination with food debris and blockage of canals
3. The need for unnecessary follow-up appointments to close the tooth

In addition, it is more difficult to close a tooth after it has been left open for several days. Some studies have shown that there may be a positive correlation between the length of time a tooth has been left open (if more than 1 or 2 weeks) and the number of attempts before a closed tooth remains symptom free.[3] However, if a practitioner chooses to leave a tooth open, the following should be considered:

1. Measure the exact working length of the tooth.
2. Completely clean and shape the canals, using copious irrigation (NaOCl).
3. Prescribe vigorous saline rinses to keep the access opening and pulp chamber patent.
4. See the patient within 48 hours, and if the symptoms have abated, isolate the tooth, irrigate copiously with NaOCl, dry the canals with measured paper points, and close the tooth.

This approach will relieve the discomfort, remove the inciting factors within the canal system, minimize the time available for bacteria to colonize in the canals, prevent pushing of debris past the apex before closure, and establish a closed environment as soon as possible. If the patient is still not comfortable after 48 hours, the tooth may be left open an additional day or two. However, if the symptoms have not abated after this time, other etiologic factors have been overlooked and the case must be reassessed to determine the course of treatment.

ANALGESICS

If prescription analgesics are routinely used to manage endodontic emergencies, accurate diagnoses and proper technique may be lacking. For most emergency cases, mild analgesics are sufficient. In fact, if the proper diagnosis is made and treatment is rendered at the emergency visit, analgesics are probably not necessary at all.

Most often a patient will have continued pain after emergency treatment because of improper diagnosis and failure to address the causes of pain or perhaps because new causes of pain have been added by the practitioner, such as overinstrumentation or failure to seal the access opening properly.

With the advent of over-the-counter ibuprofen and other nonsteroidal antiinflammatory agents, most patients do not need prescription drugs. On the other hand, if a prescription analgesic is necessary, the best medications are combination narcotic and antiinflammatory drugs. These may be aspirin-codeine or aspirin–synthetic codeine combination drugs, or a variety of other analgesic-antipyretic narcotic combinations if the patient cannot tolerate aspirin. The use of these medications should be limited to 1 or 2 days postoperatively. If the pain has not subsided significantly by that time, the practitioner should see the patient to assess the nature of the problem.

In situations where a vital pulp (inflamed or noninflamed) has been extirpated and the canals have been instrumented, the patient may experience slight swelling or a swollen sensation after treatment. In these cases the swelling usually is not attributable to an infectious process but to histamine release resulting from inflammation at the root apex.[45] This will usually resolve without the use of any medication, though aspirin or a nonsteroidal antiinflammatory agent may be considered. In rare cases an antihistamine may be prescribed. In cases of acute pain subsequent to vital pulp extirpation, the use of locally placed corticosteroids has been advocated.[53] Although potentially effective, this treatment tends to mask the underlying cause of the pain. In addition, it may alter the necessary inflammatory process required for healing, making the periradicular tissues more susceptible to bacterial and toxin invasion.[45]

> **Therefore the routine use of corticosteroids in this manner is strongly discouraged.**

ANTIBIOTICS

Antibiotics are often misused in the management of endodontic emergencies. At the same time, they have been the saving grace for improper diagnosis and treatment. In general, there are only five dental indications for prescribing antibiotics for the endodontic emergency patient. These indications are:

1. Prophylactic use when medical reasons dictate
2. Diffuse swelling (cellulitis)
3. Lymphadenopathy
4. Fever
5. Avulsion or luxation injuries (see Chapter 10)

> **Pain is not an indication for antibiotic coverage, nor should antibiotics be prescribed for such. Pain before or after an emergency appointment does not necessarily indicate an infection and the need for antibiotic coverage. Antibiotics are not indicated when a diagnosis cannot be determined, or as a panacea for poor technique. Therefore the routine use of antibiotics in endodontic treatment is contraindicated and should be discouraged.**

If the patient is to be given antibiotics, the ideal regimen is penicillin or a derivative thereof (amoxicillin), at least 1 to 2 g stat., followed by 500 mg q6h for 5 to 7 days. If the patient is allergic to penicillin but has taken one of the cephalosporins without an allergic reaction, these may be cautiously prescribed. There is a 10% cross-reactivity to the cephalosporins in penicillin-allergic patients. These drugs should not be prescribed indiscriminately. If the patient must be given some alternative antibiotic regimen, erythromycin is the next drug of choice. For diffuse swelling, a loading dose of 1 to 2 g is recommended, followed by 500 mg q6h. Other considerations include clindamycin 300 mg stat., followed by 150 mg tid for 5 days. Metronida-

zole has also been used in combination with amoxicillin for any stubborn infectious process. Although effective in specific situations, its routine use, however, is discouraged.

Patients taking antibiotics must be closely evaluated at least every 24 to 48 hours and should be told to drink plenty of liquids and to monitor their temperature. Oral antibiotic coverage usually will not demonstrate its effect for at least 24 to 48 hours, and swelling may increase over this latent period. Even though the swelling may not diminish in this time, it is not an indication to change antibiotic coverage. In addition, culture and sensitivity tests may be performed, if possible, with the results available in 2 days. Therefore, changing antibiotic within the first 48 hours of treatment before the laboratory test results become available is contraindicated.

> **Astute attention to the patient's chief complaint, proper gathering of clinical data, and rendering the appropriate treatment to remove the cause will ensure a minimal number of problems in the management of endodontic emergencies.**

References

1. August D: Managing the abscessed tooth: instrument and close? *J Endod* 3:316-318, 1977.
2. Auslander WP: The acute apical abscess, *NY State Dent J* 36:623-630, 1970.
3. Bence R, Meyers R, Knoff R: Evaluation of 5,000 endodontic treatments: incidence of the opened tooth, *Oral Surg Oral Med Oral Pathol* 49:82-84, 1980.
4. Birchfield J, Rosenberg PA: Role of anesthetic solution in intrapulpal anesthesia, *J Endod* 1:26-27, 1975.
5. Bremer G: Measurements of special significance in connection with anesthesia of the inferior alveolar nerve, *Oral Surg Oral Med Oral Pathol* 5:966-988, 1952.
6. Byers MR, Taylor PE, Khayat BG, Kimberly CL: Effects of injury and inflammation on pulpal and periapical nerves. *J Endod* 16:85-91, 1990.
7. Carter RB, Keen EN: The intramandibular course of the inferior alveolar nerve, *J Anat* 108:433-440, 1971.
8. Casey DM: Accessory mandibular canals, *NY State Dent J* 44:232-233, 1978.
9. Chapnick L: Nerve supply to the mandibular dentition: a review, *J Can Dent Assoc* 46:446-448, 1980.
10. Clem WK: Post-treatment endodontic pain, *J Am Dent Assoc* 81:1166-1170, 1970.
11. Cook WA: The cervical plexus and its probable role in the oral operators field, *Dent Items Int* 73:356-361, 1951.
12. deJong RH, Cullen SC: Buffer-demand and pH of local anesthetic solutions containing epinephrine, *Anesthesiology* 24:801, 1963.
13. Dorn S: Treatment of the endodontic emergency: a report based on a questionnaire. Part I. *J Endod* 3:94-100, 1977.

14. Elliott JA, Holcomb JB: Evaluation of a minimally traumatic alveolar trephination procedure to avoid pain, *J Endod* 14:405-407, 1988.

15. Evers H, Haegerstam G: *Introduction to dental local anesthesia,* Fribourg, 1990, Mediglobe, SA, p 91.

16. Flood TR, Samaranayake LP, MacFarlane TW et al: Bacteraemia after incision and drainage of dento-alveolar abscesses, *Br Dent J* 169:51-53, 1990.

17. Frommer J, Mele FA, Monroe CW: The possible role of the mylohoid nerve in mandibular posterior tooth sensation, *J Am Dent Assoc* 85:113-117, 1972.

18. Gardner ED, Gray DJ, O'Rahilly R: *Anatomy: a regional study of human structure,* ed 4, Philadelphia, 1975, Saunders, pp 630-632, 662-673.

19. Grover PS, Lorton L: Bifid mandibular nerve as a possible cause of inadequate anesthesia in the mandible, *J Oral Maxillofac Surg* 41:177-179, 1983.

20. Gutmann JL: Endodontic emergency treatment, *J Calif Dent Inst Contin Educ* 42:3-48, 1992.

21. Gutmann JL, Harrison JW: *Surgical endodontics,* St Louis, IEA [Ishiyaku EuroAmerica] Publishers Inc, 1991, pp 387-396.

22. Haveman CW, Tebo HG: Posterior accessory foramina of the human mandible, *J Prosthet Dent* 35:462-468, 1976.

23. Heaseman PA: Clinical anatomy of the superior alveolar nerves, *Br J Oral Maxillofac Surg* 22:439-447, 1984.

24. Heaseman PA: Variation in the position of the inferior dental canal and its significance to restorative dentistry, *J Dent* 16:36-39, 1988.

25. Heyeraas KJT: Vascular reactions in the dental pulp during inflammation, *Acta Odontol Scand* 4:247-256, 1983.

26. Jablonske NG, Cheng CM, Cheng LC, Cheung HM: Unusual origins of the buccal and mylohyoid nerves, *Oral Surg Oral Med Oral Pathol* 60:487-488, 1985.

27. Loetscher CA, Melton DC, Walton RE: Injection regimen for anesthesia of the maxillary first molar, *J Am Dent Assoc* 117:337-340, 1988.

28. Loetscher CA, Walton RE: Patterns of innervation of the maxillary molar: a dissection study, *Oral Surg Oral Med Oral Pathol* 65:86-90, 1988.

29. Loizeaux AD, Devos BJ: Inferior alveolar nerve anomaly, *J Hawaii Dent Assoc* 12:10-11, 1981.

30. Madeira MC, Percinoto C, Silva MGM: Clinical significance of supplementary innervation of the lower incisor teeth: a dissection study of the mylohyoid nerve, *Oral Surg Oral Med Oral Pathol* 46:608-614, 1978.

31. Malamed SF: The periodontal ligament (PDL) injection: an alternative to the inferior alveolar block, *Oral Surg Oral Med Oral Pathol* 53:117-121, 1982.

32. Malamed SF: The management of pain and anxiety. In Cohen S, Burns R, editors: *Pathways of the pulp,* ed 6, St Louis, Mosby, 1994, pp 612-627.

33. Malamed SF, Trieger NT: Intraoral maxillary nerve block: an anatomical and clinical study. *Anesth Prog* 30:44-48, 1983.

34. Malamed SR: *Handbook of local anesthesia,* ed 3, St Louis, Mosby, 1990.

35. Natkin E: Treatment of endodontic emergencies, *Dent Clin North Am* 18:243-255, 1974.

36. Nicholson ML: A study of the position of the mandibular foramen in the adult human mandible, *Anat Rec* 212:110-112, 1985.

37. Najjar TA: Why can't you achieve adequate regional anesthesia in the presence of infection? *Oral Surg Oral Med Oral Pathol* 44:7-13, 1977.

38. Phillips WH: Anatomic considerations in local anesthesia, *J Oral Surg* 1:112-121, 1943.

39. Quinn CL, Malamed SF: Local anesthetic considerations in dental specialties. In Malamed SF: *Handbook of local anesthesia,* ed 4, Mosby, St Louis, 1997, pp 233-242.

40. Roda RS, Blanton PL: The anatomy of local anesthesia, *Quintessence Int* 25:27-38, 1994.

41. Rood JP: The analgesia and innervation of mandibular teeth, *Br Dent J* 140:237-239, 1976.

42. Rood JP: The nerve supply of the mandibular incisor region, *Br Dent J* 143:227-230, 1976.

43. Rood JP: Some anatomical and physiological causes of failure to achieve mandibular analgesia, *Br J Oral Surg* 15:75-82, 1977-78.

44. Seltzer S, Bender IB: *The Dental Pulp,* ed 3, Philadelphia, JB Lippincott, 1984, pp 373-386.

45. Seltzer S, Naidorf IJ: Flare-ups in endodontics: II. Therapeutic measures, *J Endod* 11:559-567, 1985.

46. Simon JHS: Periapical pathology. In Cohen S, Burns R, editors: *Pathways of the pulp,* ed 6, St Louis, Mosby, 1994.

47. Smulson MH, Hagen JC: Pulpoperiapical pathology and immunologic considerations. In Weine FS: *Endodontic therapy,* ed 5, St Louis, Mosby, 1996.

48. Smulson MH, Sieraski S: Histophysiology and diseases of the dental pulp. In Weine FS, editor: *Endodontic therapy,* ed 5, St Louis, Mosby, 1996.

49. Torabinejad M, Walton RE, Ogilvie AL: Periapical pathosis. In Ingle JI, Taintor JF, editors: *Endodontics,* ed 3, Philadelphia, 1985, Lea & Febiger.

50. Van Hassel HJ: Physiology of the human dental pulp, *Oral Surg Oral Med Oral Pathol* 32:126-134, 1971.

51. Wallace JA, Michanowicz AE, Mundell RD, Wilson EG: A pilot study of the clinical problem of regionally anesthetizing the pulp of an acutely inflamed mandibular molar, *Oral Surg Oral Med Oral Pathol* 59:517-521, 1985.

52. Walton RE, Pashley DH, Dowden WE: Pulp pathosis. In Ingle J, Taintor JF, editors: *Endodontics,* ed 3, Philadelphia, 1985, Lea & Febiger.

53. Weine FS: *Endodontic therapy,* ed 5, St Louis, 1989, Mosby.

54. Weiner S, McKinney R, Walton R: Characterization of the periapical surgical specimen, *Oral Surg Oral Med Oral Pathol* 53:293-302, 1982.

55. Wong MKS, Jacobsen PL: Reasons for local anesthesia failures, *J Am Dent Assoc* 123:69-73, 1992.

56. Yamaura Y: Immunohistochemical investigation on the nerve fibers of the dental pulp after cavity preparation, *Jpn J Conserv Dent* 30:824-838, 1987.

Problems in the Management of Tooth Resorption

Eric J. Hovland
Thom C. Dumsha

"I have seen resorption of apical cementum progressing, with such attending conditions, while on the opposite surface of the same root there was a marked hyperplasia of cementum. In fact, it seems quite common to find these processes going on at the same time."[*]

Tooth resorption is a perplexing problem for all dental practitioners. The etiologic factors are vague, diagnoses are educated guesses, and often the chosen treatment does not prevent the rapid disappearance of the calcified dental tissues. Although the occurrence of resorption cannot always be predicted, resorption can be identified radiographically. However, even this diagnostic tool has limitations because resorption on the buccal or lingual surface of the tooth usually cannot be discerned until 20% to 40% of the tooth structure has been demineralized.[1] The diagnostic dilemma is further compounded by the need to differentiate internal resorption (resorption initiated within the pulp tissue) from external resorption (resorption initiated in the periodontium). Since the etiologic factors, diagnosis, treatment, and prognosis differ for these various types of resorptive defects, the practitioner must be able to diagnose resorption radiographically or clinically, distinguish internal from external resorption, and commence appropriate treatment to halt the resorptive processes. This chapter examines ways to prevent, identify, and manage problems associated with tooth resorption.

*From Blayney JR: *Dent Items Int* 49:681-708, 1927.

INTERNAL RESORPTION

Internal resorption is initiated within the pulp chamber or root canal of the tooth (Fig. 10-1). Although the predisposing factors are unknown, the process appears to be associated with pulpal inflammation[55] and the presence of bacteria.[58, 63] It has been postulated that internal resorption is sustained by infection of necrotic pulp tissue coronal to the area where the resorption is occurring.[59] The byproducts of the necrotic pulpal tissue reach the resorbing area through the dentinal tubules. It is further theorized that this communication requires a special and unusual tubule route to lead from an area of infected necrotic tissue to vital tissue and may explain why internal resorption is rare.[59] Internal resorption of dentin is preceded by disappearance of the odontoblastic layer of cells, followed by an invasion of macrophage-like dentin-resorbing cells.[33] The inflammation and subsequent resorption can result from trauma,[53] partial pulp removal,[45] caries,[36] pulp capping with calcium hydroxide,[18] or a cracked tooth.[61]

> **Internal resorption is usually asymptomatic and is discovered on routine radiographic evaluation.**

The resorptive process may progress slowly, rapidly, or intermittently, with periods of activity and inactivity. Since it is difficult to determine the rate of activity, treatment must be initiated immediately after the diagnosis has been made. If the

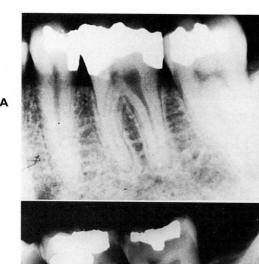

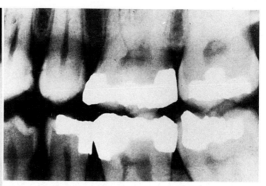

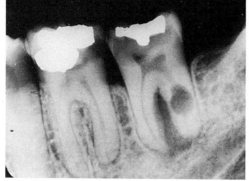

Fig. 10-1 *A, Internal resorptive defect at orifice of distal canal of mandibular molar. **B,** Bite-wing radiograph demonstrating mesial extent and size of defect. **C,** Internal resorption in middle third of distal root of mandibular molar. Notice size and shape of defect and extensive carious involvement.*

resorption continues, it will most likely result in perforation of the tooth wall. Management consists of removing the pulpal tissue, followed by root canal treatment. The prognosis is excellent once the inflamed tissue has been removed. There are, however, problems that may be encountered in the diagnosis and management of internal resorption; these are considered below.

Identification and Differentiation: Radiographic Analysis

Initially, internal resorption must be differentiated from external resorption. The key diagnostic tool is a good radiograph (often a combination of periradicular and bite-wing films are appropriate). The differential radiographic guidelines are as follows[27]:

1. The margins of the internal resorptive defect are smooth and well defined; by contrast, the margins of an external resorption are rough, vary in density, and have a "moth-eaten" appearance (Fig. 10-2).
2. Most internal resorptive defects are symmetrical, though they may be eccentric. External resorptive defects are usually asymmetrical.
3. The anatomic configuration of the root canal is altered and increases in size with internal resorption. In external resorption the canal is

unaltered, and its outline can be followed through the resorptive defect (Fig. 10-3), unless the resorption is deep and has extensively invaded the canal.

4. Radiographs exposed at different horizontal beam angles can aid in distinguishing internal from external resorption. If the defect is internal, the relationship of the canal to the defect will remain the same, regardless of the angle. If the defect is external, the relationship of the defect to the canal will shift as the horizontal angle of the beam is altered. This difference exists because the internal resorptive defect is an expansion of the canal, whereas external resorption is separate and is often superficial on the root surface, lateral to the canal.

CLINICAL PROBLEM: A 60-year-old homeless male presents to the dental school for treatment. During the initial examination a large resorptive defect is identified in the area of the apical third of the root of the maxillary right central incisor (Fig. 10-4, *A*). There is also a large periapical radiolucency. The resorptive defect is symmetrical and appears to have smooth walls, which suggest internal resorption. However, the main root canal

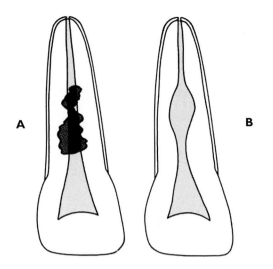

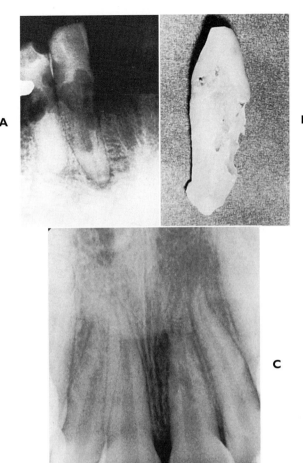

Fig. 10-2 *Radiographic characteristics of external,* ***A,*** *and internal,* ***B,*** *resorption. Notice irregularity of external resorption versus the smooth, symmetric outline of internal resorption.*

appears visible through the defect, which suggests external resorption.

Solution: To determine the diagnosis of external or internal resorption, a second radiograph was taken (Fig. 10-4, *B*). The tooth was exposed from a more severe distal angle. The resorptive defect remained stable in its relationship to the root canal which indicates it is internal resorption rather than external. If the defect had moved in relationship to the root canal, it would have indicated external resorption. Root canal treatment, using techniques that enhance débridement and three-dimensional obturation are indicated to manage this tooth (see Chapters 5 and 6).

Management: Pulp Removal and Canal Preparation

Removal of all the inflamed tissue in the resorptive defect can sometimes be difficult. Since it may not be possible to use routine filing techniques for cleaning and shaping the root canal in the resorbed areas, chemical agents[36,58] or ultrasonic cleaning[57] must be used.

Initially, copious irrigation with 5.25% sodium hypochlorite (NaOCl) should be used to loosen and dissolve attached pulpal remnants in areas of the resorptive defect inaccessible to filing procedures. NaOCl is a strong antimicrobial agent, an excellent solvent of necrotic tissue, and the most effective endodontic irrigant for removing pulpal debris from the root canal system.[35]

Fig. 10-3 ***A,*** *Mandibular canine with severe external resorption. Canal can be followed through the tooth.* ***B,*** *Extracted tooth. There is significant irregular loss of tooth structure.* ***C,*** *Maxillary left central incisor with external resorption. The resorption is irregular and the canal can be followed through the resorptive defect.*

Ultrasonic instrumentation coupled with high-volume flushing can also be effective in cleaning the resorbed areas. The cavitation effect of scrubbing and dislodging inaccessible debris, along with the bactericidal effects of the NaOCl, promotes optimal cleaning of the resorbed areas.[44] The coronal access to the root canal may have to be modified or enlarged to allow greater penetration of the NaOCl (see Chapter 3). Failure to do so may leave vital tissue remnants or necrotic tissue debris, which may interfere with the subsequent root canal treatment. Should these tissue remnants

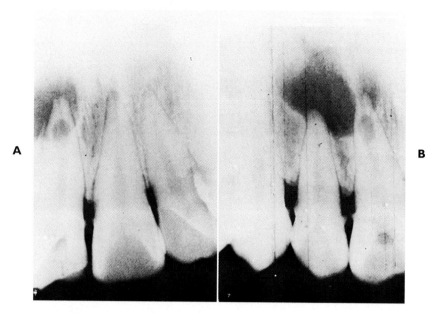

Fig. 10-4

persist or be difficult to remove mechanically at the first visit, an interim calcium hydroxide dressing may be placed after the initial canal cleaning.[58] At the next visit the calcium hydroxide and tissue debris are flushed from the canal, and obturation proceeds as described in the next section.

Management: Canal Obturation

Because of the size, irregularity, and inaccessibility of internal resorptive defects, obturation of the canal may be technically difficult. If the resorptive defect is sufficiently coronal to the apex, the portion of the canal apical to the resorption can be obturated with a solid core of gutta-percha and any of the available techniques (see Chapter 6). The resorptive area, however, must be filled with a material that will flow into the irregularities of the defect. Obturation techniques such as vertical compaction with warm gutta-percha, thermoplasticized gutta-percha, or pressure syringe injection are indicated (Fig. 10-5). If the defect is moderate in size, these techniques will fill the void completely; however, if the defect is large, greater compaction pressures may be required during obturation to fill the resorbed area satisfactorily. If the resorption is located entirely within sound tooth structure, this approach is straightforward and effective.

In cases of expansive internal resorption in which a perforation or near-perforation of the tooth wall exists, excessive vertical or lateral forces must be avoided during compaction to prevent the extrusion of filling material into the periodontium. In these cases the use of a calcium hydroxide–based root canal sealer (Sealapex, Kerr Manufacturing Co., Romulus, Mich.; Calciobiotic Root Canal Sealer, Hygenic Corp, Akron, Ohio) should be considered in conjunction with the gutta-percha filling material. Calcium hydroxide has the potential to stimulate an osseous reparative response, should a perforation in the root wall become evident subsequent to obturation.

Perforating Internal Resorption

When internal resorption has progressed through the tooth into the periodontium, the practitioner is faced with the additional problems of periodontal inflammation, bleeding, and difficulty in obturating the canal. The presence of a perforation cannot always be determined radiographically unless a lateral radicular lesion is found adjacent to the resorptive defect (Fig. 10-6). Clinically, there will usually be continued hemorrhage in the canal after all the pulp has been removed. In addition, when the canal is dried with paper points, hemorrhage may be visible only at the point of perforation. In some cases of long-standing perforation, a sinus tract may be evident on the oral mucosa adjacent to the defect.

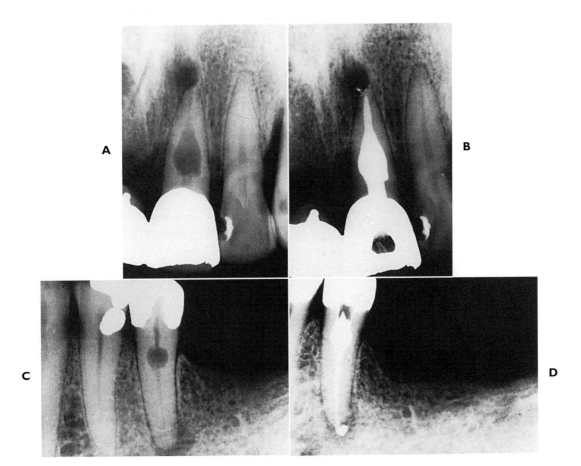

Fig. 10-5 *A, Preoperative radiograph of large internal resorptive defect in midroot of a maxillary central incisor. B, Postoperative radiograph of same tooth. Canal was obturated with warm gutta-percha. C, Mandibular second premolar with internal resorptive defect. D, Postoperative radiograph of same tooth. Canal was obturated using the vertical condensation technique in the coronal third. The canal orifice has been greatly enlarged to accommodate this obturation technique.*

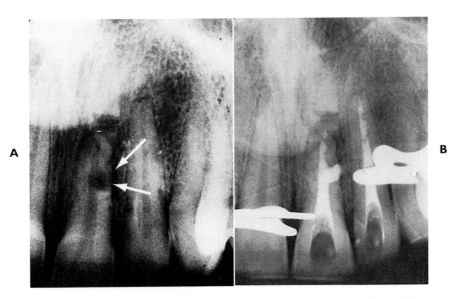

Fig. 10-6 *A, Internal resorptive defect in a maxillary central incisor. Notice the radiolucent semicircle (arrows) in the periodontium adjacent to the defect, indicating a perforation. B, Obturation with calcium hydroxide shows extruded material into the periodontium, confirming the perforating internal resorption.*

A clinical tool to enhance the radiographic detection of perforation is the placement of a highly radiopaque calcium hydroxide–barium sulfate paste in the root canal. If a perforation exists, the paste will move into the periodontal ligament at the point of perforation and will be visible radiographically.[25] Conveniently, this method of diagnosis is also the method of treatment and is accomplished as described below.

Nonsurgical Repair

In cases of minimal internal resorptive perforation, the placement of calcium hydroxide paste into the canal may stimulate periodontal repair and result in sufficient osseous tissue regeneration to allow a subsequent permanent root canal obturation.[26] Calcium hydroxide powder is mixed with a sterile solution, either saline or anesthetic, until it has a puttylike consistency. Since calcium hydroxide has approximately the same radiodensity as dentin, one part of barium sulfate is added to four parts of calcium hydroxide to enhance the radiographic appearance of the mixture. The paste is placed in an amalgam plugger, carried to the tooth, and condensed into the canal with a vertical condensing plugger, gutta-percha cone, large paper point, lentula, or McSpadden condenser.[23,40] A fortified zinc oxide–eugenol cement, such as IRM (L.D. Caulk, Milford, Del.), composite resin, or amalgam restoration is placed to prevent interappointment leakage. The patient is recalled approximately 8 weeks later for evaluation and replacement of the calcium hydroxide paste. Three-month recall visits are scheduled until there is radiographic or clinical evidence of a hard-tissue barrier at the perforation site. The canal is then obturated with gutta-percha and root canal sealer, and a permanent restoration is placed.

During obturation of the canal system subsequent to perforation repair, the use of a root canal sealer containing calcium hydroxide should be considered to enhance the apposition of calcified tissue.

The reparative tissue barrier that forms is usually incomplete, exhibiting voids or porosity,[28,31] hence the need to stimulate further healing. The nonsurgical management of perforating internal resorption with calcium hydroxide should be attempted only if the defect is not extensive, if the defect is apical to the epithelial attachment (since exposure of the defect to salivary contaminants will result in failure), and if hemorrhage in the canal can be controlled.[20]

Surgical Repair

If calcium hydroxide treatment is unsuccessful or not feasible, surgical repair of the defect may be considered.[20] The defect is exposed with a full mucoperiosteal flap to allow good access to and good vision of the entire root.[30] The resorptive defect is curetted, cleaned, and restored with an alloy, or, if aesthetics dictate, a composite resin or glass ionomer restoration. The root canal must be obturated before the procedure (Fig. 10-7). If that is not possible, a silver or gutta-percha cone may be temporarily placed in the canal before the defect is filled. This keeps the external filling from blocking the canal and provides an internal matrix onto which the external filling can be condensed.

Surgical repair is possible only if there is adequate access to the resorptive area.

If the resorption is extensive or occurs on the proximal or lingual surfaces of the root, surgical repair is often impossible, and the tooth may have to be extracted, resected (if multirooted), extruded (see Chapter 8), or intentionally replanted.[19]

Root and Tooth Resection

If the resorbed area is located in the radicular third, the root may be resected coronally to the defect and the apical segment is removed. If one root of a multirooted tooth is affected, root or tooth resection may be considered based upon anatomic, periodontal, and restorative parameters (see Chapter 8).

Intentional Replantation

If perforating resorption with minimal root damage occurs in an inaccessible area, intentional replantation may be considered if all other options short of extraction are unfeasible.

CLINICAL PROBLEM: A 53-year-old male patient presents with a complaint of pain and bleeding in the gingiva when brushing in the area of the mandibular right first molar. Periodontal probings revealed a 5 mm horizontal probing directly into the buccal root of the first molar (Fig. 10-8, *A*). A bitewing radiograph reveals a radiolucent area mesial to the pulp chamber (Fig. 10-8, *B, arrow*). A working diagnosis of perforating internal-external resorption was made.

Solution: A surgical tissue flap was reflected and substantiated that there was a resorptive defect that reached to the pulp chamber from the external surface of the mesial root (Fig. 10-8, *C*). The defect was cleaned, and osseous recontouring was performed (for crown lengthening see Chapter 8)

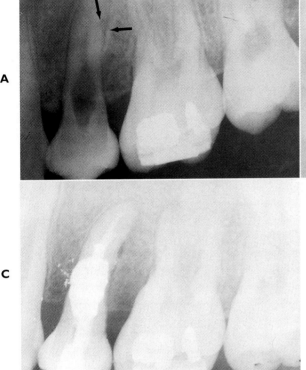

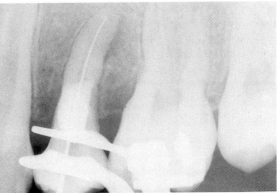

Fig. 10-7 A, *Significant perforating internal resorption in the cervical third of a maxillary second premolar. Notice also the presence of a lateral defect on the distal of the root in the apical third (arrows). This is either an external resorptive defect or a large lateral canal.* **B,** *Defect was temporarily sealed while the root canal treatment was completed.* **C,** *Root canal was obturated. Notice the large lateral canal exiting in the apical third. The resorptive defect was sealed with amalgam. The patient is symptom free.*

(Fig. 10-8, *D*). A pulpectomy was performed during the surgical procedure, a silver cone was placed into the mesiobuccal canal to protect the canal space (Fig. 10-8, *E*), and an amalgam was placed into the resorptive defect from the buccal (Fig. 10-8, *F, arrows*). The soft tissue was replaced and sutured (Fig. 10-8, *G*). Root canal treatment was begun within 10 days after the surgery, and the case was obturated with gutta-percha and sealer (Fig. 10-8, *H, I*). The patient presented for a 2-year recall and was symptom free and without evidence of periodontal disease or periapical pathosis (Fig. 10-8, *J*). Recognition of this type of defect and treatment before or during the root canal treatment is essential for overall success.

EXTERNAL RESORPTION

External resorption is initiated in the periodontium and often results in significant loss of hard tooth structure. Histologically it is characterized by a scalloped border along the root surface with the hard-tissue lacunae lined with osteoclasts. Radiographically the defect has a rough, asymmetrical, moth-eaten appearance. The outlines of the root canal anatomy are generally intact. The differentia-tion from internal resorption is based primarily on the radiographic appearance.

External root resorption can result from a variety of causes:

1. Traumatic damage to teeth
2. Periradicular inflammation
3. Excessive forces during orthodontic movement
4. Conditions associated with impacted teeth
5. Bleaching of nonvital teeth

Each of these causes poses unique problems in prevention, identification, and management.

Traumatic Damage to Teeth

> **External root resorption is a common and serious complication subsequent to avulsion or luxation injuries.**

Avulsion injuries

An avulsed tooth is one that has been completely displaced from its alveolar socket. Since varying degrees of external resorption will most likely affect all avulsed teeth,[6] the major problems are to prevent, limit, or reverse the resulting resorptive process. In these cases, two major clinical types

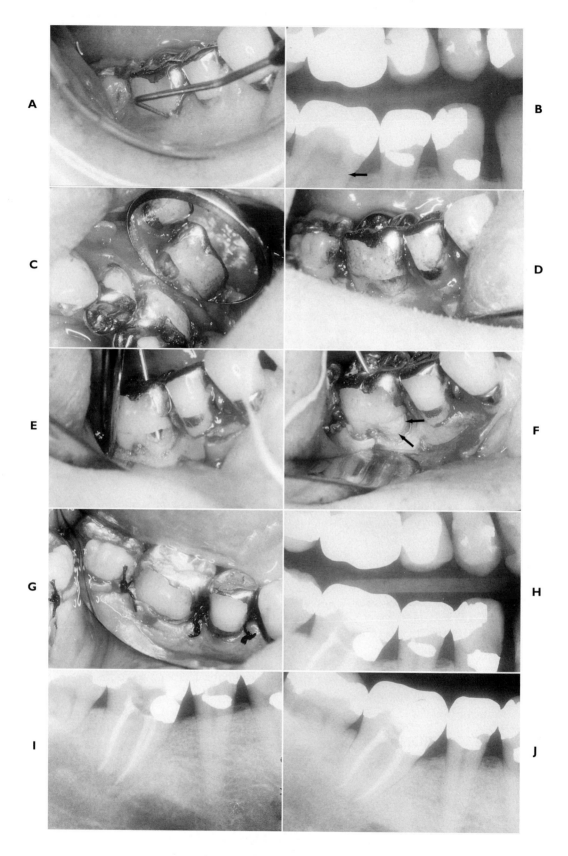

Fig. 10-8

of external resorption—replacement and inflammatory—are particularly problematic.

Replacement Resorption. Replacement resorption, or ankylosis, is characterized by osseous ingrowth into the resorbed areas of the root (Fig. 10-9). Replacement resorption may be progressive, in which case the entire root is eventually lost (Fig. 10-10), or transient, in which case bone-filled areas are later remodeled and resorbed by cells in the adjacent normal periodontium. In most cases, regardless of treatment rendered, progressive replacement root resorption results in eventual tooth loss. Therefore, it is essential that every effort be made to preserve the periodontal ligament and thus halt or limit the resorptive process. This is best accomplished by preserving the periodontal ligament cells and fibers.

CLINICAL PROBLEM: A radiograph reveals minor external resorption associated with a maxillary left central incisor that had previous root canal treatment (Fig. 10-11, *arrows*). The patient's history revealed that the tooth was avulsed 2 years previously and replanted by a dentist 45 minutes later. The root canal treatment was subsequently completed on the 36-year-old patient. The patient still has a temporary filling in the access opening.

Solution: First, the temporary restoration must be replaced with a permanent restoration to prevent potential leakage. Some authorities would suggest that the root canal be retreated because of the high incidence of potential coronal leakage over time through temporary fillings. The resorption that is occurring is the replacement type subsequent to the avulsion injury. Since there does not appear to be active inflammatory resorption, the coronal seal is probably still intact. There is neither a cure nor a treatment for replacement resorption. Since the patient is older (36 years), the resorption will most likely be slow and occur over decades. Younger patients demonstrate a much greater rate of resorption. The following factors, crucial to the management of traumatic avulsion injuries, have a direct influence on the viability of the cells and fibers in question.

The interval from injury to replacement of the tooth is a major factor in the maintenance of ligament viability and subsequent root resorption.

Time. Teeth replanted within 30 minutes have been reported to exhibit root resorption in only 10% of cases, whereas 95% of teeth replanted after 2 hours show root resorption.[13] Teeth replanted as soon as possible, particularly at the time of injury, or those that receive immediate professional care will have the best prognosis.

If the tooth cannot be immediately replanted, proper storage of the tooth can favorably influence periodontal ligament viability.

Storage Medium. Although additional research is needed, the preferred storage media for maintaining the viability of periodontal cells and fibers seem to be saliva,[5] physiologic saline,[5] milk,[17,51] or Hanks balanced salt solution.[37] The most recent literature regarding storage media suggest that Hanks and milk are probably least damaging to the periodontal ligament cells present on the root surface. Maintaining the tooth in these media will mitigate some of the problems encountered when there is a delay in replantation. On the other hand, the root that is allowed to dry will show the maximum amount of resorption.[15] If saline is not available, tap water, though not so effective as the other media in preserving the viability of the cells and fibers, is preferable to dry storage. In addition, rinsing for 10 seconds in tap water, as well as storage in saline, appears to dilute or wash out some of the autolytic enzymes and toxic material from degenerating tissue and bacteria.[7,15] If the tooth will be out of the socket for an extended period of time (longer than 2 hours), milk appears to be the ideal storage medium for long-term preservation of cells and fibers.[17]

Tooth Socket. Preserving the viability of the periodontal cells and fibers in the alveolar socket as well as on the root surface is an important aspect for preventing resorption.[48] Therefore the socket lining must be protected and should not be damaged by curettage or forceful replantation. If the alveolar socket has been fractured, progressive replacement resorption is almost a certainty.[8]

Stabilization. The length of time a splint is in place[2] and the rigidity of the splint[2] have been shown to influence the occurrence of replacement resorption. Excessive splint time or rigidity does not allow functional stimulation of the periodontal ligament, which prevents remodeling of the initial ankylosis after trauma and its repair with cemental replacement.[2] For avulsion injuries in which there are no alveolar or root fractures, a splint that allows physiologic movement of the tooth is placed for 7 to 10 days, which will provide the best conditions for preventing progressive root resorption.

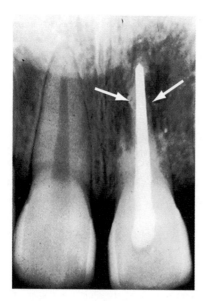

Fig. 10-9 *Maxillary central incisor with replacement resorption subsequent to traumatic injury.*

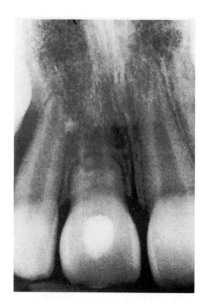

Fig. 10-10 *Maxillary central incisor with severe replacement resorption. Approximately 70% of the root has been replaced with bone.*

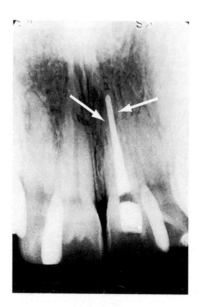

Fig. 10-11

However, in situations where an alveolar or root fracture is present, a rigid splint must be placed for a period of 6 to 8 weeks to prevent tooth movement (see Chapter 11).

Root Surface. Removal of or damage to the periodontal ligament on the root surface will lead to extensive replacement resorption.[14] Large areas of denuded root surface are subjected to excessive osteoclastic action and subsequent osseous replacement. Therefore the root should not be scraped, dried, or manipulated with caustic chemicals. Once replacement resorption has begun it will likely continue until the tooth is lost. There is limited evidence that placing calcium hydroxide in the root canal may retard or eliminate the resorptive process.[62] Short- and long-term evaluation of this phenomenon is necessary before this procedure can be recommended.

Antibiotic Coverage. The administration of antibiotics at the time of replantation has been reported to significantly alter the resorptive process in laboratory animals.[32] (The antibiotics prevented inflammatory resorption while replacement resorption was still present. However, this response is considered more favorable than the rapid loss of tooth structure in inflammatory resorption.) An alteration in the bacterial population appears to be the key issue in controlling both the potential infective and the subsequent inflammatory processes that normally accentuate the resorptive process.

Calcium hydroxide has been advocated for various types of traumatic injuries. It has been the mainstay for treatment of both luxation and avulsion injuries. However, few studies have actually examined its efficacy under laboratory conditions.

Calcium Hydroxide. For the most part it has been convention to utilize this medicament in avulsion injuries and many luxation injures. Andreasen[9-12] examined its efficacy in a human population; however, this was a retrospective study of 400 avulsed teeth. Only one study has examined its ability to control resorption under long-term and controlled laboratory conditions. In this study with monkeys, calcium hydroxide failed to elicit any therapeutic effect on either inflammatory or replacement resorption.[24] Calcium hydroxide will continue to be used based primarily on historical attitudes. Additional research under controlled conditions is highly warranted to determine its true efficacy or lack thereof.

Tooth Management. The American Association of Endodontists has recently published updated guidelines (October, 1995) for treatment of the avulsed tooth. Section V, Endodontic Treatment, of these guidelines is presented:

A. Tooth with open apex (divergent apex) and less than one hour extraoral dry time:
   1. Replant in an attempt to revitalize the pulp.
   2. Recall patient every 3-4 weeks for evidence of pathosis.
   3. If pathosis is noted, thoroughly clean and fill the canal with calcium hydroxide (apexification procedure).
B. Tooth with open apex (divergent apex) and greater than one hour extraoral dry time:
   1. Thoroughly clean and fill canal with calcium hydroxide.
   2. Recall the patient in 6-8 weeks.
   3. Because of poor prognosis, consider alternative treatment options.
C. Tooth with partially to completely closed apex and less than one hour extraoral dry time:
   1. Biomechanically clean the root canal system in 7-14 days.
   2. Medicate the canal with calcium hydroxide for as long as practical, usually 6-12 months.
   3. Then, obturate canal with gutta percha and sealer unless complications are apparent.
D. Tooth with partially to completely closed apex and greater than one hour extraoral dry time:
   1. Perform root canal therapy either intraorally or extraorally.
   2. Before replantation, remove tissue tags from the root surface and soak the tooth in an accepted dental fluoride solution.

After obturating the canal with gutta-percha, the access opening must be sealed with a composite resin, dentin bonding agent, or other suitable permanent restoration to eliminate potential leakage into the root canal.

Inflammatory Resorption. Inflammatory resorption is characterized by bowl-shaped areas of resorption involving both cementum and dentin (Fig. 10-12). The resorbed areas contain multinucleated cells within the inflamed granulation tissue. This type of resorption is rapidly progressive and will continue if treatment is not instituted. In many cases, extensive root resorption is evident after as little as 6 weeks (Fig. 10-13). Development of this type of resorption after replantation is dependent on at least five known factors[4]:
   1. Injury to the periodontal ligament
   2. The initial external resorptive process progressing through the cementum and exposing dentinal tubules
   3. The presence of necrotic, contaminated pulp tissue that communicates with the resorbed areas through the tubules
   4. The possible presence of bacterial contamination on the root surface after replantation
   5. The age and maturation of the tooth

Thus, with inflammatory resorption, the periodontal ligament is damaged, resulting in external root resorption, which then progresses, exposing dentinal tubules. If the pulp is necrotic and the dentinal tubules are both wide and patent, the bacterial and necrotic tissue-breakdown products may leak through the tubules and stimulate extensive osteoclastic activity.[3] This pulpally stimulated resorption will rapidly and irreversibly destroy the tooth. The problem is to prevent and manage this type of resorptive process.

Treatment of Inflammatory Resorption. Since both a necrotic pulp and the presence of bacteria are necessary components of inflammatory resorption, the process can be arrested by immediate root canal treatment. The tooth is opened, and the canal is cleaned and shaped. Although this will inhibit or prevent continued inflammatory resorption, a slower progressive replacement resorption may continue. Also, as previously mentioned, antibiotics may assist in controlling the inflammatory resorptive process. *If the root is completely formed, treatment must be initiated within 1 to 2 weeks after replantation.* Most pulps of replanted teeth with closed apices will become necrotic.[13] Therefore it is good preventive management to remove the tissue before inflammatory resorption begins. The 1- to 2-week delay will give the periodontal ligament time to heal before root canal treatment is begun.[3]

If inflammatory resorption has already become a significant problem, longer term use of calcium hydroxide may be warranted.[60] However, the use of calcium hydroxide in the treatment of resorption in avulsion injuries has recently been questioned.[24]

Since many pulps in teeth with open apices may remain partially vital, it is best to observe these teeth for signs or symptoms of pulpal necrosis or resorption.

Because of the potential for rapid and destructive inflammatory root resorption, periodic recall evaluation is imperative. Wide patent dentinal tubules in immature teeth of young patients serve as direct pathways for leakage of bacterial products to the resorbed tooth surface, which will significantly enhance the resorptive process. Therefore it is recommended that the patient be seen every 3 months, followed by recall evaluation over the next 5 years.

CLINICAL PROBLEM: A 30-year-old male patient was skateboarding when he fell and avulsed his maxillary right central incisor. The patient arrived at your office 45 minutes later with the tooth in a cup of water. A radiograph of the injured area is immediately exposed to see that there is no debris in the socket nor any apparent alveolar fractures (Fig. 10-14, *A*). The prognosis would have been more favorable if the tooth had been stored in milk or saline rather than tap water.

Solution: Time is of the essence to minimize further damage to the periodontal ligament cells of the tooth. The tooth should be handled only by the crown. The root should be briefly rinsed in saline (10 seconds) and immediately replanted. A passive splint is then placed to hold the tooth in position, and the patient is given an appointment for a return visit in 7 to 10 days (Fig. 10-14, *B*). It is critical that the patient return in 7-10 days to have the pulp removed (Fig. 10-14, *C*). Delay in the extirpation can lead to extensive inflammatory root resorption. After extirpation of the pulp and cleaning of the root canal system, the splint is removed and calcium hydroxide is placed. The patient is then given another appointment to complete root canal treatment (see avulsion treatment guidelines).

Luxation Injuries

Luxation injuries may be categorized as follows[8]:
1. Concussion: an injury without abnormal loosening or displacement of the tooth
2. Subluxation: an injury resulting in loosening but not displacement of the tooth (Fig. 10-15)
3. Extrusive luxation: an injury resulting in partial displacement of the tooth from the alveolar socket along its long axis (Fig. 10-16)
4. Lateral luxation: an injury resulting in partial displacement of the tooth from the alveolar socket in a horizontal (mesial, facial, distal, lingual) direction (Fig. 10-17)
5. Intrusive luxation: an injury resulting in displacement of the tooth into the socket (Fig. 10-18).

External resorption is usually not a sequela of concussion or subluxation injuries, occurring in only about 10% of extrusively luxated teeth. Intrusive luxation injuries, however, are followed by replacement resorption in over 50% of cases.[1] It is in these cases that proper treatment is imperative to prevent ankylosis and significant loss of root structure.

Since most (98%) intrusively luxated teeth with closed apices become necrotic,[1] root canal treatment must be instituted as soon as possible after the injury. The canals must be thoroughly cleaned and shaped and calcium hydroxide placed. Root canal treatment can decrease the incidence of inflammatory resorption to a minimum. After 1 to 2 weeks the canal can be permanently obturated with guttapercha. However, because of the traumatic damage to the periodontal ligament, varying degrees of replacement resorption may ensue.

CLINICAL PROBLEM: A 20-year-old male patient presents to your office with an extrusively luxated left maxillary central incisor. The tooth is repositioned, a splint is placed, and the patient has been advised to return in 10 days. Since the tooth has a closed apex, root canal treatment is indicated. After completion of the treatment, the patient inquires about the long-term prognosis for the tooth. The patient's friend told him that root resorption could be a problem.

Solution: Root resorption is rarely a problem with extrusively luxated teeth. Root resorption occurs in less than 10% after the extrusive luxation injury, and if it does occur, it is usually minimal and progresses slowly. The patient should be told that minimal root resorption may occur, but that it is usually not a problem with extrusively luxated teeth.

Periradicular Inflammation

Inflammation arising from chronic pulpal inflammation or the direct contamination of the periradicular tissues through poorly filled root canals or leaking restorations may stimulate cementoclastic and dentinoclastic activity, resulting in the resorption of hard dental tissues (Fig. 10-19). Root canal

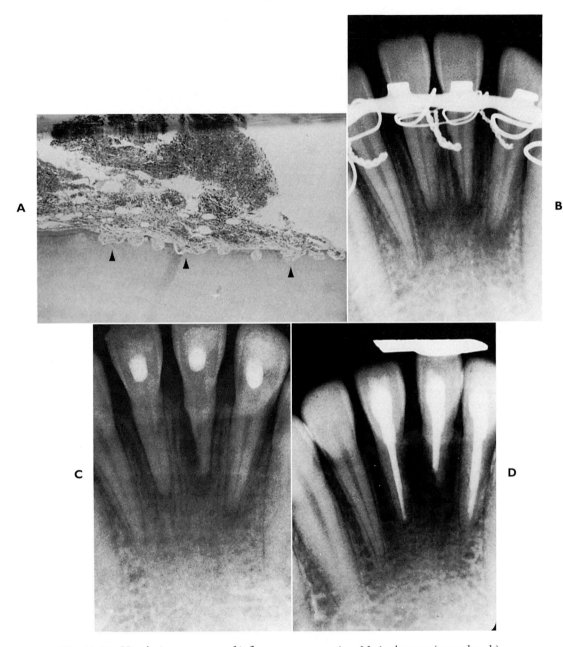

Fig. 10-12 *Histologic appearance of inflammatory resorption. Notice lacunae (arrowheads) filled with clastic cells. (Hematoxylin and eosin, original magnification 40×.)* **B,** *Mandibular incisors subsequent to trauma. Teeth are splinted but necrotic pulps have been removed. Notice the initial inflammatory resorption.* **C,** *Severe inflammatory resorption on mesial aspect of mandibular central incisor immediately before placement of calcium hydroxide.* **D,** *Three-year recall radiograph. Defect has been replaced with osseous tissue.*

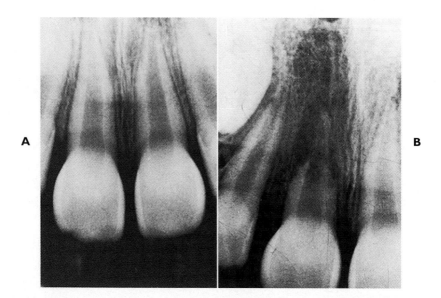

Fig. 10-13 *A, Postoperative radiograph immediately after central incisor was replanted. B, Appearance 6 weeks after replantation. Severe inflammatory resorption has destroyed most of the root.*

débridement, disinfection, and obturation will usually arrest the process; however, the apical resorptive process is uneven and often results in an open apex. This creates a problem in determining the apical extent of canal instrumentation and obturation. In addition, radiographic interpretation of the extent and location of the apical resorption is limited to a two- dimensional view of a three-dimensional process (Fig. 10-20).

Locating the Apical Foramen or Canal Exit

In some situations the radiograph will provide a good depiction of the apical foramen or canal exit, whereas in other cases radiographic interpretation is difficult. The following may provide some clues in determining the location of the canal exit into the periodontal tissues when apical resorption is present.

1. Carefully examine the root canal on the radiograph to determine if it remains intact through the resorbed area. If it appears unaltered, it is more likely that the resorbed area has not exposed a large portion of the canal. If altered, the canal probably leaves coronally to the affected area.

2. Paper points can be used to determine the canal exit. The practitioner observes the position of dampness or hemorrhage on the tip of the point. If the canal is dry, the point will become moistened by tissue fluids, blood, or pus when it reaches inflamed periradicular tissues. This procedure, however, may be inac- curate because of fluid in the canal or lack of fluid in the periradicular tissues. The technique is more reliable if it is performed after the canal has been debrided, flushed, and dried in the previous appointment.

3. The use of an electronic apex locator may be of value when the exit or foramen is not excessively large. However, apex locators are unreliable in teeth with large open apices, or in the presence of blood, pus, or other fluids. When apical resorption is present, the best results are obtained in a dry canal and using a file that fits snugly in the apical portion of the canal.

4. The practitioner may have to rely on experience, tactile sensation, and judgment in estimating the position of the apical foramen. If the foramen cannot be determined, it is usually wise to obturate short of the resorbed area rather than risk extruding excess cement and gutta-percha into the periodontium.

5. Refer to Chapter 5 for the discussion on instrumentation past the apex and loss of apical constriction, as management of the apically resorbed root is quite similar.

Sealing the Irregular Resorbed Apex

1. The key to complete obturation of the irregular apex is to establish a dentin matrix or apical stop against which to condense the gutta-percha. If the apical opening is not ex-

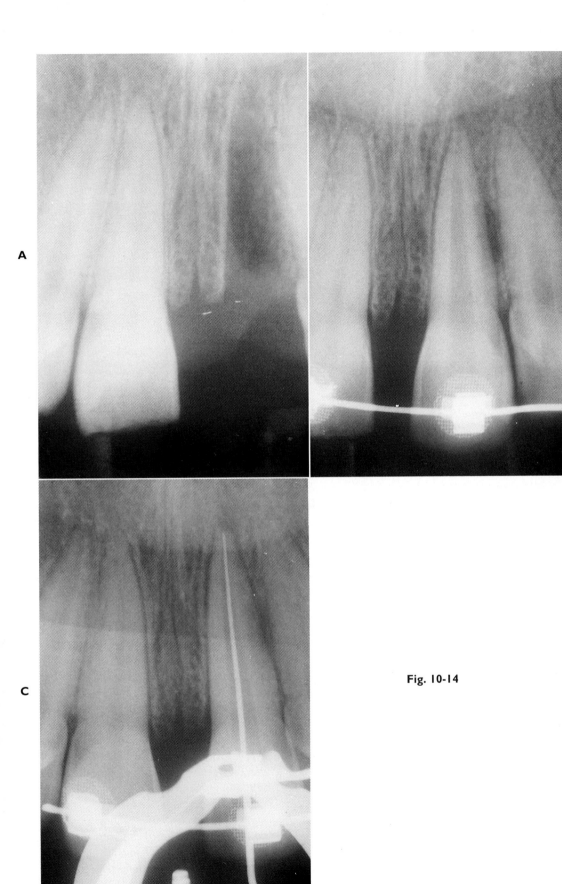

Fig. 10-14

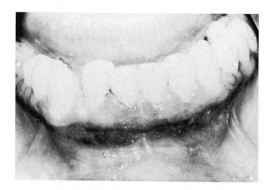

Fig. 10-15 *Subluxation of mandibular central incisor. Note hemorrhagic exudate in sulcus.*

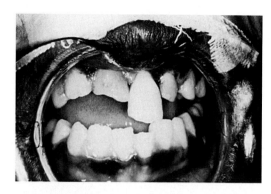

Fig. 10-16 *Extrusive luxation of maxillary central incisor. Notice degree of displacement.*

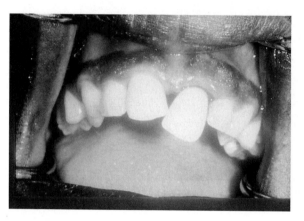

Fig. 10-17 *Lateral luxation of maxillary left central incisor.*

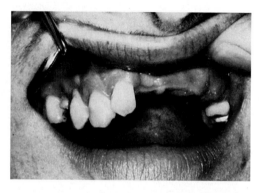

Fig. 10-18 *Intrusive luxation of maxillary lateral incisor 3 months after trauma. The tooth did not reerupt into a normal occlusal position.*

cessively large, a stop or apical dentin matrix can be created by stepping back 1 to 2 mm from the apical foramen and instrumenting to a size approximately two to three file sizes greater than the apical opening. The gutta-percha is fit to and condensed against this stop.

2. If the open apex is excessively large or irregular, a master cone of gutta-percha is custom fabricated and adapted against the apical barrier or constriction.[16,50] Do this by dipping the apical portion of a snugly fit master cone into methylchloroform, eucalyptol, or hot water to soften the gutta-percha (see Chapter 6). The softened cone is then placed to the apical stop and moved up and down several times in the canal to conform to the canal anatomy. It is wise to do this in a moist canal containing the endodontic irrigant. It prevents adherence of the softened cone to the walls of the canal and serves to limit the softening action of the chemical solvent. Once the cone is removed,

let it dry, coat it with root canal sealer (again, consider a calcium hydroxide–based sealer), place in the canal, and carefully condense with lateral or vertical compaction.

3. If neither of the previous techniques is possible, it may be necessary to establish a calcified tissue barrier at the apex before obturation. This is best accomplished by cleaning and shaping the canal and placing calcium hydroxide to the determined canal length. Replace the calcium hydroxide approximately every 3 months until a calcified apical stop is demonstrated either radiographically or clinically. Subsequently the root canal is obturated with gutta-percha and sealer. Recent studies have reported favorable healing of the periradicular tissues after the placement of a calcium hydroxide plug.[52] In addition, enhanced apical sealing has been noted when an apical plug of calcium hydroxide has been used before root canal obturation.[64]

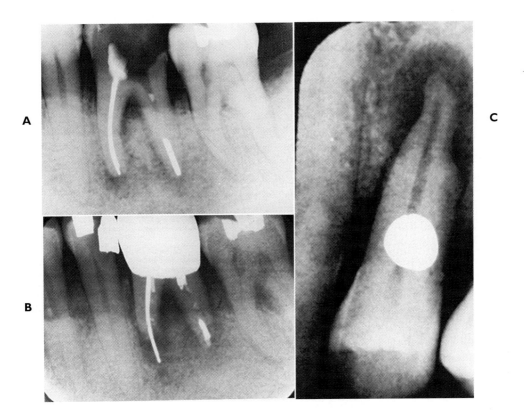

Fig. 10-19 *A, Failing root canal treatment in mandibular first molar. Silver cones are present. B, Several years later the tooth was found to be unsalvageable because of extensive root resorption and bone loss in the furcation. C, External root resorption arising from chronic periradicular inflammation.*

4. Clean dentin chips can also be packed in the apical one third to serve as an apical barrier or stop for the compaction of gutta-percha.[16] When the canal is properly cleaned, shaped, and dried, fresh dentin chips are generated with large (No. 50 to 70) Hedström files or rotary instruments (Gates-Glidden burs or Peeso reamers) in the middle and coronal portions of the canal. Once a reasonable number of dentin chips are visible around the orifice and in the canal, the chips are pushed apically with a small plugger. Continue this procedure until the master apical K-file can be inserted short of the working length with the tactile sensation of a sound, hard apical barrier. Generally, 0.5 to 2 mm of dentin chips will suffice, based on the size of the irregular apical opening.

5. If a nonsurgical approach is impossible or has proved unsuccessful, periradicular surgery is indicated to remove the resorbed portion of the root apex and to seal the apical foramen properly. In most cases, however, the nonsurgical approach is the treatment of choice.

CLINICAL PROBLEM: A 40-year-old female patient presents with persistent discomfort and occasional swelling around the root of the mandibular right second premolar. She cannot understand why this tooth hurts her because root canal treatment has already been performed. Clinical examination reveals a cast restoration on this tooth, and the soft tissues around the tooth are inflamed and tender to palpation. The tooth is also painful to percussion. A radiograph reveals a previously root-filled tooth, a poorly adapted root filling in the apical half of the tooth, a large radiolucency, and apical invasive resorption (Fig. 10-21, *A*). The diagnosis is failed root canal treatment with acute periradicular periodontitis concomitant with apical resorption.

Solution: The primary cause of the patient's problem is the poorly obturated (and cleaned?) root canal. The primary practitioner challenge is the

A   B   C

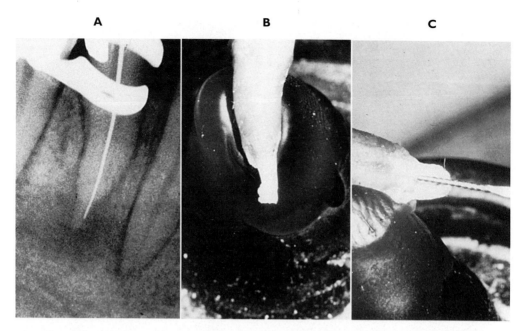

Fig. 10-20 *A,* *External root resorption caused by periradicular inflammation. This working length radiograph is a two-dimensional view and determination of the canal exit is difficult. **B,*** *Extracted tooth showing same view as the radiograph. **C,*** Extracted tooth showing the third dimension of the resorbed root. Notice that the canal exits several millimeters short of the radiographic apex.*

management of the resorbed root. Nonsurgical root canal retreatment is indicated. The tooth was accessed, and the root canal was retreated (see Chapter 7). Hedström files were used to carefully remove debris on the canal walls in the apical portion of the root. Calcium hydroxide was used in the apical portion to assist in an apical stop. Although the gutta-percha obturation looks acceptable, it may very well be beyond the end of the resorbed root (Fig. 10-21, *B*). A 9-year reevaluation shows the periradicular tissues are stable even though the apical portion of the root does not seem to have a well-adapted filling (Fig. 10-21, *C*). The patient is symptom free.

CLINICAL PROBLEM: A 48-year-old male patient presents with pain to chewing on the mandibular left first molar. Occasionally he has a fullness or pressure sensation in the tooth. At times the tooth is very tender to touch. He believes he has had a root canal on the tooth but is not sure. Clinical examination reveals that the first molar is tender to percussion and palpation. A localized swelling is present over the distal root, and the patient identifies that as being tender during palpation. Probings are within normal limits. A radiograph shows that previous root canal treatment had

been performed (Fig. 10-22, *A*). The quality of the filling is questionable, large radiolucencies are present, there is apical resorption on the distal root, and there is a circumscribed area of focal sclerosis apical to the distal root. The diagnosis is failed root canal treatment with acute periradicular periodontitis, apical resorption, and chronic focal sclerosing osteitis.

Solution: The main cause of failure may very well be lack of a quality root canal obturation, though the poor obturation in itself usually does not cause failures. Generally the canals have not been properly cleaned or coronal leakage is present. Either of these two etiologic factors can stimulate the apical resorption or the sclerotic response. In this case, nonsurgical root canal retreatment is indicated. The retreatment was completed (Fig. 10-22, *B*). Three-year reevaluation reveals a good healing response with significant reduction in the radiolucencies and attempts to remodel the sclerosis (Fig. 10-22, *C*). The patient is symptom free.

Excessive Forces during Orthodontic Movement

Although external root resorption occurs in nearly all patients undergoing orthodontic tooth movement, in most cases the resorption is clinically insignificant. Factors that influence the resorption of orthodontically moved teeth may include the magnitude of the forces applied, the type of tooth movement, the patient's age and sex, dietary or systemic complications, genetic factors, immunological reactions, the character of root cementum, or the periodontal microvasculature.[46,56] Most root resorption associated with orthodontic tooth movement is minimal and ceases after the orthodontic appliances are removed. However, in a few cases the root resorption can be severe or can continue after active treatment, resulting in shortened root length and tooth mobility (Fig. 10-23).[56] Since the resorptive process will most likely stop after cessation of the orthodontic forces, the treatment, once root resorption is recognized, is to eliminate the excessive forces being applied to the roots of the teeth.

Conditions Associated with Impacted Teeth

External root resorption caused by an adjacent impacted tooth has been reported to occur in approximately 1 of every 12 cases (Fig. 10-24).[43] The resorption ceases after the impacted tooth is removed and repair of the resorbed area usually occurs. The treatment of external root resorption associated with impacted teeth has been classified as described below.[38]

Type I

Type I external root resorption involves the periodontium only or minor root surface resorption. Treatment consists of removing the impacted tooth and observing the affected tooth structure. Should further resorption be evident at a later time, appropriate treatment to manage external root resorption is indicated.

Type II

The periodontium and dentin are involved in Type II resorption. If the resorptive process affects the cervical portion of the teeth, treatment is by surgical extraction of the impacted tooth and appropriate restorative, periodontal, or orthodontic treatment to manage the resorbed area (see Chapter 8). If the resorption is apical to the epithelial attachment and cannot be probed, the suggested treatment entails surgical extraction of the impacted tooth and observation of the resorbed area.

Type III

The periodontium, dentin, and pulp are involved in the resorptive process. Root canal treatment should be initiated, but if it is not feasible or fails and the tooth is multirooted, a root or tooth resection may be considered (see Chapter 8).

Type IV

Periodontium, dentin, pulp, and adjacent structures are involved. This resorption, in rare cases, may progress so rapidly that endodontic treatment of the affected tooth is futile and both teeth must be extracted.

Bleaching of Nonvital Teeth

Numerous reports have shown external cervical resorption after the use of Superoxol (30% hydrogen peroxide) (UBECO, Long Island City, N.Y.) in the bleaching of discolored, nonvital teeth[29,34,41,42,47] (Fig. 10-25). It is quite possible that the Superoxol seeps through patent dentinal tubules and initiates an inflammatory resorptive response in the cervical area.[34] Another theory suggests that damage to the periodontium, caused by the bleaching agent at the time of treatment, may heal or be followed by ankylosis. When the situation is complicated by bacterial contamination of the gingival sulcus, progressive root resorption associated with persistent inflammatory changes in the periodontium is possible (Fig. 10-26).[22]

It has been reported that the use of heat with Superoxol may cause or increase the potential for external cervical resorption. It has been postulated that this occurs by heat driving the Superoxol through the dentinal tubules, thereby altering the cementum.[43] *It is therefore recommended that the bleaching technique of choice should be the use of sodium perborate and Superoxol (walking bleach) rather than heat and Superoxol (thermocatalytic).* The Superoxol and sodium perborate powder are mixed into a paste and placed in the chamber, which is sealed with a strong temporary restoration (zinc oxide–eugenol cement). The patient is asked to return in 1 week for evaluation and possible replacement of the bleaching paste. This procedure is continued until there is no further improvement or the desired result is obtained.

The treatment of cervical root resorption is quite difficult, since both periodontal and restorative treatment are necessary. In advanced cases, root extrusion or extraction may be indicated. Therefore prevention of this process is the key to effective management. This is accomplished by minimizing the use of heat and protecting the gingival attachment of the tooth with a base of zinc oxide–eugenol placed in the access opening in the area of the cervical margin (Fig. 10-27). This should prevent the movement of the bleaching agent through the patent dentinal tubules to the dentin-cementum junction, or directly to the peri-

Fig. 10-21

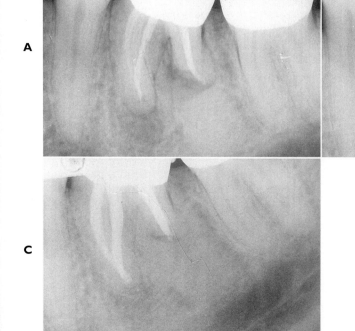

Fig. 10-22

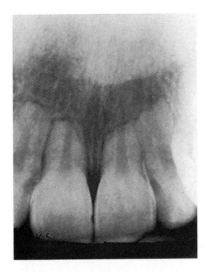

Fig. 10-23 *External resorption secondary to orthodontic procedures.*

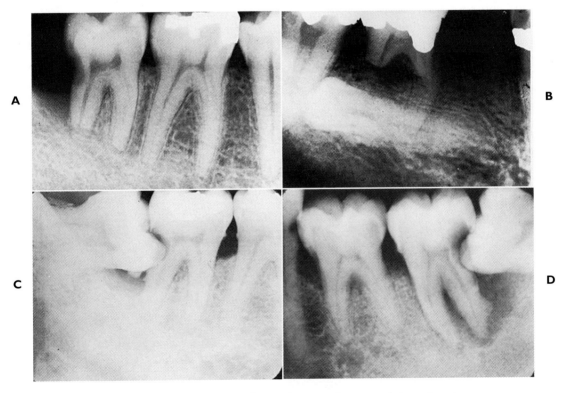

Fig. 10-24 *Various types of resorption secondary to tooth impaction.*

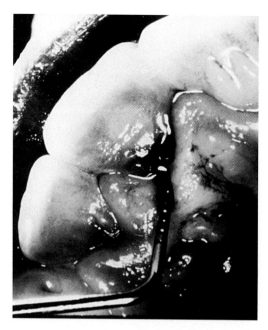

Fig. 10-25 *External cervical root resorption manifested as a defect in the cervical area of the tooth, one year after bleaching.*

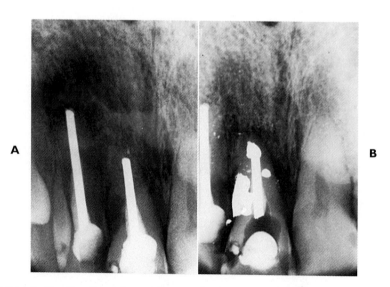

Fig. 10-26 *A, Recall radiograph several years after bleaching of maxillary central incisor. Note severe defect on mesial root surface adjacent to the cementoenamel junction. B, Postoperative radiograph showing repair of defect with alloy.*

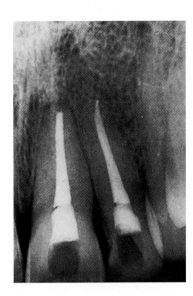

Fig. 10-27 *Maxillary central and lateral incisor prepared for bleaching. Temporary restorative material has been placed in the orifice of the canals to prevent bleaching solution from penetrating into the dentinal tubules at the cementoenamel junction.*

odontium in areas devoid of cementum. Recently it has been recommended that a sealant (Barrier, produced by Teledyne Getz, Elk Grove Village, Ill.) be used to prevent the leakage of the bleaching agent into the apical portion of the root and laterally into the periodontal tissues.[21] Although *in vitro* studies have indicated that a thick paste of calcium hydroxide placed in the cervical portion of the pulp canal space after bleaching may alter the pH and promote a favorable environment for repair of any damage to the cervical periodontal ligament,[39] recent *in vivo* studies could not confirm the efficacy of calcium hydroxide for this use.[54]

References

1. Andreasen JO: Luxation of permanent teeth due to trauma: a clinical and radiographic follow-up study of 184 injured teeth, *Scand J Dent Res* 78:273-286, 1970.
2. Andreasen JO: The effect of splinting upon periodontal healing after replantation of permanent incisors in monkeys, *Acta Odontol Scand* 33: 313-323, 1975.
3. Andreasen JO: The effect of pulp extirpation or root canal treatment on periodontal healing after replantation of permanent incisors in monkeys, *J Endod* 7:245-252, 1981.
4. Andreasen JO: Relationship between surface and inflammatory resorption and changes in the pulp after replantation of permanent teeth, *J Endod* 7:294-301, 1981.
5. Andreasen JO: Effect of extra-alveolar period and storage media upon periodontal and pulpal healing after replantation of permanent incisors in monkeys, *Int J Oral Surg* 10:43-53, 1981.
6. Andreasen JO: External root resorption: its implications in dental traumatology, pedodontics, periodontics, orthodontics, and endodontics, *Int Endod J* 18:109-118, 1985.
7. Andreasen JO: Root fractures, luxation and avulsion injuries—diagnosis and management, In Gutmann JL, Harrison JW, editors: Proceedings of an International Conference on Oral Trauma. Chicago, 1986, American Association of Endodontists.
8. Andreasen JO, Andreasen FM: *Essentials of traumatic injuries to the teeth,* Copenhagen, Munksgaard, 1991, pp 77-131.
9. Andreasen JO, Borum MK, Andreasen FM: Replantation of 400 avulsed permanent incisors: factors related to root growth, *Endod Dent Traumatol* 11:69-75, 1995.
10. Andreasen JO, Borum MK, Jacobsen HL, Andreasen FM: Replantation of 400 avulsed permanent incisors: diagnosis of healing complications, *Endod Dent Traumatol* 11:51-58, 1995.
11. Andreasen JO, Borum MK, Jacobsen HL, Andreasen FM: Replantation of 400 avulsed permanent incisors: factors related to pulpal healing, *Endod Dent Traumatol* 11:59-68, 1995.
12. Andreasen JO, Borum MK, Jacobsen HL, Andreasen FM: Replantation of 400 avulsed permanent incisors: Factors related to periodontal ligament healing, *Endod Dent Traumatol* 11:76-89, 1995.
13. Andreasen JO, Hjorting-Hansen E: Replantation of teeth: I. Radiographic and clinical study of 110 human teeth replanted after accidental loss, *Acta Odontol Scand* 24:263-286, 1966.
14. Andreasen JO, Kristerson L: The effect of limited drying or removal of the periodontal ligament: periodontal healing after replantation of mature permanent incisors in monkeys, *Acta Odontol Scand* 39:1-13, 1981.
15. Andreasen JO, Schwartz O: The effect of saline storage before replantation upon dry damage of the periodontal ligament, *Endod Dent Traumatol* 2:67-70, 1986.
16. Beatty RG, Zakariasen KL: Apical leakage associated with three obturation techniques in large and small root canals, *Int Endod J* 17:67-72, 1984.
17. Blomlöf L, Lindskög S, Anderson L et al: Storage of experimentally avulsed teeth in milk prior to replantation, *J Dent Res* 62:912-916, 1983.
18. Cabrini RI, Maisto OA, Manfredi EE: Internal resorption of dentine: histopathologic control of eight cases after pulp amputation and capping with calcium hydroxide, *Oral Surg Oral Med Oral Pathol* 10:90-96, 1957.
19. Chivian N: Intentional replantation, *J NJ Dent Soc* 38:247-250, 1967.
20. Chivian N: Root resorption. In Cohen S, Burns R, editors: Pathways of the pulp, ed 5, St Louis, 1991, Mosby, pp 504-547.
21. Costas F, Wong M: Intracoronal isolatin barriers: effect of location on root leakage and effectiveness of bleaching agents, *J Endod* 17:365-368, 1991.
22. Cvek M, Lindvall AM: External root resorption following bleaching of pulpless teeth with oxygen peroxide, *Endod Dent Traumatol* 1:56-60, 1985.
23. Dumsha TC, Gutmann JL: Clinical techniques for the placement of calcium hydroxide, *Compend Cont Dent Educ* 6:482-489, 1985.

24. Dumsha TC, Hovland EJ: Evaluation of long-term calcium hydroxide treatment in avulsed teeth—an in vivo study, *Int Endod J* 28:7-11, 1995.

25. England MC: Diagnostic procedure for confirmation of a suspected resorptive defect of the root, *J Endod* 3:157-159, 1977.

26. Frank AL, Weine FS: Non-surgical therapy for the perforation defect of internal resorption, *J Am Dent Assoc* 87:863-868, 1973.

27. Gartner AH, Mack T, Somerlott RG et al: Differential diagnosis of internal and external root resorption, *J Endod* 2:329-334, 1976.

28. Goldberg F, Massone EJ, Spielberg C: Evaluation of the dentinal bridge after pulpotomy and calcium hydroxide dressing, *J Endod* 10:318-320, 1984.

29. Goon WY, Cohen S, Borer RF: External cervical root resorption following bleaching, *J Endod* 12:414-418, 1986.

30. Gutmann JL: Principles of endodontic surgery for the general practitioner, *Dent Clin North Am* 28:895-908, 1984.

31. Ham JW, Patterson SS, Mitchell DF: Induced apical closure of immature pulpless teeth in monkeys, *Oral Surg Oral Med Oral Pathol* 33:438-449, 1972.

32. Hammarström L, Blomlöf L, Feiglin B et al: Replantation of teeth and antibiotic treatment, *Endod Dent Traumatol* 2:51-57, 1986.

33. Hammarström L, Lindskög S: Resorption of teeth and alveolar bone, *Int Endod J* 18:93-108, 1985.

34. Harrington GW, Natkin E: External resorption associated with bleaching of pulpless teeth, *J Endod* 5:344-348, 1979.

35. Harrison JW: Irrigation of the root canal system, *Dent Clin North Am* 28:797-808, 1984.

36. Heithersay GS: Clinical endodontic and surgical management of tooth and associated bone resorption, *Int Endod J* 18:72-92, 1985.

37. Hiltz J, Trope M: Vitality of human lip fibroblasts in milk, Hanks balanced salt solution and Viaspan storage media, *Endod Dent Traumatol* 7:69-72, 1991.

38. Holcomb JB, Dodds RN, England MC: Endodontic treatment modalities for external root resorption associated with impacted mandibular third molars, *J Endod* 9:335-337, 1983.

39. Kehoe JC: pH reversal following in vitro bleaching of pulpless teeth, *J Endod* 13:6-9, 1987.

40. Kleier DJ, Averbach RE, Kawulok TC: Efficient calcium hydroxide placement within the root canal, *J Prosthet Dent* 53:509-510, 1985.

41. Lado EA, Stanley HR, Weisman MI: Cervical resorption in bleached teeth, *Oral Surg Oral Med Oral Pathol* 55:78-80, 1983.

42. Latcham N: Postbleaching cervical resorption, *J Endod* 12:262-264, 1986.

43. Madison S, Walton R: Cervical resorption following bleaching of endodontically treated teeth, *J Endod* 16:570-574, 1990.

44. Martin H: Ultrasonic disinfection of the root canal, *Oral Surg Oral Med Oral Pathol* 42:92-99, 1976.

45. Masterton JB: Internal resorption of the dentin: a complication arising from unhealed pulp wounds, *Br Dent J* 118:241-249, 1965.

46. Mattison GD, Gholston LR, Boyd P: Orthodontic external root resorption: Endodontic considerations, *J Endod* 9:253-256, 1983.

47. Montgomery S: External cervical resorption after bleaching a pulpless tooth, *Oral Surg Oral Med Oral Pathol* 57:203-206, 1984.

48. Morris ML, Moreinis A, Patel R et al: Factors affecting healing after experimentally delayed tooth transplantation, *J Endod* 7:80-84, 1981.

49. Nitzen D, Kernan T, Marmany Y: Does an impacted tooth cause root resorption of the adjacent one? *Oral Surg Oral Med Oral Pathol* 51:221-224, 1981.

50. Oswald RJ: Procedural accidents and their repair, *Dent Clin North Am* 23:593-616, 1979.

51. Patil S, Dumsha TC, Sydiskis, RJ: Determining periodontal ligament (PDL) cell vitality from exarticulated teeth stored in saline or milk using fluorescein diacetate, *Int Endod J* 27:1-5, 1994.

52. Pitts DJ, Jones EL, Oswald RJ: A histological comparison of calcium hydroxide plugs and dentin plugs used for the control of gutta-percha root canal filling material, *J Endod* 10:283-293, 1984.

53. Rabinowitch BZ: Internal resorption, *Oral Surg Oral Med Oral Pathol* 10:193-206, 1957.

54. Rotstein I, Friedman S, Mor C et al: Histological characterization of bleaching-induced external root resorption in dogs, *J Endod* 17:436-441, 1991.

55. Seltzer S, Bender IB: *The dental pulp,* ed 3, Philadelphia, JB Lippincott, 1984, p 266.

56. Sims MR, Weekes WT: Resorption related to orthodontics and some morphological features of the periodontal microvascular bed, *Int Endod J* 18:140-145, 1985.

57. Stamos DE, Stamos DG: A new treatment modality for internal resorption, *J Endod* 12:315-319, 1986.

58. Tronstad L: Pulp reactions in traumatized teeth. In Gutmann JL, Harrison JW, editors: Proceedings of an International Conference on Oral Trauma. Chicago, 1986, American Association of Endodontists.

59. Tronstad L: Root resorption—etiology, terminology, and clinical manifestations, *Endod Dent Traumatol* 4:241-252, 1988.

60. Trope M, Moshonov J, Nissan R, Bust P, and Yesilsoy C: Short vs. long-term calcium hydroxide treatment of established inflammatory root resorption in replanted dog teeth, *Endod Dent Traumatol* 11:124-128, 1995.

61. Walton RE, Leonard LA: Cracked tooth: an etiology for "idiopathic" internal resorption? *J Endod* 12:167-169, 1986.

62. Webber R: Traumatic injuries and the expanded endodontic role of calcium hydroxide. In Gerstein H, editor: *Techniques in clinical endodontics.* Philadelphia, 1983, WB Saunders.

63. Wedenberg C, Lindskög S: Experimental internal resorption in monkey teeth, *Endod Dent Traumatol* 1:221-227, 1985.

64. Weisenseel JA, Hicks ML, Pelleu GB: Calcium hydroxide as an apical barrier, *J Endod* 13:1-5, 1987.

Chapter 11

Problems Encountered with Fractured Teeth

James L. Gutmann
Gerald N. Glickman

"The teeth are liable to be fractured by blows, which may be inflicted either by accidents, or from malicious intentions. The incisors of the upper jaw are the most exposed to these accidents: boys, in their various amusements, occasionally receive blows in the mouth, which not unfrequently occasion fractures of the front teeth."[*]

The concept of problem solving in the area of fractured teeth poses a unique challenge from the aspects of prevention, identification, and management. Although fractures that involve posterior teeth are usually slow to develop and manifest as a variety of intertwined variables, fractures of the anterior teeth are primarily the result of trauma.[10] In both regions fractures may involve the crown, root, or both, in addition to being horizontal, vertical, or angulated. Likewise, although some types of fractures can be anticipated and prevented, others result from unforeseen or unexpected causes and must be dealt with on an emergency basis.

The purpose of this chapter is to highlight, in a problem-solving mode, the prevention, identification, and management of commonly encountered situations in which tooth structure is fractured. The prevention of fractures will be highly dependent not only on the patient examination and diagnosis, but also on the identification of those factors that can contribute to fractures and the control of these factors by the practitioner.

[*]From Fox J: London, James Swan, 1806.

Success regarding the identification and management of traumatic fractures will be predicated on the thoroughness of the patient examination and the appropriateness and timeliness of treatment.

CORONAL FRACTURES
Prevention, Identification, and Management

The active prevention of coronal fractures in normal day-to-day living is unrealistic and is a moot point. Prevention, however, during hazardous activities, such as job-related activities (as during sports), may occur in the form of mouth protection and on-the-job training to avoid circumstances that may predispose to traumatic incidents. Although such incidents are uncommon, the major result of these types of fractures is dental trauma, whether direct or indirect, and these accidental injuries remain the predominant type that is reported.[23] This implies that management of the crown fracture will usually fall in the category of a dental emergency and principles cited in Chapter 9, including diagnosis, treatment planning, anesthesia, analgesics, and antibiotics, should be integrated into the total case management.

In cases in which an acute trauma accident has resulted in a crown fracture (Fig. 11-1), pulpal preservation is crucial when root formation is incomplete. Pulpal protection with calcium hydroxide, zinc oxide–eugenol cement, and acid-

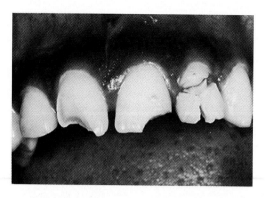

Fig. 11-1 *Facial trauma resulting in varied types of crown fracture, from a simple uncomplicated enamel-dentin fracture* (left central incisor) *to a deep dentin fracture without pulp exposure* (right central incisor) *to a complicated fracture with exposed pulp* (lateral incisor).

etched, dentin-bonded composites is the treatment of choice.[1,2,21]

CLINICAL PROBLEM: An 8-year-old female patient presents after school with fractured maxillary central incisors. She suffered a blow to her mouth during the afternoon recess. Pain is present but minimal. Both teeth exhibit uncomplicated coronal fractures with the deeper fracture in the right central incisor. The teeth are tender to percussion and palpation, but mobility is minimal. Thermal sensitivity is present, especially with the right central. A radiograph reveals incomplete root formation on both teeth (Fig. 11-2, *A*).

Solution: The most important aspect of this case is to ensure the continued vitality of the pulp tissue to enable the root apices to close and to enhance the amount of secondary dentin on the root walls. Protection of the exposed dentin is essential. Fig. 11-2, *B to D,* show reevaluations at 3 months, 9 months, and 15 months respectively. Attempts to keep the fractured surfaces protected routinely failed. However, ultimate root-end closure had been achieved as has thickening of the root walls.

When root formation is complete, nonsurgical root canal treatment results in a very high degree of success and should be considered as the treatment of choice. Table 11-1 highlights the identification and management of crown fractures.

In the process of preserving the pulp after a crown fracture, periodic assessment of the pulp will be necessary. Hence the need to perform initial pulp sensibility tests is imperative, as is follow-up evaluation every 6 to 8 weeks for approximately 6 months.[14] Likewise, patient symptoms and func-

tion, as well as radiographic evaluation as to the status of root development, linear calcification of the pulpal space, diffuse calcification of the pulp, internal or external resorption, or the development of a periradicular radiolucency, are also essential to the successful management of these potential untoward sequelae to tooth trauma.

Early recognition and intervention are key elements in the preventive aspect of managing all traumatic injuries, especially crown fractures.

CLINICAL PROBLEM: A 25-year-old male was referred for emergency endodontic treatment of a maxillary left central incisor after a sporting accident 24 hours earlier. He had received a blow to the mouth with a football. He said the tooth was painful to touch and said that he had to avoid thermal changes. Clinical examination revealed the coronal segment to be mobile and extremely tender to palpation. The adjacent teeth were not tender to palpation or percussion. A periradicular radiograph was taken, and a horizontal radiolucent line was evident in the middle of the crown and cervically (Fig. 11-5, *A, arrows*). The injury was classified as a complicated crown fracture because the transverse fracture line had perforated the pulp chamber and hemorrhagic fluid was evident along the fracture line (Fig. 11-5, *B, arrow*). Diagnosis was irreversible pulpitis and acute periradicular periodontitis subsequent to a complicated crown fracture.

Solution: After anesthesia, the cervical segment of the crown was carefully isolated (Fig. 11-5, *B*), and the coronal segment was gently removed using a spoon excavator (Fig. 11-5, *C*). Notice the transverse nature of the fracture and the palatal extent of the fracture that was visible on the radiograph as the cervical radiolucent line (Fig. 11-5, *A*). A 3 mm exposure of a viable pulp was evident. Since the tooth had complete root formation and the pulp had been exposed to oral fluids via the fracture line, pulp extirpation and root canal treatment were completed during the same appointment to facilitate the restorative plan (Fig. 11-5, *D*). The patient was scheduled for periodic recall to monitor the status of the adjacent teeth as well as the endodontically treated tooth.

VERTICAL TOOTH FRACTURES

First of all, many factors that predispose to vertical fractures of teeth cannot be altered or controlled by the practitioner.[16] These include masticatory accidents,[5-7,24,32] natural tight cusp-fossa relationships

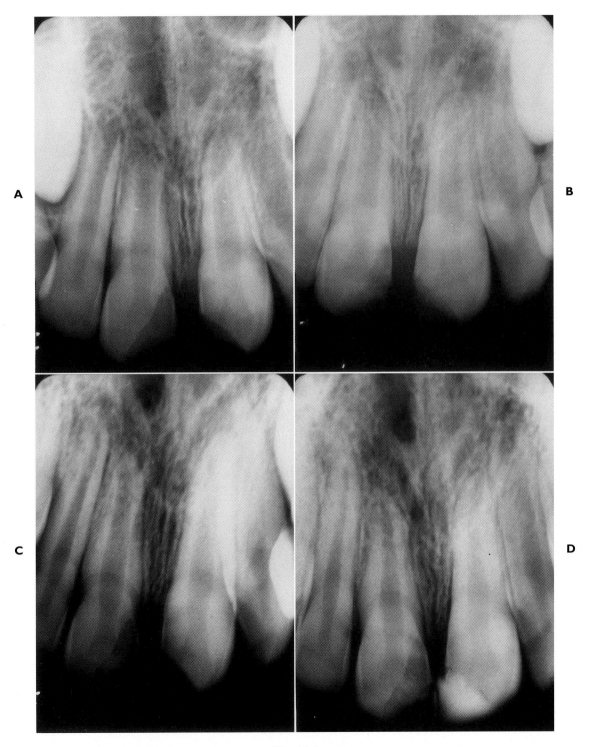

Fig. 11-2

▼ **Table 11-1** Identification and management of crown fractures

TYPE OF CROWN FRACTURE	IMPORTANT CLINICAL FINDINGS AND TREATMENT OPTIONS
Infraction—crack without loss of structure	Visualize with fiberoptic or intense light source directed parallel to the vertical axis of the tooth.
	Highly possible that pulp has been damaged; therefore baseline sensibility testing with continued evaluation every 6 to 8 weeks is recommended. Evaluate for other structural damage.
	Explain to the patient the possible pulpal sequelae and need for evaluation and treatment. Consider drawing a picture of the tooth in the patient's chart with the position and direction of the cracks or craze lines noted.
Uncomplicated—fracture of enamel and dentin but not the pulp	Often associated with luxation injuries or commonly involves a fracture of the mesial incisal of maxillary central incisors (Fig. 11-3).
	Do sensibility testing as a point for future reference.
	If confined to the enamel, selectively grind and smooth the fractured edge.
	If dentin exposed, place calcium hydroxide liner over the dentinal tubules and restore with an acid-etch, light-cured composite resin. In some cases a temporary crown is appropriate.[1,2,21]
	If dentin deeply exposed, examine for a pulp exposure. Check in 6 to 8 weeks.
	If associated with a more extensive tooth injury, e.g., luxation, a splint will be necessary (see Chapter 10).
Complicated—fracture of enamel, dentin, and pulp	Bleeding will be present if pulp is viable (Fig. 11-4).
	Pulp cap if less than 6 hours since trauma. Partial pulpotomy or complete pulpotomy if the root has not completed its formation. Pulpectomy is indicated based on the degree of root closure and extent of damage to the tooth structure (Fig. 11-4).
	If associated with a more extensive tooth injury, e.g., luxation, a splint will be necessary (see Chapter 10).

or steep intercuspation,[3,5,6,26] bruxism, and thermal cycling.[5,17] Second, clinical detection of fractures can be exceedingly difficult, especially in their initial stages of development or beneath extensive restorations. Additionally, radiographs are of little value in these initial stages.[18] In some cases surgical intervention may actually be necessary for fracture identification (Fig. 11-6).[11] Third, the patient's symptoms may mimic many other possible diagnoses, such as temporomandibular joint syndrome, sinus problems, vague headaches, and ear pain.[27] Fourth, the efficacious management of fractured teeth is highly dependent on a complete set of variables that are often not controllable by the practi-

tioner, such as extent of fracture, tooth and root anatomy, position of fracture, masticatory function, and previous dental intervention.

Prevention

Prevention of vertical tooth fractures is difficult because many are already present before diagnosis or treatment, are predisposing in nature, and are initially overlooked as etiologic factors. However, other contributing factors can be controlled and many fractures can be prevented.[27] These factors reside primarily in the nature of the restorative and endodontic procedures performed and must be considered by all practitioners. Likewise, additional

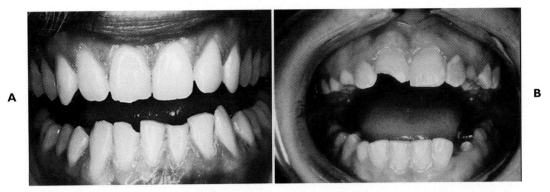

Fig. 11-3 *A, Simple enamel fractures (infractions) with minimal or no exposed dentin. Often selective grinding or acid-etched, bonded composite is indicated. B, Complicated coronal fracture involving the deeper dentinal tissues*

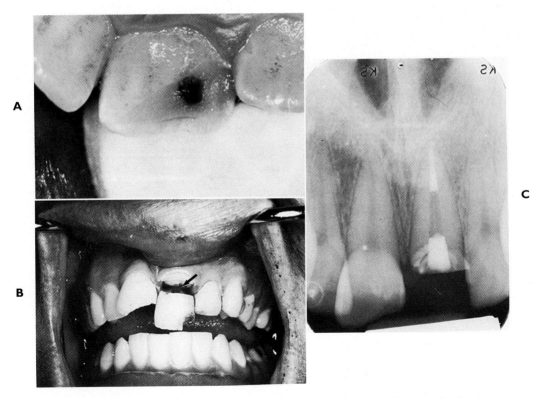

Fig. 11-4 *A and B, Examples of complicated coronal fractures that are deep into the dentin with exposed pulps. C, Tooth in B treated with complete pulpectomy and root canal filling.*

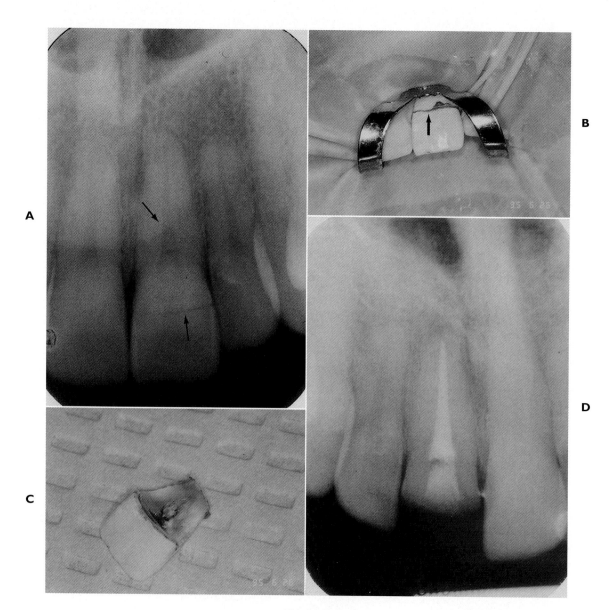

Fig. 11-5

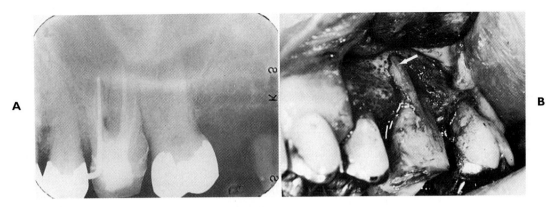

Fig. 11-6 A, *Significant probing in narrow channel along the mesiobuccal root of the maxillary first molar.* **B,** *Tissue has been reflected, and a vertical fracture is evident* (arrow).

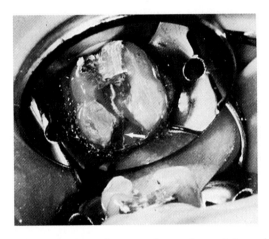

Fig. 11-7 *Presence of a crown fracture* (arrow) *beneath a gold inlay; the patient had experienced severe pulpitis. (From Schweitzer JL, Gutmann JL, Bliss RQ:* Int Endod J *22:64-74, 1989.)*

factors that may predispose to fracture may interplay in specific cases.

Contributing restorative factors
1. Soft gold inlays (Fig. 11-7)
2. Large amalgams undermining tooth structure (Fig. 11-8)
3. Excessive instrumentation and removal of tooth structure
4. Reinforcing pins
5. Intraradicular posts and dowels (Fig. 11-9)
6. Insertion (hydrostatic) pressures during post placement[26]
7. Failure to properly restore endodontically treated teeth
8. Improper occlusal adjustments

Contributing endodontic factors
1. Excessive compaction forces (Fig. 11-10)

2. Excessive canal preparation
3. Wedging of filling materials and instruments (silver cones, spreaders, pluggers)
4. Excessive use of straight rotary instruments, such as Gates-Glidden burs or Peeso reamers in thin roots (Fig. 11-11)
5. Excessive use of sonic or ultrasonic instruments during cleaning and shaping of the canal or during post or fractured-instrument removal

Other predisposing factors
1. Periodontal disease with significant bone loss
2. Pathological entities
3. Traumatogenic occlusion
4. Corrosion of intraradicular posts (implies coronal or apical leakage in canal)
5. Occlusal discrepancies, such as open anterior bites, posterior cross-bites, or edge-to-edge occlusion (Fig. 11-12)
6. Anatomic tooth form
7. Tooth abrasion or erosion

Identification

Identification of vertical tooth fractures can also be exceedingly difficult because their initiation, in the form of cracks or craze lines, is not always readily discernible (Fig. 11-13).[6] In addition, some teeth having an internal structural weakness at calcification sites that fail to coalesce are impossible to predict.[13] Finally, fractures that began beneath large amalgam or cast metallic restorations are virtually impossible to detect until extensive signs or symptoms appear, the restoration is removed (Fig. 11-14), or a significant periodontal defect is identified.

The difficulty encountered in the identification and diagnosis of vertically fractured teeth has led to the clinical diagnosis of *cracked-tooth syndrome*.[5]

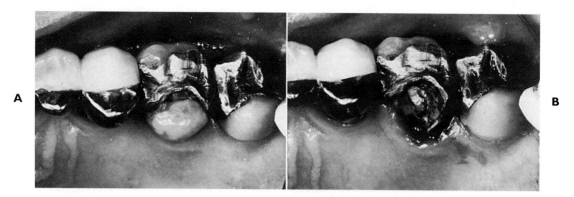

Fig. 11-8 *A, Maxillary first molar with large multiple-surface amalgam. Fracture of palatal cusp is evident. **B,** Removal of fractured segment shows extensive undermining of the cusp by the restoration.*

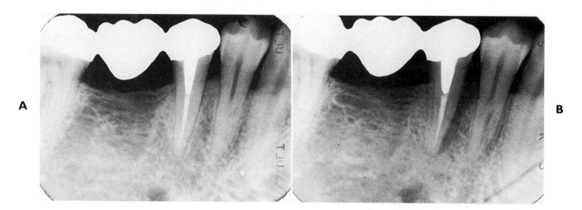

Fig. 11-9 *A, Tapered cast post in mandibular premolar. Most of the post is coronal to root-supported bone. **B,** Angular bone loss on mesial is characteristic of vertical fracture, presumed to be a result of the wedging effect of the post.*

Other terms used to identify this entity have been *cuspal-fracture odontalgia,*[9] *incomplete tooth fracture,*[19,22] *split-root syndrome,*[27] *greenstick fractures of the tooth crown,*[30] *vertical root fracture,*[16,17,20] *incomplete crown-root fractures,*[13] and *adult root fracture.*[3] In those cases where the fracture has been identified and attributed to dental procedures, the term *dentistogenic,*[3] or *odontiatrogenic,* tooth fracture[27] (of dentist origin) has been cited.

Clinical Findings

Clinical signs and symptoms are often elusive or bizarre in nature and may be difficult to detect or reproduce during patient examination. Subjective symptoms may often be predicated on the extent and duration of fracture, coupled with the pulpal response and associated degenerative changes and periodontal involvement, if any. The following symptoms may appear singly or in concert:

1. Sustained pain during biting pressures
2. Pain only upon release of biting pressures
3. Occasional momentary sharp pain during mastication
4. Sensitivity to thermal changes
5. Sensitivity to mild stimuli, such as sweet or acidic foods
6. Persistent dull pain

Clinical examination

A wide array of clinical findings characterizes the patient with a tooth fracture, whether it is complete or incomplete, such as:

1. Pain to selective percussion on specific tooth margins or cusps. The percussion may be done along the long axis of the tooth or angled against a labial surface or cuspal slope.
2. Generalized discomfort to percussion.
3. Presence of craze or fracture lines on facial (Fig. 11-15) or lingual surfaces or marginal ridges. Lighter lines, which are more difficult

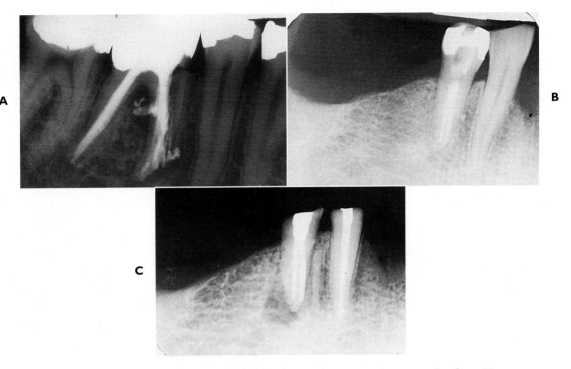

Fig. 11-10 *A, Immediate recognition of a root fracture due to excessive compaction forces. Even though the patient was anesthetized, he felt a sharp pain and heard a "crack" during the compaction procedure.* **B,** *Long-term recognition of a tooth fracture. Mandibular premolar with two canals obturated.* **C,** *Same tooth at 6-month evaluation; fracture of roots is evident, presumably a result of the wedging force of compaction.*

to visualize, are often more recent in occurrence, whereas darker, stained cracks are generally older in origin.

4. Significant gaps between old restorations and tooth structure.

5. Cracked restorations.

6. Narrow-channel sinus tracts along the periodontium that are identified with a careful circumferential, small incremental probing technique; or sinus tracts that do not heal.

7. Radiographic evidence of a thickened periodontal ligament space.

8. A diffuse, longitudinal radiolucency (see Fig. 11-11).

9. Radiolucent fracture line with or without segment separation (Figs. 11-11 and 11-16). In some of these cases there will be no evidence of root canal treatment. This has been referred to as an "adult root fracture."[3]

10. Radiopaque lines visible in the treated root canal. These represent the movement of gutta-percha or root canal sealer into the fracture.

11. Pulpal necrosis in a virgin tooth.

12. Surgical root-end fillings that have become displaced from their root-end cavities. This may also include surgical root-end fillings that have a characteristic "tail" or line of material extending from the body of the filling material. Also during the surgical procedure, if blood from the field is wiped across the resected root face and then rinsed off the root with water, blood will be retained in the fracture line if present.[22]

13. Commonly observed fractured teeth include the mandibular second molar, followed by the mandibular first molar and maxillary premolars.

Sensibility tests (tooth response to electrical or thermal stimulation) are generally not helpful in identifying or diagnosing a fractured tooth.

Radiographic findings are generally more discernible in the latter stages of fracture development, when not of traumatic origin.

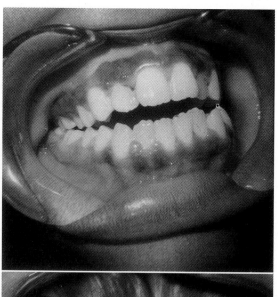

Fig. 11-11 *Excessive use of Peeso reamers in mandibular canine resulted in a thinning of the root and fracture, presumably occurring during the condensation. Notice the diffuse longitudinal radiolucency on the distal. Also there is a dark (radiolucent) line along the distal border of the root canal filling material (arrowheads).*

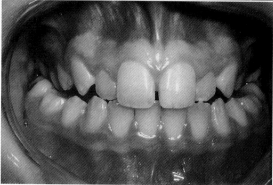

Fig. 11-12 *A, Anterior open bite places excessive forces into the central fossae and marginal ridges of the mandibular teeth. B, Posterior cross-bite places shearing forces against the lingual walls of the mandibular molars.*

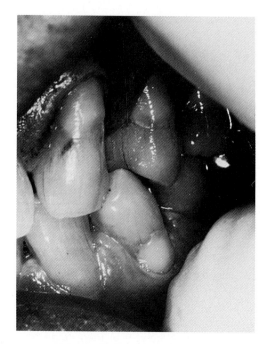

Fig. 11-13 *Marginal ridge of the maxillary first premolar occludes with the distal slope of the buccal cusp of the mandibular first premolar. Notice the fracture line on the mesial wall of the maxillary premolar. This is a common finding and must be identified during examination.*

CLINICAL PROBLEM: A 72-year-old male patient presents with low-grade discomfort in a mandibular central incisor. The discomfort has been vague for 2 or 3 months and now is more focused on this particular tooth. He claims to have seen some pus coming from around the tooth when he pushes on the gum tissue overlying the tooth. Clinical examination reveals a small sinus tract at the mucogingival junction overlying the severely worn mandibular right central incisor. The tooth is slightly tender to percussion and is definitely tender to palpation. A radiograph reveals a previously root-treated tooth with a large radiolucency. Two canals are obturated in the tooth, and the filling appears adequate (Fig 11-17, *A*).

Solution: A diagnosis of subacute to acute suppurative periradicular periodontitis is appropriate subsequent to apparently adequate root canal

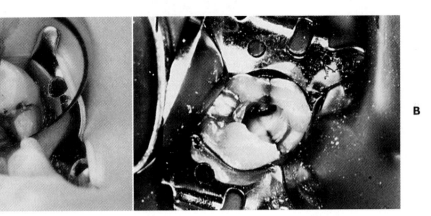

Fig. 11-14 A, *Angular fracture line under old amalgam restoration. Fracture is in all dimensions, running both mesiodistally and down the buccal and palatal surfaces.* **B,** *Fracture lines are visible after large amalgam restoration was removed. Notice fracture on the buccal and mesial walls.* (**B** *From Schweitzer JL, Gutmann JL, Bliss RQ:* Int Endod J *22:64-74, 1989. Case courtesy Dr. David Parkins.*)

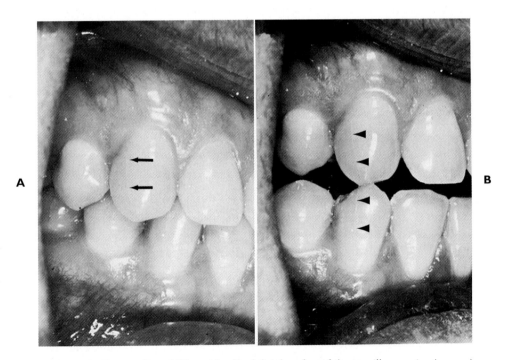

Fig. 11-15 A, *Fracture line visible on the distal facial surface of the maxillary canine* (arrows). **B,** *When patient moves jaw into lateral excursion, notice the alignment of fracture lines* (arrowheads) *in both the maxillary and mandibular canines. These findings are usually indicative of other dental problems, which can be addressed in an attempt to prevent further tooth fracture.*

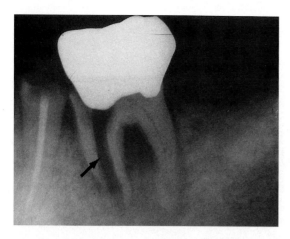

Fig. 11-16 *Complete vertical fractures can occur without previous root canal treatment and may be referred to as "adult root fractures." Causes for this demise are usually multiple and complex.*[3]

treatment. Therefore further investigation is essential to try to identify the etiologic factor for this failure. Incremental probing on the mesial and distal line angles indicates a sound periodontal attachment (Fig. 11-17, *B* and *C*). Probing in the center of the tooth reveals a deep, narrow channel pathognomonic of a vertical fracture (Fig 11-17, *D*). Extraction is the treatment of choice in this case. This case emphasizes the careful use of probing to assess teeth that appear to have failed root canal treatment.

Clinical assessment

During the clinical examination, specific dental treatment may be necessary to aid in the identification of a fractured tooth (complete or incomplete). These procedures compose a set of evaluative procedures that extend the problem-solving concept beyond that of a mere oral examination. These procedures include:

1. Biting tests on specific cusps, using a rubber wheel, orangewood stick, or instrument designed to focus biting pressures (Fig. 11-18) (Tooth Slooth, Professional Results, Laguna Niguel, Calif.).
2. Removal of crowns or old restorations with or without subsequent staining of the tooth structure with 1% to 2% methylene blue (Fig. 11-19).
3. Fiberoptic disclosure of fractures lines (Fig. 11-20).
4. Surgical exposure of root structure. When this approach is used, a full mucoperiosteal flap

is indicated. Also, the patient should be advised that this is a diagnostic procedure (see Fig. 11-6).

Management

The creative management of vertically fractured teeth is a crucial part of the problem-solving process. This implies that the choice of extraction may often be the wisest course of treatment, provided that all other possibilities have been considered and the patient is cognizant of both the dilemma and the prognosis. The ultimate course chosen is dependent on multiple factors that are intimately interrelated, such as level of discomfort, pulpal status, extent and location of the fracture, restorative needs, periodontal status, tooth position, patient function, overall treatment plan, and economics. Valiant attempts to retain fractured teeth have met with both success and failure.[12]

CLINICAL PROBLEM: A 45-year-old male patient presents with pain to pressure on the mandibular left second molar. There are 7 mm probings on the distal of the tooth. A crown preparation was initiated 1 month previously, but the patient chose not to have the restoration completed because of the pain. A year previously the tooth was diagnosed as having a fracture line on the distal marginal ridge. Symptoms of continuous, long-term discomfort tend to indicate that an irreversible pulpitis exists. Radiographic assessment reveals normal anatomical relationships (Fig. 11-21, *A*).

Solution: Root canal treatment was initiated on this tooth. After an access opening was performed, a crack was noted along the distal wall of the opening to the level of the orifice of the distal canal. Root canal treatment was completed, using a softened gutta-percha technique and vertical condensation (Obtura). Space was left in the coronal portion of the canal (Fig. 11-21, *B*). After removal of the smear layer in the coronal canal space and pulp chamber with citric acid, a glass-ionomer cement was injected to serve as a core (Fig. 11-21, *C*). The tooth was subsequently crowned, and the patient is presently symptom free at an 8-month reevaluation (Fig. 11-21, *D*). (Case courtesy Dr. Hedley Rakusin.)

Tables 11-2 and 11-3 will provide considerations and options in management; however, each case is uniquely challenging in both treatment and outcome. Additionally, these directives cannot begin to anticipate the multitude of variables that will affect each case, hence the need for intuitive, integrated and creative problem-solving approaches to management.

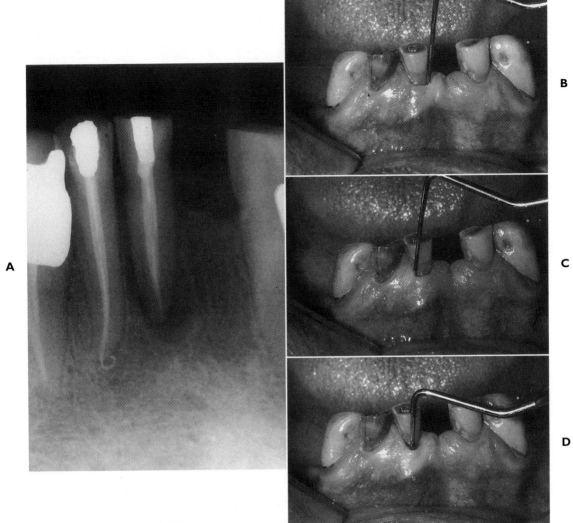

A

B

C

D

Fig. 11-17

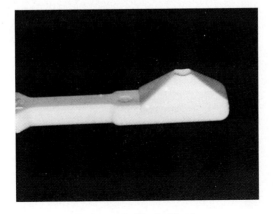

Fig. 11-18 *Tooth Slooth.*

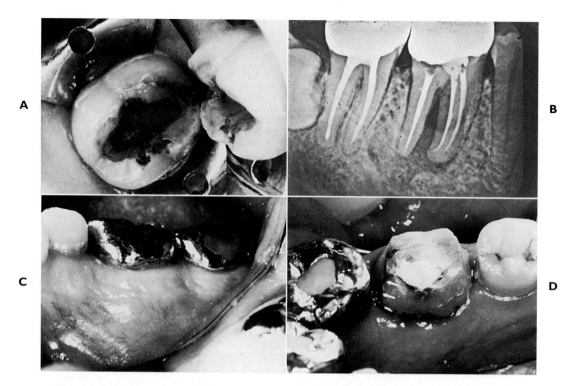

Fig. 11-19 A, *One-percent methylene blue was used to disclose multiple craze lines in the pulpal roof of a mandibular molar. A major fracture line is visible across the distal marginal ridge.* **B,** *Significant furcation bone loss adjacent to mandibular first molar.* **C,** *Clinical appearance of tooth, crown, and tissues.* **D,** *After crown removal a fracture line is visible down the distal surface of the molar (arrows). (From Schweitzer JL, Gutmann JL, Bliss RQ: Int Endod J 22:64-74, 1989.)*

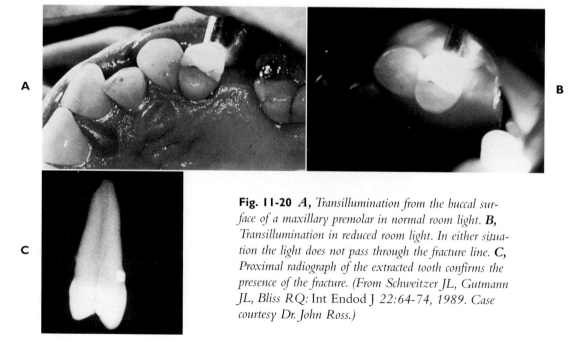

Fig. 11-20 A, *Transillumination from the buccal surface of a maxillary premolar in normal room light.* **B,** *Transillumination in reduced room light. In either situation the light does not pass through the fracture line.* **C,** *Proximal radiograph of the extracted tooth confirms the presence of the fracture. (From Schweitzer JL, Gutmann JL, Bliss RQ: Int Endod J 22:64-74, 1989. Case courtesy Dr. John Ross.)*

▼ **Table 11-2** Treatment considerations in the management of vertically fractured teeth—crown/crown-root fractures

INCOMPLETE FRACTURES	
PULPAL STATUS	**TREATMENT OPTIONS**
Asymptomatic or reversible pulpitis	Remove individually fractured cusp(s)—crown tooth. Splint with an orthodontic band and observe. Prepare for crown—place sound temporary crown and observe before placing permanent crown. Immediately place permanent crown. Relieve occlusion, place sedative restoration (zinc oxide–eugenol) and observe. If asymptomatic place permanent crown.
Symptomatic irreversible pulpitis or necrosis with subacute or acute periradicular periodontitis	Root canal treatment, minimizing the removal of tooth structure in canal preparation. The use of a softened gutta-percha technique with minimal condensation force is preferred. If sufficient tooth structure remains, place a glass-ionomer† or acid-etched, dentin-bonded core without post and restore with permanent crown. Core material can be placed 2-3 mm into the canal orifices. If insufficient tooth structure remains, consider a passively placed post along with an acid-etched, dentin-bonded core and permanent crown with margins of 2 mm or more of sound tooth structure. Crown lengthening and/or extrusion may be necessary.

▼ **Table 11-3** Treatment considerations in the management of vertically fractured teeth—crown/crown-root fractures

COMPLETE FRACTURES	
CROWN-ROOT STATUS	**TREATMENT OPTIONS**
Complete crown fracture—root and periodontium intact	Root canal treatment followed by acid-etched, dentin-bonded core and permanent crown
Complete crown fracture with root fracture 1 to 3 mm deep into one root of a multirooted tooth or single root tooth	Root canal treatment followed by a glass-iontomer core into the canal to the depth of the fracture; permanent crown; meticulous oral hygiene essential. Alternative—acid-etch, bonded composite. Consider crown lengthening or tooth extrusion, or both, prior to restoration to include the depth of the fracture line (see Chapter 8)
Complete crown fracture with root fracture beyond 3 mm deep in one root of a multirooted tooth or single root	Consider root extrusion with crown lengthening (see Chapter 8) Extraction or root or tooth resection (see Chapter 8)
Fracture of tooth through the furcation	Tooth resection or extraction, depending on root anatomy, position of furcation, and amount of supporting bone

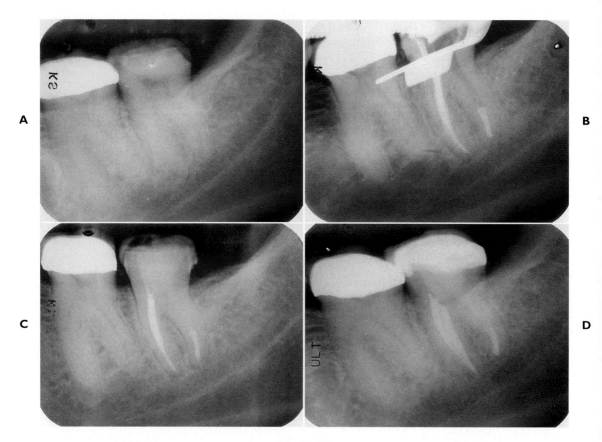

Fig. 11-21

CLINICAL PROBLEM: A 77-year-old man presented with recurrent pain and swelling on the palatal aspect of a maxillary left premolar. The tooth in question was the middle peer abutment of a five-unit fixed prosthesis. A review of the patient's record disclosed a radiograph taken immediately before the placement of the bridge (Fig. 11-22, *A*). Bone and tooth structure were sound. Fig. 11-22, *B,* shows the fixed prosthesis 1 year after placement. Notice that root canal treatment was performed on the premolar and the tooth was restored with a post, core, and crown. At this appointment the patient complained of a dull ache around the premolar. Probings revealed a pocket beginning to form on the mesiopalatal aspect of the premolar. During the next 3 years multiple osseous grafting procedures were performed to manage the pocket that had formed. Fig. 11-22, *C,* shows the present status of the abutment tooth at a total of 4 years after the placement of the fixed prosthesis. Fig. 11-22, *D* and *E,* shows the clinical placement of a periodontal probing marker and the radiographic position of the point.

All information indicates the presence of a vertical fracture in the premolar.

Solution: The best way to demonstrate the presence of the fracture and to determine a plan of treatment is to reflect the palatal soft tissue and examine the tooth. Upon tissue reflection a vertical fracture was evident (Fig. 11-22, *F, arrows*). Treatment options were limited, and the stable nature of the fixed prosthesis along with an atraumatic occlusal pattern led to the surgical resection of the root from beneath its coronal retainer (Fig. 11-22, *G*). A 6-month clinical view of the prosthesis demonstrates good tissue healing (Fig. 11-22, *H, black arrows*) with cleanable embrasure spaces *(white arrow)* and reasonable adaptation of the soft-tissue ridge to the newly created pontic.

HORIZONTAL ROOT FRACTURES
Identification and Management
As with crown fractures, horizontal root fractures can be a result of dental trauma and must be addressed primarily in an emergency setting.

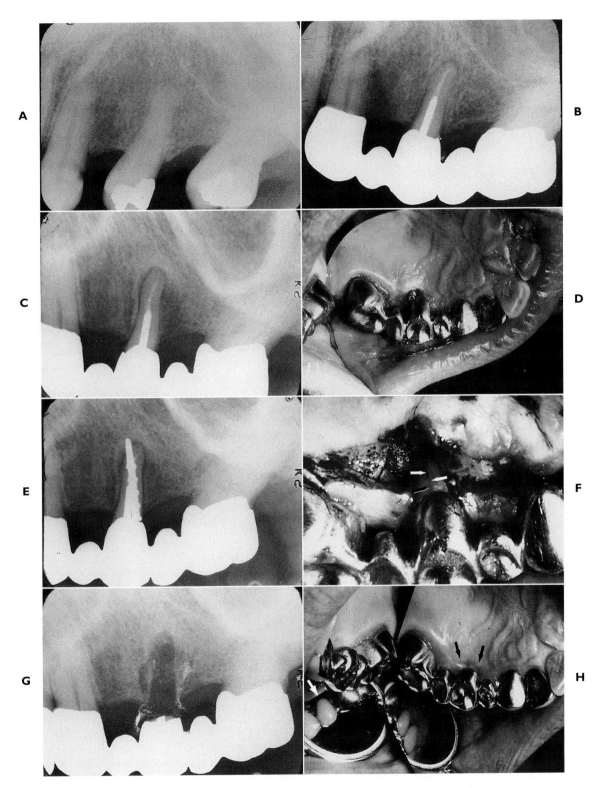

A

B

C

D

E

F

G

H

Fig. 11-22

293

▼ **Table 11-4** Treatment considerations in the management of horizontal fractured roots

POSITION OF FRACTURE	FRACTURED SEGMENTS IN APPOSITION TREATMENT OPTIONS
Apical third	If asymptomatic and no signs of osseous breakdown, keep under observation.
	Adjust occlusion if tooth mobile.
	If symptoms or signs of pulpitis or necrosis or apical resorption present, treat with nonsurgical root canal treatment in both segments if possible. If symptoms continue, especially upon biting or percussion, surgically remove the apical segment.
Middle third	If asymptomatic and no signs of osseous breakdown, keep under observation.
	Splinting and occlusal adjustment may be necessary.
	If symptoms of an irreversible pulpitis are present, it may be possible to treat both segments or just the coronal segment, whereas the apical segment may retain its viability. If apical segment exhibits pulpal necrosis and cannot be successfully treated nonsurgically, treat the coronal segment and surgically remove the apical segment. In some cases titanium oxide or aluminum oxide ceramic implants in the end of the root have been successful (Fig. 11-23).
Coronal third	If fracture does not communicate with the gingival sulcus and coronal segment is stable, adjust occlusion and observe. If segment is mobile, stabilize with splint. Observe.
	If fracture communicates with gingival sulcus, remove coronal segment and evaluate for crown lengthening, extrusion and lengthening, root submersion or extraction, depending on other treatment factors. Perform root canal treatment as a part of total treatment if tooth retained.

Because these fractures are designated as horizontal, intraalveolar, or transverse in nature, often they will appear angular and multiple during radiographic assessment (see Fig. 11-5). Hence it is imperative that multiple radiographs be taken to ascertain the exact nature of the fracture or fractures present.[4,15] For example, recommended for an anticipated radicular fracture of a maxillary central incisor are radiographs taken at 45 degrees (elongated), 110 degrees (foreshortened), and 90 degrees (periapical) to delineate the nature of the fracture.

Clinical examination in these cases may reveal a variety of possibilities, and treatment, if any, will be dependent not only on signs and symptoms, but also on the position of the fractured segments in the alveolus[8] (Tables 11-4 and 11-5). Under ideal circumstances, it is not uncommon for a horizontally fractured root to require no treatment (Fig. 11-25). Since many patients experience little or no discomfort after a horizontally fractured root, dental care may not even be sought, and evidence of a healed fracture is identified on routine radiographic examination. Along with the healed fracture, however, may be evidence of crown discoloration, linear calcification in one or both segments, internal or external resorption, and symptom-free pulpal necrosis.

CLINICAL PROBLEM: A 16-year-old male patient presents with a 2-week-old history of trauma to the maxillary left central incisor. Sensibility tests were nonresponsive on this tooth and normal on the adjacent teeth. A horizontal fracture is present at the junction of the apical and middle thirds of the root. The segments are in reasonable apposition, and the tooth is splinted at the incisal contacts (Fig. 11-26, A). One month later the patient was still symptom free; however the tooth was slightly discolored. There is no radiographic evidence of significant

▼ **Table 11-5** Treatment considerations in the management of horizontally fractured roots

POSITION OF FRACTURE	FRACTURED SEGMENTS NOT IN APPOSITION TREATMENT OPTIONS
Apical third	Perform root canal treatment if signs or symptoms dictate. Root tip may have to be surgically removed if signs or symptoms present, such as pain, sinus tract, or radiolucency.
Middle third	Try to reposition and splint for approximately 8 to 12 weeks. Observe. Anticipate root canal treatment on the coronal segment and possibly the apical segment if it can be negotiated. Apical segment may have to be removed surgically if signs or symptoms dictate. Remove apical segment and place titanium oxide or aluminum oxide ceramic implant. Intraradicular splint after root canal treatment in both segments.
Coronal third	If fracture communicates with sulcus, remove coronal segment and evaluate for crown lengthening, root extrusion with crown lengthening, root submergence or extraction (Fig. 11-24). (see Chapter 8) If fracture does not communicate with sulcus, reposition, splint for 8 to 12 weeks, adjust occlusion, and observe for signs or symptoms of pulpal necrosis. If fracture present, try root canal treatment on both segments if root is stable as a singular entity. If not, extract coronal segment and evaluate.

changes (Fig. 11-26, *B*). Sensibility tests have not changed. Five weeks later the patient presented with significant radiographic changes (Fig. 11-26, *C*). Resorption is evident at the borders of the fracture, and sensibility tests indicate no response.

Solution: A diagnosis of a necrotic pulp, along with the radiographic changes, indicates the need for immediate intervention. The root canal was accessed, measured, and cleaned and shaped (Fig. 11-26, *D*). Inflammatory resorption is evident (see Chapter 10) and must be managed with both the removal of the inciting cause and the placement of calcium hydroxide in an attempt to arrest the inflammatory resorption. Six months after canal cleaning and shaping and with evidence of a halt in the resorptive process, the root canal was obturated with a gutta-percha core-carrier technique (Fig. 11-26, *E*) (Thermafil plastic, see Chapter 6). Long-term recall evaluation is necessary. (Case courtesy Dr. Hedley Rakusin.)

Clinical Problem: A 28-year-old male patient was referred for evaluation and treatment of a maxillary right central incisor. The patient's chief complaint was "pain upon biting and the tooth was always draining." The patient stated that the tooth

was injured during a basketball game about 8 years previously and that a dentist performed "some type of root canal treatment" on the tooth at that time. Over the past 2 months, however, he noticed a bad taste in his mouth and that the tooth was becoming tender to biting. Clinical examination revealed a draining sinus tract in the alveolar mucosa near the apex of tooth of the right central incisor and a 9 mm narrow-based periodontal defect at the midfacial. It was also apparent that the temporary filling in the palatal access opening was leaking. A periradicular radiograph showed a transverse root fracture in the apical third of the root with extensive osseous breakdown at level of the fracture (Fig. 11-27, *A*). Notice the depth of probing and the traced sinus tract. A diagnosis of pulp necrosis with acute suppurative periradicular periodontitis subsequent to an apical transverse root fracture was made.

Solution: After administration of local anesthetic, the tooth was isolated with a ligated rubber dam. After the palatal temporary filling was removed, the canal was debrided to the apical extent of the coronal root segment with use of 2.5% NaOCl and Hedström files (Fig. 11-27, *B*). Calcium

A   B   C

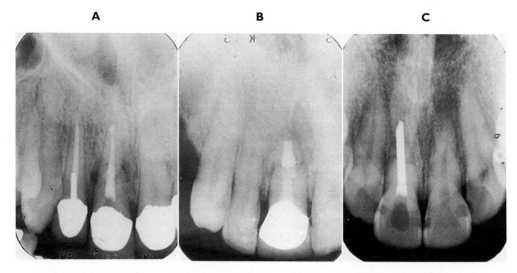

Fig. 11-23 **A,** *Root canal treatment of both segments of a horizontally fractured tooth. Segments were in apposition, and pulp became necrotic with presence of lateral radiolucencies. Calcium hydroxide sealer (Sealapex) was used. Notice movement of sealer into the fracture line.* **B,** *Alternative way of managing a horizontal fracture. The apical segment is filled with gutta-percha and sealer, whereas the coronal segment is filled with calcium hydroxide. Periodic evaluation will be necessary.* **C,** *Endodontic endosseous implant was used after the removal of the apical half of the fractured tooth. Nine-month recall shows good osseous healing.*

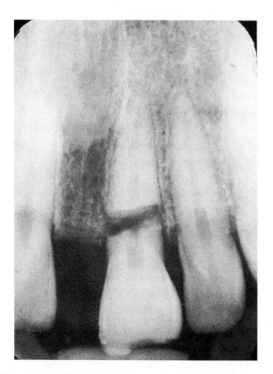

Fig. 11-24 *Coronal third fracture with separated segments and communication with the gingival sulcus. Extraction of both segments is indicated.*

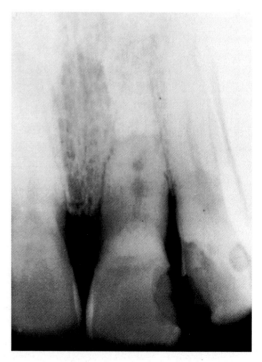

Fig. 11-25 *Symptomless tooth 2 years after horizontal fracture. Notice partial calcification or possible internal resorption. The edges of the fracture have undergone some remodeling. Case may be characterized as a "union" type of healing with a combination of calcific and connective tissue.*

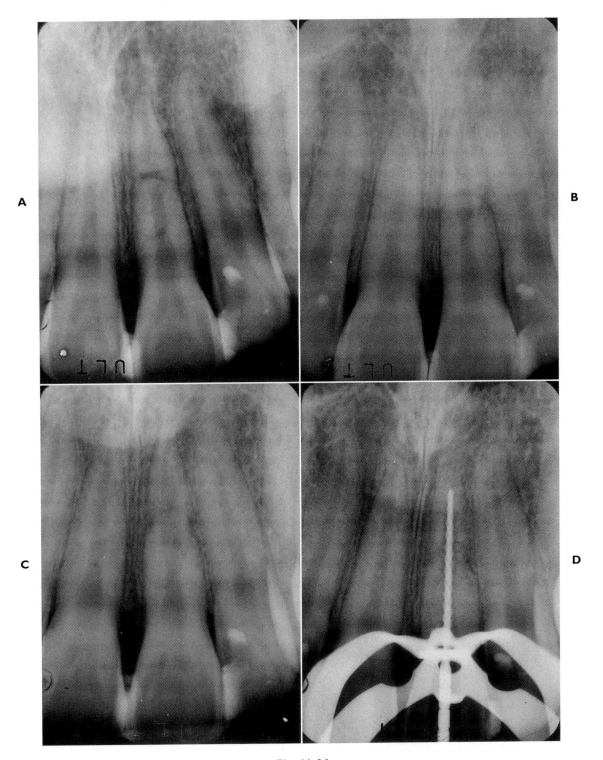

Fig. 11-26

Continued.

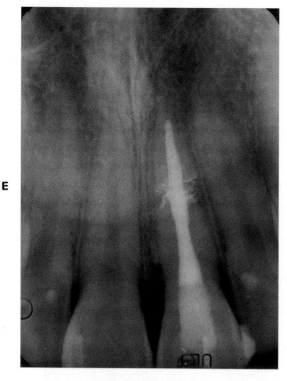

E

Fig. 11-26 cont'd.

hydroxide was placed as an interim dressing before tooth closure. At the following visit (2 weeks later), the patient was symptom free, but the sinus tract was still present. The tooth was reopened, and the canal was completely cleaned, shaped, and obturated with gutta-percha and sealer using lateral compaction (Fig. 11-27, *C*). The patient was requested to return in 1 month to determine the status of the sinus tract. At the 1 month follow-up exam, the patient was symptom free, but the sinus tract had not healed. Periradicular surgery was scheduled to remove the fractured apical root segment. The displaced apical segment most likely contained necrotic, infected tissue and thus the cause of the persistent sinus tract and periodontal defect. At the surgery appointment, the apical segment was removed (Fig. 11-27, *D*), the osseous defect was curetted, and the apical segment of the coronal root segment was lightly beveled to smooth any resorptive irregularities. A postoperative radiograph was taken (Fig. 11-27, *E*). At the 4 month follow-up exam, the sinus tract had healed, the periodontal probing depth at the midfacial was 4 mm, and incomplete osseous healing was evident (Fig. 11-27, *F*). The patient was scheduled for periodic reevaluation to monitor further healing.

Healing of Root Fractures

The ability of the practitioner to anticipate or predict healing of fractured roots is predicated on the following circumstances.

1. Close adaptation of the fractured segments
2. Stability of the segments in the alveolus
3. Absence of factors that would prevent healing, that is, infection, compromised healing potential of the patient, periodontal disease, and so forth
4. The more apical the fracture, the better the prognosis[3,33]

Although healing occurs primarily through bony union or fibrous union, multiple investigators have identified the specific nature of healing that does occur. A brief review of these concepts will assist the practitioner in the ultimate "problem-solving" assessment of these cases, which must occur on a regular basis to determine the success or failure of treatment (see Chapter 1). It is important for the clinician to be primarily concerned with union versus nonunion, as opposed to the actual histologic findings during posttreatment assessment.

Calcific healing ("union" type of healing)
The following description refers to Fig. 11-28:
1. Occurs primarily when segments are in close apposition.
2. Callus formation occurs along the lateral borders of the fracture.
3. Partial linear calcification of the canal is present in the region of the fracture and in the apical segment.
4. Pulp is viable with reduced level of responsiveness.
5. Percussion will be painless.
6. Mobility will be within physiologic limits.
7. Seen most often in teeth with immature root formation at the time of fracture.

Connective tissue healing ("union" type of healing)
The following description refers to Fig. 11-29:
1. Comparable to fibrous healing of bone.
2. Segments may or may not be separated.
3. Edges of fracture have been remodeled and appear rounded.
4. Mobility is within physiologic limits.
5. Percussion may give varied but not a painful response to percussion.
6. Fracture line appears radiolucent.
7. Pulp canal space often exhibits extensive calcification.

Bone and connective tissue healing ("union" type of healing)
The following description refers to Fig. 11-30:

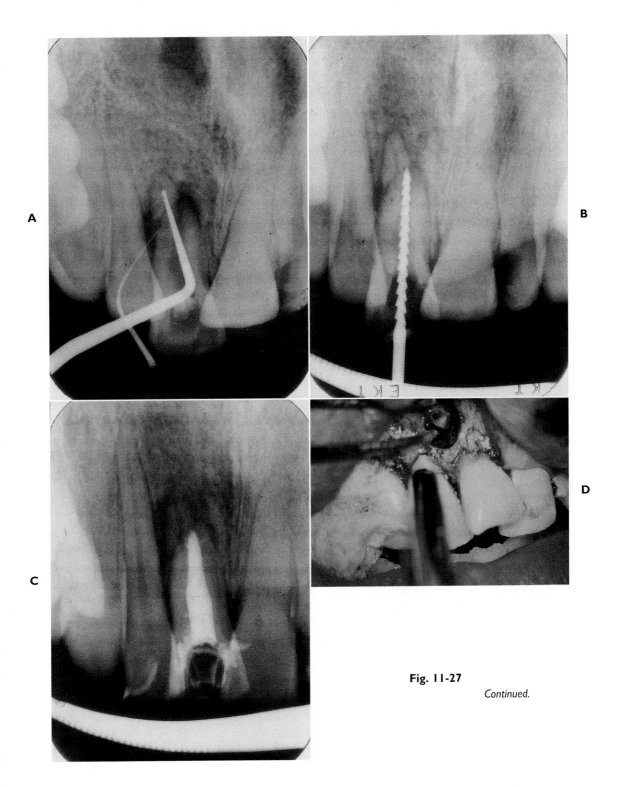

Fig. 11-27

Continued.

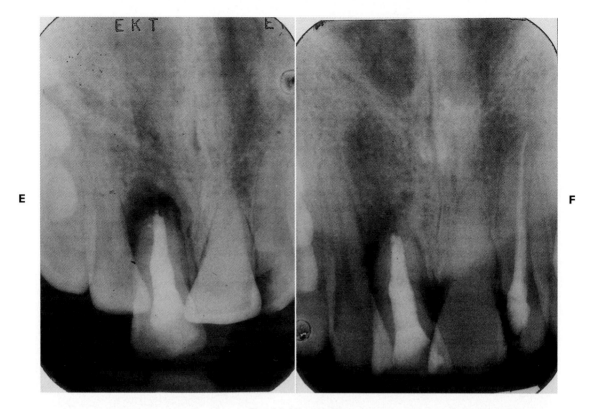

E

F

Fig. 11-27 cont'd.

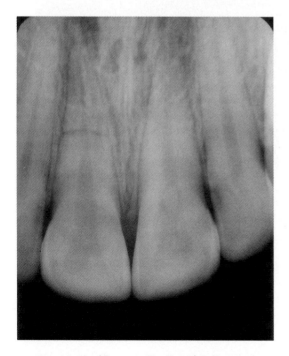

Fig. 11-28 *(Courtesy Dr. David P. Rossiter.)*

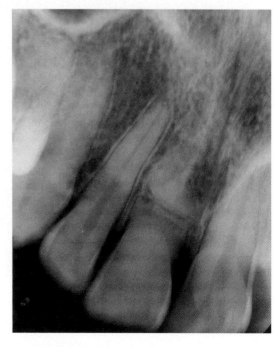

Fig. 11-29 *(Courtesy Dr. David P. Rossiter.)*

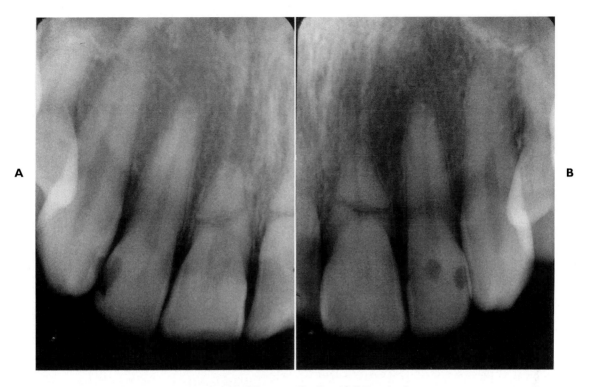

Fig. 11-30 *(Courtesy Dr. David P. Rossiter.)*

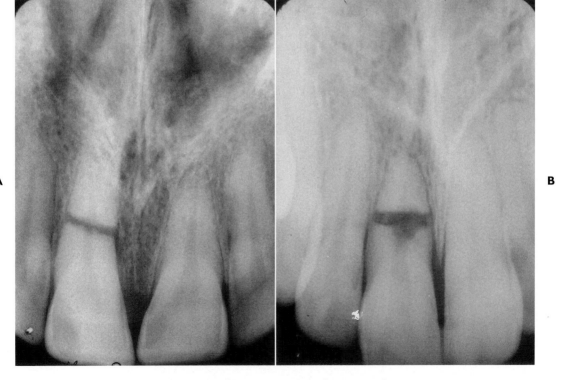

Fig. 11-31 *(Courtesy Dr. David P. Rossiter.)*

1. Occurs when there is greater separation of fractured segments.
2. Interposition of bone and connective tissue into fracture.
3. Periodontal ligament space commonly seen between and around both fractured segments.
4. Pulp space calcification extensive.
5. Pulp viable but at reduced levels of responsiveness.
6. Mobility within physiological limits; coronal segment often continues eruption.

"Nonunion" of segments with granulation tissue

The following description refers to Fig. 11-31:

1. Primarily resulting from pulpal contamination during trauma.
2. Occurs in cases of severe dislocation.
3. Apical segment retains vitality; coronal segment undergoes pulpal necrosis.
4. Wide gap seen between fractured segments.
5. Tooth will be loose and sensitive to percussion.
6. Tooth may be slightly extruded and exhibit color changes.
7. Sinus tract may be present at level of fracture line.

When applying the concepts of success and failure highlighted in Chapter 1, the first three modes of healing of horizontally fractured roots can be considered as clinically, radiographically, and histologically acceptable. Nonunion healing with the interposition of granulation tissue is considered as histologically unacceptable but depending on the signs and symptoms may be considered as clinically or radiographically acceptable or questionable, or any combination thereof. Management of these specific categories can be found in Tables 11-4 and 11-5.

References

1. Andreasen FM, Daugaard-Jensen J, Munksgaard EC: Reinforcement of bonded crown fractured incisors with porcelain veneers, *Endod Dent Traumatol* 7:78-83, 1991.
2. Andreasen JO, Andreasen FM: *Textbook and color atlas of traumatic injuries to the teeth,* ed 3, Copenhagen, 1994, Munksgaard, pp 279-314.
3. Bender IB, Freedland JB: Adult root fracture, *J Am Dent Assoc* 107:413-419, 1983.
4. Bender IB, Freedland JB: Clinical considerations in the diagnosis and treatment of intra-alveolar root fractures, *J Am Dent Assoc* 107:595-600, 1983.
5. Cameron CE: Cracked-tooth syndrome, *J Am Dent Assoc* 68:405-411, 1964.
6. Cameron CE: The cracked-tooth syndrome: additional findings, *J Am Dent Assoc* 93:971-975, 1976.
7. Caufield JB: Hairline tooth fracture: a clinical case report, *J Am Dent Assoc* 102:501-502, 1981.
8. Feiglin B: Clinical management of transverse root fractures, *Dent Clin North Am* 39:53-78, 1995.
9. Gibbs JW: Cuspal fracture odontalgia, *Dent Dig* 60:158-160, 1954.
10. Gutmann JL, Everett Gutmann MS: Cause, incidence, and prevention of trauma to teeth, *Dent Clin North Am* 39:1-14, 1995.
11. Gutmann JL, Harrison JW: *Surgical endodontics,* Boston, 1991, Blackwell Scientific Publications, pp 360, 368.
12. Gutmann JL, Rakusin H: Endodontic and restorative management of incompletely fractured molar teeth, *Int Endod J* 27:343-348, 1994.
13. Hiatt WH: Incomplete crown-root fracture in pulpal-periodontal disease, *J Periodontol* 44:369-379, 1973.
14. Josell SD: Evaluation, diagnosis, and treatment of the traumatized patient, *Dent Clin North Am* 39:15-24, 1995.
15. Lindahl B: Transverse intra-alveolar root fractures: roentgen diagnosis and prognosis, *Odontol Revy* 9:10-24, 1958.
16. Lommel TJ, Meister F, Gerstein H et al: Alveolar bone loss associated with vertical root fractures: report of six cases, *Oral Surg Oral Med Oral Pathol* 45:909-919, 1978.
17. Luebke RG: Vertical crown-root fractures in posterior teeth, *Dent Clin North Am* 28:883-894, 1984.
18. Matusow RJ: Endodontic complications of root fractures, *J Am Dent Assoc* 114:766, 1987.
19. Maxwell EH, Braly BV: Incomplete tooth fracture—prediction and prevention, *Calif Dent Assoc J* 5(10):51-55, 1977.
20. Meister F, Lommel TJ, Gerstein H: Diagnosis and possible causes of vertical root fractures, *Oral Surg Oral Med Oral Pathol* 49:243-253, 1980.
21. Munksgaard EC, Højtved L, Jørgensen EHW et al: Enamel-dentin crown fractures bonded with various agents, *Endod Dent Traumatol* 7:73-77, 1991.
22. Pitts DL, Natkin E: Diagnosis and treatment of vertical root fractures, *J Endod* 1983. 9:338-346,
23. Rauschenberger CR, Hovland EJ: Clinical management of crown fractures, *Dent Clin North Am* 39:25-52, 1995.
24. Ritchey B, Mendenhall R, Orban B: Pulpitis resulting from incomplete tooth fracture, *Oral Surg Oral Med Oral Pathol* 10:665-670, 1957.
25. Rosen H: Cracked tooth syndrome, *J Prosthet Dent* 47:36-43, 1982.
26. Ross RS, Nicholls JI, Harrington GW: A comparison of strains generated during placement of five endodontic posts, *J Endod* 17:450-456, 1991.
27. Schweitzer JL, Gutmann JL, Bliss RQ: Odontiatrogenic tooth fracture, *Int Endod J* 22:64-74, 1989.
28. Silvestri AR: The undiagnosed split-root syndrome, *J Am Dent Assoc* 92:930-935, 1976.
29. Stewart GG: Clinical application of glass ionomer cements in endodontics: case reports. *Int Endod J* 23:172-178, 1990.
30. Sutton PRN: Greenstick fracture of the tooth crown, *Br Dent J* 112:362-363, 1962.
31. Trope M, Tronstad L: Resistance to fracture of endodontically treated premolars restored with glass ionomer cement or acid etch composite resin, *J Endod* 17:257-259, 1991.
32. Weibusch FB: Hairline fracture of a cusp: report of a case, *J Can Dent Assoc* 38:192-194, 1972.
33. Zachrisson BU, Jacobsen I: Long term prognosis of 66 permanent anterior teeth with root fracture, *Scand J Dent Res* 83:345-354, 1975.

▼

Chapter 12

Problems Encountered with Pulpal-Periodontal Interrelationships

James L. Gutmann
Paul E. Lovdahl

". . . I have never found a pulp removed from a pyorrhetic tooth to be normal . . . where a pathologic pulp is present, a pyorrhetic condition cannot be cured by treatment applied exclusively to the external surface of the root, with no treatment of the pulp itself."[*]

". . . interradicular periodontal lesions can be initiated and perpetuated by inflamed or necrotic pulps. Extension of the inflammatory lesions from the dental pulp apparently occurs through accessory or lateral canals situated in the furcation regions of premolars and molars . . ."[†]

Although interrelationships between pulpal and periodontal disease have been both confirmed and denied for over 100 years,[3,7,9] during this time little was written concerning the diagnosis and management of these interrelated entities, other than indicating that teeth having these problems were often extracted based on a poor prognosis for retention. This was especially true if a periodontal pocket united with a periradicular lesion of pulpal origin. The various diagnostic and clinical aspects of this problem still face practitioners who attempt to accurately manage these cases. The purpose of this chapter is to provide a thoughtful and contemporary review of the basis for and against the presence of interrelated pulpal and periodontal disease states, to examine the pathways that may contribute to this interrelationship, to integrate this information into a problem-solving approach to management, and to address commonly asked questions and clinical dilemmas regarding these relationships.

PULPAL-PERIODONTAL INTERACTIONS

Pulp tissue degenerates after a multitude of insults, such as caries, restorative procedures, chemical and thermal insults, trauma, and some periodontal treatment. When products from pulp degeneration reach the supporting periodontium, rapid inflammatory responses characterized by bone loss, tooth mobility, and sinus tract formation can ensue. If this occurs in the apical region, a periradicular lesion forms. If this occurs with crestal extension of the inflammation, a periodontitis of pulpal origin is formed.[29] However, the lesion formed has little anatomic similarity to a periodontally induced defect.

Periodontal disease, on the other hand, is generally a slow-developing process that may have a gradual atrophic effect on the dental pulp. Reports have identified the presence of inflammation, localized tissue infarction, fibrosis, a decrease in cells, resorptions, localized coagulation necrosis, and dystrophic calcification in the pulps of teeth with surrounding and influencing periodontal disease.[18,21,23,25,27,30-32] Complete pulpal necrosis caused by periodontal disease, however, is uncommon.[21] Additionally, periodontal procedures such as deep scaling and curettage,[33] with the use of localized medicaments, and gingival injury or wounding[32] may enhance further pulpal inflammation and perpetuate the interrelated disease process.

---

[*]From Cahn LR: *Dent Item Int* 49:598-617, 1927.
[†]From Seltzer S, Bender IB, Nazimov H: *J Periodontol* 38:124-129, 1967.

Pulpal and periodontal disease states have been created and studied experimentally in the teeth of monkeys, dogs, and man over the past 30 years. However, a true and unquestionable consensus has not been identified regarding the relationship of these disease processes, especially as it applies to the human model.

The most intimate and demonstrable relationship between the two tissues is by means of the vascular system[2,10,20,26,33] as demonstrated anatomically at the apical foramen and adjacent to aberrant, accessory communications.[6,9,13,22,25] These channels, when patent, may serve as potential routes of inflammatory interchange (Fig. 12-1). Still other channels, covered by cementum, may be exposed during scaling or other periodontal therapeutic procedures.[33] A major concern, however, is the fact that is it unknown to what extent these vascular communications must be disrupted to cause a resultant, overwhelming inflammatory process.[21]

Although the focus of communication between the pulp and periodontium focuses on the vascular route, many other valid avenues exist. The following anatomic entities or pathways must be considered in the exchange of inflammatory products and bacteria. Each has been addressed in the literature in isolated situations, but seldom if ever have they all been identified as potentially contributing to this dynamic interchange.[12]

1. Dentinal tubules
2. Lingual grooves
3. Root or tooth fractures
4. Cemental agenesis or hypoplasia
5. Root anomalies
6. Intermediate bifurcation ridges
7. Fibrinous communications
8. Cervical enamel projections
9. Damage to the cementum or a trauma-resorption process

Although the consensus supports the influence that a degenerating or inflamed pulp can have on the periodontium, not all investigators are in agreement about the influence of periodontal disease on the pulp.

In 1964 Mazur and Massler suggested that there was no relationship between the severity of periodontal disease (as measured by the amounts of exposed root) and changes in the pulp.[24] Teeth from the same patient with a wide variety of periodontal compromises demonstrated pulps to be histologically similar. Some pulps varied within the same

patient from nearly normal to that of advanced degeneration, and it was believed that these changes were related more to the systemic condition of the patient than to chronologic age or status of the periodontium (Fig. 12-2).

Bender and Seltzer, in 1972, found no relationship between pulp disease and the (1) depth of the periodontal pocket, (2) extent of bone loss, and (3) extent of periodontal disease.[2] The greatest pulpal reactions that were observed in the presence of periodontal disease appeared to be related to excessive accessory communications.

Hattler and associates, in 1977, using a rice rat model with induced periodontal disease, could not demonstrate any concomitant pulpal changes.[16] However, no accessory communications were identified in the rat teeth.

Bergenholtz and Lindhe, in 1978, placed ligatures around the necks of teeth in six adult rhesus monkeys to induce inflammation and periodontal destruction.[4] Subsequent plaque accumulation after 5 to 7 months caused loss of 30% to 40% of the tissue supporting the roots. One group of teeth received no further treatment. Another group was subjected to scaling and root planing. After treatment, plaque was allowed to accumulate for 2, 10, and 30 days on the freshly planed root surfaces. Histologic examination showed that in comparison to teeth with a normal periodontium, 57% of the teeth with a diseased periodontium had pathologic pulp tissue alterations. These changes within the pulp were not of an extreme nature, and only one tooth showed signs of total pulp necrosis. Aggravation of increased incidence of pulpal pathosis was essentially the same for the group of teeth with periodontitis alone and the group subjected to scaling and plaque accumulation. The study concluded that, in the monkey, (1) periodontal disease is limited to the cervical half of the root and (2) plaque accumulation on exposed root surfaces did not cause severe changes in the pulp of the roots involved.

Czarnecki and Schilder, in 1979, investigated the pulps of 46 human teeth that evidenced varying degrees of periodontal disease.[11] Pulpal changes in these teeth were within normal limits, and severe caries or extensive coronal restorations were identified with pulpal changes regardless of the degree of periodontal involvement. Correlations could not be made between the presence or severity of periodontal disease and histologic pulpal changes. Similar findings were reported by Torabinejad and Kiger.[34]

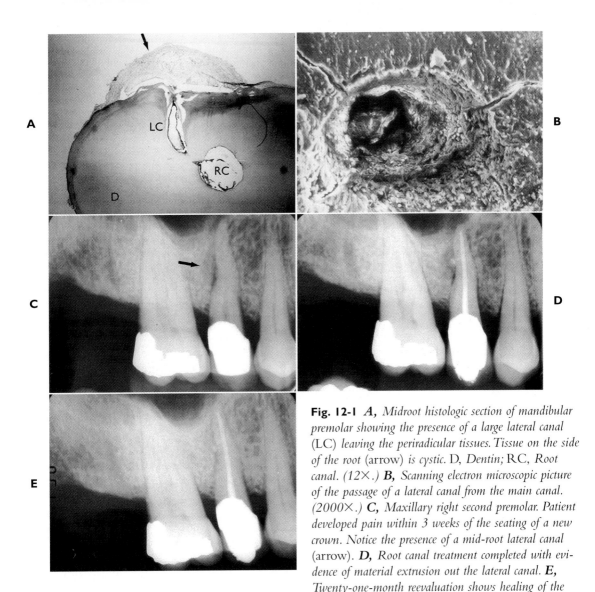

Fig. 12-1 **A,** *Midroot histologic section of mandibular premolar showing the presence of a large lateral canal (LC) leaving the periradicular tissues. Tissue on the side of the root (arrow) is cystic. D, Dentin; RC, Root canal. (12×.)* **B,** *Scanning electron microscopic picture of the passage of a lateral canal from the main canal. (2000×.)* **C,** *Maxillary right second premolar. Patient developed pain within 3 weeks of the seating of a new crown. Notice the presence of a mid-root lateral canal (arrow).* **D,** *Root canal treatment completed with evidence of material extrusion out the lateral canal.* **E,** *Twenty-one-month reevaluation shows healing of the lateral lesion with root canal treatment only.* (**C** to **E** *Courtesy Dr. Jordan Schweitzer)*

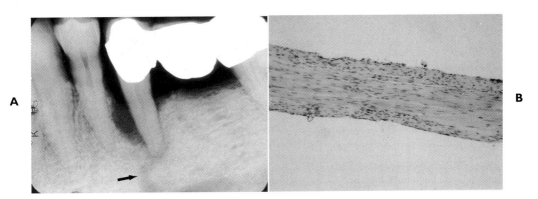

Fig. 12-2 **A,** *Mandibular left second premolar showing a deep angular defect on the mesial of the root. Notice the extension of the mental foramen (arrow). Pocketing is also evident on the distal. The case was originally diagnosed as a combined pulpoperiodontal lesion.* **B,** *Pulp tissue from this tooth is normal with no evidence of inflammatory cells or significant degeneration. (10×.)*

305

Although most of the studies before 1979 were done under the assumption that periodontal disease directly affects the pulp and the histologic observations from such studies may support that concept, conclusions cannot be drawn solely on the basis of such observations. These studies often fail to include an evaluation of teeth that previously received periodontal therapy or teeth that were periodontally normal. The lack of inclusion of age-matched teeth and variations in the anatomical pathways of communication between these two tissues in different human and animal subjects also adds to the disparate findings.[17]

Recent studies have focused more on the role played by an infected or degenerating pulp on the supporting periodontium.[5,8,17] Hirsch et al and Clark and Hirsch have identified a strong association between pulpal pathosis and localized, severe angular alveolar defects that are commonly identified as primary lesions of periodontal origin caused by specific oral bacteria. It was believed that periodontal disease of pulpal origin has the potential to occur in the early states of pulpal disease. An extension of this disease by the path of least resistance with a rapid breakthrough to the gingival sulcus could account for the sudden and severe deepening of localized areas of periodontal pathosis. Influenced by additional communication from the compromised pulp by alternative anatomic pathways, a further inflammatory reaction is encouraged in the periodontium with increased granulation tissue formation and osteoclastic activity. Colonization of these defects by organisms suited to exploit these pathologic conditions accounts for the presence of the periodontopathogens and the antibodies directed against them.[8] Although potentially plausible, this theory is highly speculative, and further studies are warranted. Therefore, before one approaches pulpal-periodontic relationships from a clinical standpoint, two very important issues might be highlighted.

Pulpal disease and its extension into the periodontium causes a localized periodontitis with the potential for further extension into the oral cavity. Periodontal disease and its extension has little short-term effect on the dental pulp.

CLINICAL PARAMETERS AND CLASSIFICATIONS

Previously an accurate diagnosis of the interrela-

tionship of pulpal and periodontal disease states was hampered by the absence of contributions to the dental literature that provided clinically relevant and biologically substantiated classifications for this relationship. A workable classification for pulpal-periodontal disease entities that was based on possible cause, diagnosis, and prognosis was introduced in 1970.[28] The essential elements of this classification are as follows with more specific characteristics, diagnostic criteria, and projected treatment or prognosis identified in Charts 1 to 6.

1. The primary pulpal lesion in which inflammatory or infective processes in the dental pulp extended into the periodontium causing loss of the supporting apparatus: After root canal treatment alone, rapid healing of the periodontium occurred (Chart 1 and Fig. 12-3).

2. The primary pulpal lesion that has extended to the periodontium becomes chronic in nature, with the ultimate superimposition of true periodontal disease: Prognosis is highly dependent on the successful treatment of both entities (Chart 2) (Fig. 12-4).

3. The primary lesion of periodontal origin that is totally dependent on periodontal therapy for resolution: The pulp remains unaffected (Chart 3 and Fig. 12-5).

4. The primary periodontal lesion that is chronic in nature and may influence the degeneration of the pulp by encompassing all major radicular pulpal foramina: Successful treatment is dependent on the management of both disease processes (Chart 4 and Fig. 12-6).

5. The combined pulpal-periodontal lesion in which the two disease processes are independently initiated and ultimately join in the surrounding periradicular tissues: The progression of each may influence the other (Chart 5 and Fig. 12-7).

The essentials of this classification have been of significant value to the practice of both endodontics and periodontics. An additional classification that may be commonly seen and may reflect the presence of two separate and distinct entities has also been proposed.[1] This is referred to as the "concomitant pulpal-periodontal lesion" (Chart 6 and Fig. 12-8). In essence, both disease states exist but with different etiologic factors and with no clinical evidence that either disease state has influenced the other. This situation often goes undiagnosed, and treatment is rendered to only one of the diseased tissues in the hopes that the other will respond favorably. In actuality, both disease processes must

CHART I
Primary Pupal Lesion (Fig. 12-3)

↓

Characteristics

Sinus tract
Tooth mobility
Localized bone loss
Narrow pocket
Swelling in attached gingiva
Sore to bite/percussion
Discomfort minimal
Large restoration
History of capping or pulpotomy
Poor root canal treatment

↓

Diagnosis

Pulp test/thermal and electric
Localized periodontal disease
Tracing of a sinus tract
Minimal to no calculus
Rapid onset
Previous pulp treatment

↓

Treatment/prognosis

Root canal treatment
Excellent prognosis

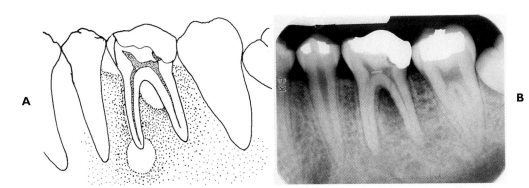

A · B

Fig. 12-3 *A, Diagram of a lesion of primary pulp origin. Long-term inflammation by recurrent decay or previous pulp cap or the pushing of debris into a pulpal exposure has resulted in a necrotic pulp with evidence of furcation bone loss.* **B,** *Radiograph of the case depicted in* **A.** *Root canal treatment only is indicated. (From Belk CE, Gutmann JL: Can Dent J 56:1013-1017, 1990.)*

CHART 2
Primary Pulpal/Secondary Periodontal
Lesion (Fig. 12-4)

↓

Characteristics

Long-standing pulpal pathoses
Superimposition of plaque/calculus
Generalized periodontal disease

↓

Diagnosis

Pulpal inflammation/necrosis based on
 exam/tests
Significant periodontal inflammation
Radiographic evidence of angular
 defects

↓

Treatment/prognosis

Root canal treatment
Periodontal treatment
Prognosis dependent on ability to treat
 both disease entities

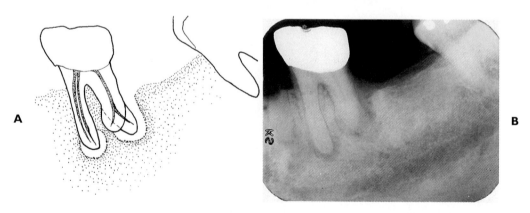

Fig. 12-4 *A,* *Diagram of a mandibular molar that exhibits pulpal necrosis affecting the surrounding bone and demonstrating crestal extension and a wide-based distal pocket.* **B,** *Radiograph of the case depicted in* **A.** *Cause is presumed to be extensive restorative procedures with possible coronal leakage. (From Belk CE, Gutmann JL:* Can Dent J *56:1013-1017, 1990.)*

CHART 3
Primary Periodontal Lesion (Fig. 12-5)

↓

Characteristics

Teeth vital
Generalized bone loss
Calculus/plaque
Soft-tissue inflammation
Broad-based pockets
Possible occlusal trauma

↓

Diagnosis

Oral exam/probing
Radiograph
Pulp testing
Patient factors

↓

Treatment/prognosis

Extent of disease/treatment
Patient compliance
Root or tooth resection or extraction

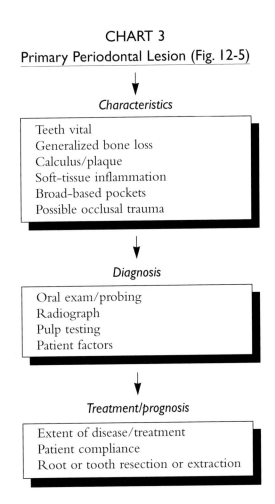

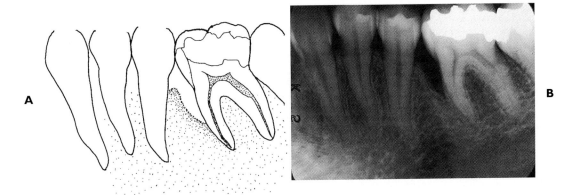

Fig. 12-5 *A, Diagram of a deep angular periodontal pocket. B, Radiograph of the case depicted in A. The singular isolated nature of this type of pocket characterizes periodontal disease. (From Belk CE, Gutmann JL:* Can Dent J *56:1013-1017, 1990.)*

CHART 4
Primary Periodontal/Secondary Pulpal Lesion (Fig. 12-6)

↓

Characteristics

Deep periodontal pockets > 6 to 8 mm
History of extensive periodontal procedures
Irreversible pulpal pathosis
Pain accentuation
Tooth needs or has large restoration

↓

Diagnosis

History of disease progression
Probing/pulp testing
Radiographic changes
Pain

↓

Treatment/prognosis

Dependent on periodontal treatment after root canal treatment

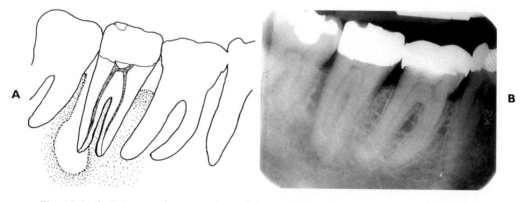

Fig. 12-6 *A, Diagram of an extensive and deep periodontal pocket that has extended to the depth of the root apex. B, Radiograph of the case depicted in A. Patient experienced symptoms of irreversible pulpitis with acute periradicular periodontitis. Biopsy of the pulp tissue was normal. (From Belk CE, Gutmann JL:* Can Dent J *56:1013-1017, 1990.)*

CHART 5
Combined Pulpal/Periodontal
Lesion (Fig. 12-7)

↓

Characteristics

Merging of apical pulpal lesion and
  progressive periodontal pocket
May mimic pulpal-only lesion
Acute or chronic in nature

↓

Diagnosis

Periodontal pocket communicates
  with apical root lesion
Pulp testing
Radiographic infraosseous pocket
Possible vertical fracture

↓

Treatment/prognosis

Root canal treatment first/periodontal
  treatment
Better prognosis with primary
  pulpal lesion
Better prognosis with short-term lesion

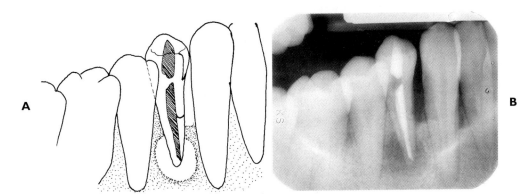

Fig. 12-7 A, *Diagram of the presence of periodontal bone loss; lateral canal at the depth of the pocket and pulpal necrosis.* **B,** *Radiograph of the case depicted in* **A** *that shows the characteristic, but rare, combined pulpoperiodontal lesion. (From Belk CE, Gutmann JL: Can Dent J 56:1013-1017, 1990.)*

CHART 6
Concomitant Pulpal-Periodontal
Lesion (Fig. 12-8)

↓

Both disease states exist with no
  evidence that either has influenced
  the other
Both entities must be treated concomitantly with prognosis dependent on
  removal of the individual causes

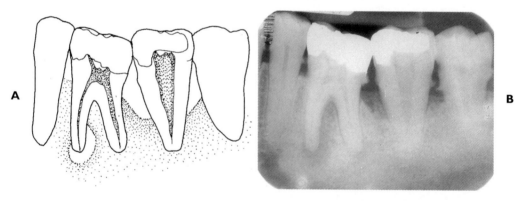

A

B

Fig. 12-8 *A, Diagram of the independent presence of a periradicular lesion of pulpal origin and periodontal disease. There is no obvious communication between the two entities. B, Radiograph of the case depicted in A. The two molars exhibit periodontal disease. The first molar shows evidence of an unrelated extension of pulpal disease to the periradicular tissues. (From Belk CE, Gutmann JL: Can Dent J 56:1013-1017, 1990.)*

be treated concomitantly, with the prognosis dependent on the removal of the individual etiologic factors and prevention of any further factors that may affect the respective disease processes. For example, perforation of the floor of a pulp chamber during root canal treatment will have an adverse effect on the diseased periodontium, which heretofore may not have been influenced by the state of the pulp tissue.

CLINICAL PROBLEM: A 55-year-old female patient presents with a long-term history of spontaneous pain in her maxillary left arch. At times she has pain to biting and often feels a pressure sensation in the area of the second premolar. She has a history of sinus problems and has been told in the past that her teeth are fine. Today she is in acute pain, especially to biting. A clinical exam reveals multiple missing teeth and an extensive restoration on the second premolar (Fig. 12-9). The missing teeth are replaced by a removable partial denture. Palpation and percussion are both abnormal on the second premolar, with the contralateral tooth being normal. Radiographically there is a radiolucency that is distally placed on the apical portion of the root *(black arrows)*. Likewise there is the beginning of a vertical periodontal defect on the distal surface *(white arrow)*. Probings are shallow on the mesial (2 to 3 mm) and deeper on the distal (4 to 5 mm).

Solution: Further pulp testing is unnecessary to make the diagnosis of pulp necrosis with acute periradicular periodontitis. Root canal treatment is indicated; however the periodontal status must also be addressed. The present findings do not reveal a communication between the two disease entities, and there is substantial support for two separate causes. However, what cannot be overlooked is the possibility of a vertical fracture that may serve as a common etiologic factor. Notice the thickened lamina dura on both the mesial and distal root surfaces. This could represent merely occlusal stresses on the tooth from the partial denture, or it may represent a reactive osseous response to a vertical fracture. Examination during root canal treatment for this latter possibility is essential (see Chapter 11). (Case courtesy Dr. James Douthitt.)

Although these classifications have been helpful in diagnosis and treatment, they may also provide unidentifiable clinical entities that challenge the clinician's ability to provide timely and successful treatment. Often erroneous treatment is rendered, or no treatment is involved, because teeth may be needlessly extracted in favor of implants or prostheses. This is true because all diagnostic states,

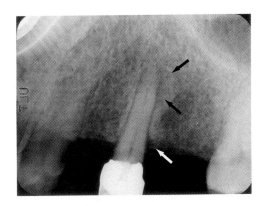

Fig. 12-9

based on succinct subjective and objective findings and limited-value pulp testing, are only probabilities relative to the true histopathologic state of the tissues.[8,17]

For the clinician, the close relationship between pulpal and periodontal disease states is reasonably established on clinical and radiographic levels. Although interpretations may vary on which came first — the proverbial "chicken or the egg" controversy — a through diagnosis and evaluation *must* ensue to determine the most probable cause, the course of disease, and the most reasonable treatment. In essence, when pulpal disease exists, the periodontium must be evaluated, and likewise, when periodontal disease is present, the clinical pulpal status must be ascertained. Should an interrelationship in disease entities exist, or if the potential for the existence is real or anticipated, appropriate treatment must be rendered to remove the true etiologic factors and enhance the prognosis for tooth retention.

CLINICAL PROBLEM: A 58-year-old male patient presented with swelling and pain to biting (percussion) and the presence of a large radiolucency that extended to the gingival sulcus around the mandibular second molar. Deep distal probings were also present. The pulp was diagnosed as being necrotic and was identified as being the cause of the patient's problem. He was told that after the root canal treatment the osseous lesion would heal and no further treatment would be necessary (Fig. 12-10, *A*). After treatment the patient's symptoms abated. However, at the 1 year reevaluation, significant bone loss was noted (Fig. 12-10, *B*), and there was a significant amount of purulence coming through the gingival sulcus.

Solution: The initial treatment plan was probably incorrect. When the patient's record was reevaluated, it was noted that upon entry into the tooth the pulp was necrotic and was in all probability the primary cause. However, with a long-term draining lesion of pulpal origin, a secondary periodontitis was superimposed. Coupled with the presence of significant deep radicular calculus (Fig. 12-10, *C*), a deep and probably unphysiologic crown margin, and a fused root, any periodontal treatment may have been futile. Ironically no periodontal treatment was even attempted. Extraction was necessary.

To identify clinically relevant situations in which the above information can be effectively integrated in a problem-solving format, commonly asked questions relative to the identification and management of pulpal and periodontal disease are addressed. Although some issues may be repetitious in nature, it is done so by design for emphasis.

Does pulpal inflammation or infection cause periodontal disease?

If the inflammation is totally within the confines of the tooth, there is little if any effect on the periodontium. The extension of pulpal inflammation or infection to the periodontium will result in localized periradicular periodontitis of pulpal origin (see Chapter 9). Strictly speaking this is not "periodontal disease." This periodontal inflammation of pulpal origin is usually reversible in nature, and healing will occur after removal of the etiologic agents by root canal treatment.

CLINICAL PROBLEM: A 64-year-old female patient presents with a chief complaint expressed as follows: "I have a toothache and it hurts when I chew on this tooth. I also have a little gumboil beside the tooth." Medically she is in good health. She indicates that the teeth in her mandibular posterior quadrant are particularly painful when the maxillary teeth come into contact with them. She has been bothered by this for over a year, but her general dentist could not see anything on the radiograph. Clinical exam reveals a draining sinus tract adjacent to the second molar. The tract was traced to the furcation region of this tooth (Fig. 12-11, *A*). No periodontal pocketing was noted. Both molars had gold crowns, and the first molar had had root canal treatment. Sensibility testing gave no response on both molars, whereas the second molar was tender to percussion and palpation. A radiolucency was present around the apices of the second molar.

Solution: Based on the subjective and objective findings, a diagnosis of pulp necrosis with acute suppurative periradicular periodontitis is appropriate (see Chapter 9). Root canal treatment is

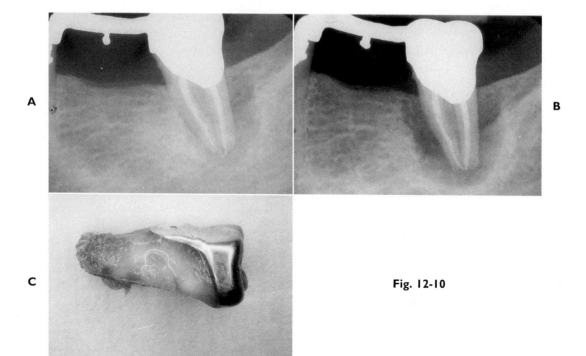

A

B

C

Fig. 12-10

indicated for the second molar. No periodontal treatment is indicated at this time. Upon obturation of the canals a large furcation canal was filled. Notice the furcation radiolucency (Fig. 12-11, *B*). Presumably the lateral canal was filled with sealer because lateral compaction was the method of obturation. A 38-month reevaluation reveals a sound periodontium and complete healing of the furcation and apical radiolucency. The patient is symptom free (Fig. 12-11, *C*). (Case courtesy Dr. Jordan Schweitzer.)

The periodontal component of any localized lesion of pulpal origin is often difficult to assess preoperatively, but it is obvious that in the presence of generalized periodontal disease the pulpal component of any so-called combined lesion may be minimal in terms of ultimate prognosis. This inflammation or infection is dissimilar to periodontal disease though there may be some common elements. Except for some furcation lesions, extensions of pulpal inflammation or infection are not capable of causing chronic periodontal disease.

Does periodontal disease cause pulpal necrosis?

There is minimal indication that periodontal disease causes complete pulpal necrosis. Although periodontal disease is common, even among patients with severe generalized bone loss, the occurrence of complete pulpal necrosis is uncommon when the pulpal disease cannot be explained by a past history of deep caries, large restorations, trauma, and so forth. Patients with severe periodontal disease commonly present with complete bone loss around one root of an intact molar (Fig. 12-12). Yet the pulp tissue is this root may evidence minimal dystrophic or degenerative changes.

CLINICAL PROBLEM: A 50-year-old female patient presents with periodic episodes of pain and swelling in the mandibular posterior right quadrant. She had been prescribed antibiotics multiple times to manage the pain and swelling (see Chapter 9). The mandibular first molar felt different to percussion and was slightly sensitive to cold. Radiographically there was a deep vertical periodontal pocket on the mesial of the first molar and loss of bone in the furcation of the second molar (Fig. 12-13, *A*). The latter tooth responded normally to all testing.

Solution: The difficult part about this case is the diagnosis and sequence of anticipated treatment. Extraction or continued treatment of the symptoms are unacceptable. Based on the subjective and objective findings, the pulp of the first molar was diagnosed as having an irreversible pulpitis with the periradicular tissues as having a subacute periradicular periodontitis. Root canal treatment was per-

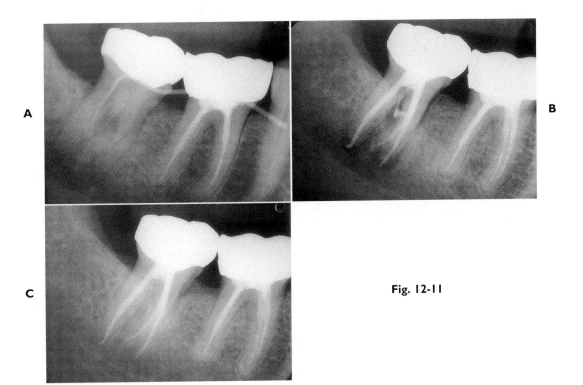

A

B

C

Fig. 12-11

formed (Fig. 12-13, *B,* and *C*) in anticipation of stimulated osseous repair using guided tissue-regenerative techniques. Interestingly the pulp tissue was necrotic in the mesial canals and viable in the distal canal. These findings would tend to support a periodontally induced pulpal degeneration. However, the strong effect of restorative procedures and occlusal leakage cannot be overlooked. (Case courtesy Dr. James Douthitt.)

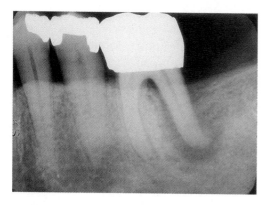

Fig. 12-12 *Complete bone loss around one root of an intact molar is common with extensive periodontal disease.*

Can periodontal treatment affect the pulp tissue, resulting in symptoms of pulpal pathosis?

Yes, periodontal treatment can affect the dental pulp. The primary mode is through severance of collateral circulation to the pulp by accessory communications. Successful periodontal treatment of infraosseous defects will usually result in root exposure either by surgical repositioning of the gingiva or in the course of healing from more conservative therapies. Root exposure is associated with increased thermal sensitivity. It is rare, however, that the degree of thermal sensitivity in these situations will require endodontic intervention unless other causes are present, the vascular supply to the pulp has been compromised, or the pulp was already undergoing degenerative changes before the periodontal surgery. In these situations it is especially important to assess the pulp status before beginning periodontal treatment. Of particular note should be any history of trauma to the teeth, episodes of pulpal symptoms, and radiographic changes indicative of pulpal degeneration, such as linear or focal calcifications, resorptions, evidence of carious lesions, or extensive restorations.

Scaling and root planing can occasionally provoke an acute pulpitis in some teeth. This may be the result of removal of the root cementum, exposure of dentinal tubules, or severing the neurovas-

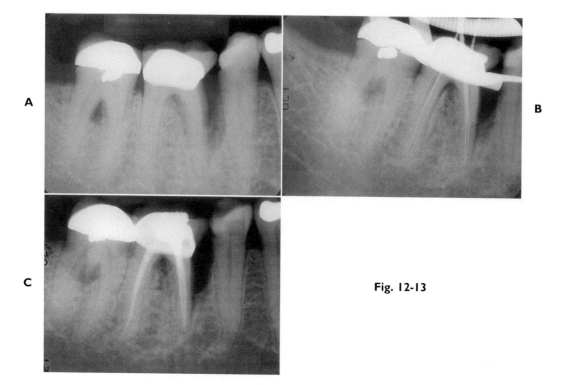

Fig. 12-13

cular bundle entering a midroot lateral canal (which might be found in a deep periodontal defect). It is still relatively rare that root canal treatment is required after deep scaling.

Finally, periodontal surgery may include scaling and root planing but often additionally involves acid etching of root surfaces as used in reattachment procedures. Etching will remove the smear layer and increase dentinal tubular exposure. Pulpal inflammation can easily result or be exaggerated. Surgery that results in root or tooth resection usually requires endodontic intervention.

On a tooth with periodontal disease and a symptomatic pulp, does it matter if the two processes are related?

No. Once pulpal symptoms begin, the decision to do root canal treatment must be based on testing and evaluation of the pulpal status. Similarly the periodontal disease must be diagnosed, and treatment must be planned according to accepted periodontal treatment standards.

It is important to remember that a thermally sensitive pulp is not an etiologic factor for any periodontal condition (except that the patient may be reluctant to clean such a tooth).

CLINICAL PROBLEM: A 58-year-old female patient presents with a chief complaint expressed as follows: "This tooth (pointing to the mandibular right quadrant) has been bothering me for a few weeks, and my general dentist doesn't seen anything on the X-ray." She has a medical history of mitral valve prolapse and requires premedication with antibiotics. The particular tooth is identified as the second molar. She indicates that it has been sensitive to hot and cold for 3 to 4 weeks and is getting progressively worse, with longer episodes of pain. Clinical examination reveals that the second molar is mesially inclined and in contact with the second premolar. There are 4 to 5 mm probings on the mesial surface. A large alloy restoration is present. Radiographically there is a significant vertical periodontal defect on the mesial with subgingival calculus along with slight widening of the periodontal ligament space apically (Fig. 12-14, *A*). Evidence of initial calcification in the pulp chamber is present. Thermal sensibility testing indicates that the second molar is hypersensitive with lingering discomfort. The tooth is also tender to percussion. All other teeth respond normally.

Solution: Based on the subjective and objective findings, the diagnosis of irreversible pulpitis with

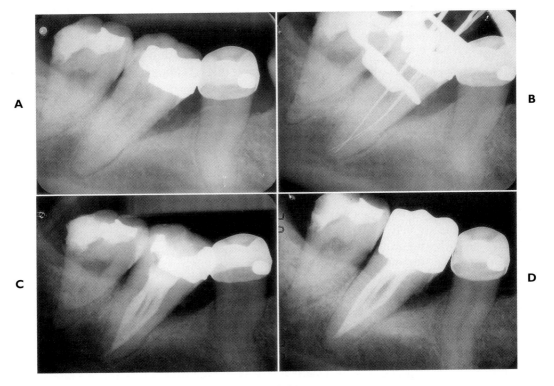

Fig. 12-14

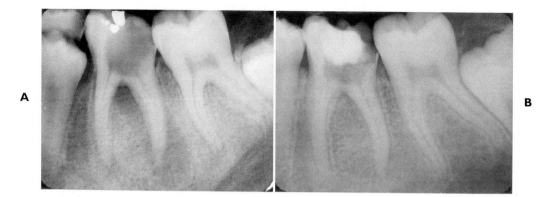

Fig. 12-15

acute periradicular periodontitis is appropriate. Root canal treatment is indicated for the immediate symptoms; however this treatment will not address the periodontal problem. Another concern should be the nature of the root canal system because the root morphology is highly suggestive of a conical or C-shaped canal (see Chapter 5). Root canal treatment was performed (Fig. 12-14, *B* and *C*), and it eliminated the patient's acute problem. A 20-month reevaluation shows normal apical periodontal tissues, a new crown, and the removal of some of the subgingival calculus. Although the vertical defect remains, it can be maintained by the patient who is symptom free and monitored by the general dentist (Fig. 12-14, *D*). (Case courtesy Dr. Jordan Schweitzer.)

> *Does an acute periradicular lesion that has resulted in soft-tissue swelling (cellulitis or acute alveolar abscess) require periodontal treatment?*

No. Although soft-tissue swelling around a tooth with acute periradicular periodontitis may even result in loss of attachment of the gingival sulcus, routine endodontic treatment will result in normal healing of the periodontium, assuming there was no preexisting periodontal defect (Fig. 12-15). Endodontic treatment for the acute abscess typically involves débridement of the canal spaces, incision and drainage, and antibiotic therapy. (See Chapter 9.)

> *Does rapid furcation bone loss alone or secondary to an acute alveolar abscess require periodontal treatment?*

No. Although there may be exceptions with respect to the furcation lesions, it is generally accepted that routine root canal treatment will result in regeneration of bone lost from the furcal exten-

sions of acute pulpal lesions or infections. No specific periodontal treatment is required. Preoperative probings confirming drainage through the gingival sulcus will usually return to normal within 2 weeks of initial endodontic treatment. However, if the probing pattern is that of a deep narrow furcation defect and is parallel to the long axis of the root, a vertical fracture must be ruled out. If this can be done, there is reasonable assurance that the probing represents a draining sinus tract of pulpal origin. If, on the other hand, the probe can be inserted horizontally into the furcation, the lesion will probably not respond to root canal treatment. Extensive periodontal treatment or extraction may be indicated.

CLINICAL PROBLEM: A 14-year-old female patient presents with acute pain and swelling. She had lost the restoration in her mandibular left first molar many months previously and failed to have it replaced. Clinical exam reveals a localized swelling adjacent to molar and a large open occlusal surface on the tooth. The cavity had food debris packed into it, and extensive decay was evident. The second molar was beginning to move anteriorly into the space created by the loss of tooth structure on the distal of the first molar. Radiographically there was evidence of significant furcation and apical bone loss (Fig. 12-15, *A*).

Solution: Subjective and objective findings indicated a diagnosis of pulpal necrosis with an acute alveolar abscess and concomitant localized cellulitis. The tooth was cleaned of its debris, and significant drainage was obtained, which reduced the localized swelling and obviated the need for an incision and drainage (see Chapter 9). The canals were superficially debrided, and the tooth was closed with cotton and a temporary filling. The patient failed to return for the next three appointments. Six months later the patient returned complaining that her temporary filling was wearing away. She was symptom free. A radiograph revealed almost complete osseous repair and reformation of normal anatomic landmarks (Fig. 12-15, *B*). This was obtained by just removing the etiologic factors of bacterial leakage and the bulk of the necrotic tissue.

Does a chronic draining sinus tract (chronic suppurative periradicular periodontitis) through the gingival sulcus require periodontal treatment?

Possibly. Occasionally a patient presents without evidence of generalized periodontal disease and a draining sinus tract in the area of the gingival margin. In molars a periapical film will confirm both apical and furcal bone loss. Pulp tests will confirm a nonresponsive pulp (nonvital). If tests did not confirm this, the defect may be either periodontal in origin or attributable to a vertical fracture.

It is important to distinguish whether the gingival attachment has been lost. In some cases there is complete attachment over the furcation and the draining tract is simply close to the gingival margin. These will usually heal within 2 to 4 weeks after root canal treatment.

Teeth that are draining through the gingival sulcus (that is, loss of attachment) will usually heal as well, but the degree of predictability is lower. In such cases it is important to advise the patient of this potential problem. From the viewpoint of pathogenesis, it is apparent that occasionally what begins as an extension of a pulpal problem gradually becomes a periodontal problem. Essentially these are drainage tracts that follow the root surface instead of leaving through the mucosa or attached gingiva. Loss of bone and attachment are the necessary consequences of this process. In this light, teeth that probe vertically along the root surface near the furcation and exhibit minimal bone loss have a more favorable chance of regaining attachment. Teeth that probe horizontally into the furcation and have extensive bone loss frequently fail to demonstrate reattachment. Treatment planning of such cases should include initial canal débridement, durable temporization, and at least 30 days of observation before a final treatment plan can be determined. Also determinable may be the presence of local factors contributing to the periodontal disease. If sulcular attachment returns, routine root canal treatment can be completed. If, on the other hand, there is no improvement, extensive periodontal management or extraction are the treatments of choice.

CLINICAL PROBLEM: A 29-year-old female patient was referred for evaluation of the mandibular left first molar. Her chief complaint was that of a gingival soreness over the tooth and an occasional bad taste in her mouth. There is a history of periodic discomfort to biting on the tooth. Clinical examination revealed pain to palpation, a normal response to percussion, and no response to thermal sensibility tests. There was deep probing in a vertical and horizontal direction on the buccal with evidence of purulent drainage (Fig. 12-16, *A*). Radiographic examination revealed a large periradicular radiolucency that extended into the furcation. Significant root resorption was also evident (Fig. 12-16, *B*).

Solution: Based on the subjective and objective findings a diagnosis of pulp necrosis with chronic suppurative periradicular periodontitis is appropriate. Root canal treatment was indicated. Within 2 weeks of initial canal débridement, probings had returned to normal. Subsequently the canals were obturated (Fig. 12-16, *C*), and reevaluations at 6 months and 18 months revealed progressive regeneration of the bone (Fig. 12-16, *D,* and *E* respectively). Root-end resorption was managed as per the guidelines in Chapter 10.

How can pulp sensibility (vitality) tests be used to confirm the presence of periodontal or pulpal disease?

Periodontal disease most often presents clinically and radiographically as a generalized disease with multiple locations of bone loss. It may also occasionally present as a localized area of severe bone loss resembling lesions of pulpal origin. A most basic principle of the extension of pulpal pathosis can readily identify periodontal lesions in most instances.

To produce periradicular bone loss of pulpal origin, the pulp must be highly inflamed or nonvital.

In the diagnosis of lesions of severe bone loss, a normal response to sensibility testing (see Figs. 1-15 and 1-16) and the absence of symptoms would rule out a pulpal cause. It follows that endodontic treatment would have no value whatsoever in the resolution of the osseous defect. Likewise, the failure of a tooth with severe bone loss to respond to sensibility tests does not necessarily confirm a nonvital pulp because there are many reasons for nonresponsiveness. However, in the presence of severe bone loss, the prognosis of the tooth is mostly dependent on the periodontal status. Periodontal probings are essential for this determination.

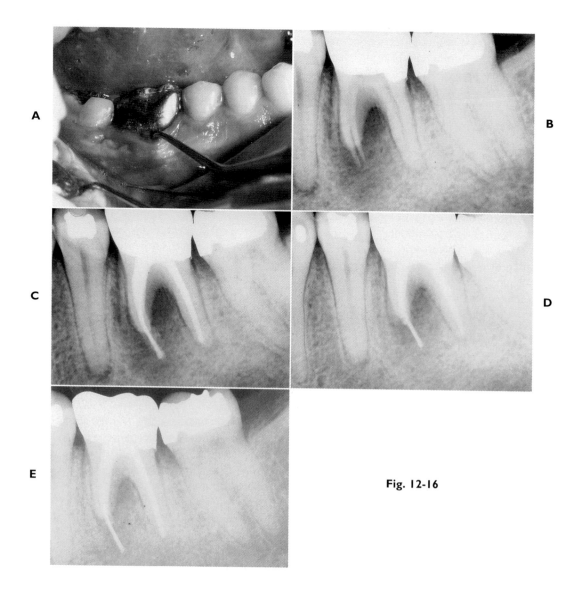

Fig. 12-16

What are the differences in periodontal probings found with a periodontal pocket, a draining sinus tract from a coronal extension of pulpal pathosis through the gingival sulcus and a vertical root fracture?

To differentiate these entities, the nature of periodontal disease and the pattern of periodontal bone loss must be considered. Infraosseous lesions of periodontal cause are rarely narrow. Calculus found on the root is usually found over a broad surface. Consequently probings will reveal wide areas of lost soft-tissue attachment and bone. Probings measured circumferentially in 0.5 to 1 mm

increments will be observed to increase gradually as the pocket is encountered. The probings will gradually decrease as the pocket is passed, and the bone level returns to normal.

The formation of a sinus tract or drainage tract occasionally will occur along the root surface leaving through the gingival sulcus. Typically probings of such tracts will be narrow in width, with a very precipitous, bony opening in the sulcus. Probing circumferentially in 0.5 to 1 mm increments will reveal normal or consistent sulcus depth until the drainage tract is reached. At this point, the probe will drop to a level equal to the full length of the root in most cases. As probings continue circumferentially, they will be normal. The radiograph of course usually reveals a periradicular lesion, with sensibility tests confirming pulpal necrosis.

In the case of vertical root fractures, the clinical presentation of periodontal probings will be the same as that for a draining sinus tract. Several distinguishing features will help to make the diagnosis. If the crack extends from one side of the root to the other, identical precipitous probing patterns will be found on opposite sides of the root. Root fractures can be found on any of the tooth surfaces (see Chapter 11). Although vertical root fractures are identified with untreated teeth, almost all will be found on teeth that have had endodontic treatment. If a precipitous probing pattern is found together with a gingival or mucosal sinus tract on the same tooth, the root is almost invariably split (see Fig. 1-23).

When the differentiation between a draining sulcular sinus tract and a vertical fracture is difficult, a mucoperiosteal tissue flap is reflected, and the root surface is inspected visually for fracture. Such a situation could occur on a tooth with failing endodontic treatment. A drainage tract could appear in the sulcus and would look like a root fracture particularly if the tooth had root canal therapy. In general, it is wise to be suspicious of drainage tracts around any tooth that has had endodontic treatment. Besides failure of the endodontic treatment and vertical root fractures, procedural errors are possible causes as well. These include instrumentation perforation, stripping perforations, access perforations, and post perforations. (See Chapters 3 to 5.)

CLINICAL PROBLEM: A 70-year-old white male presents with a draining sinus tract in the loose alveolar mucosa directly above the attached gingiva over the maxillary left canine (Fig. 12-17, *A*). The tooth serves as an abutment for a removable partial denture. Notice the impingement of the clasp design on the soft tissues *(arrows)*. The sinus tract is traced to the midroot of the tooth (Fig. 12-17, *B*). Periodontal probings are within a 3 to 5 mm range with no evidence of narrow probing. Considered as potential causes in this case are the presence of a midroot lateral canal and a vertical fracture (see Chapter 11).

Solution: Given the potential causes, surgical intervention to help establish a diagnosis is indicated. After reflection of a full mucoperiosteal tissue flap, a vertical fracture is evident (Fig. 12-17, *C*), necessitating extraction (Fig. 12-17, *D*). Immediate patient esthetic needs were addressed with the addi-

tion of a tooth to the removable partial denture (Fig. 12-17, *E*). (Case courtesy Dr. Vivian Manjarrés L.)

Is the combined pulpal-periodontic lesion a fantasy or a reality?

In order for there to be a true combined lesion certain criteria should be met.[15]

1. The tooth must have a necrotic pulp.
2. There must be destruction of the periodontal attachment apparatus from the gingival sulcus to either the apex of the root or an area of a lateral canal.
3. Both root canal therapy and periodontal therapy must be required to resolve the lesions.

In the previous discussions, several clinical problems that meet the first two criteria are seen to be endodontic problems. These include acute pulpal infections extending to the periradicular tissues with drainage through the sulcus, and a chronic sinus tract draining through the sulcus. With the possible exception of furcation bone loss, almost all of these lesions heal with routine endodontic treatment alone.

In contrast, periodontal bone loss occurs independently and well in advance of the extension of pulpal pathosis.

With a symptom-free intact pulp, root canal treatment of a periodontally involved tooth rarely if ever has any effect on the periodontal status.

As a consequence the occurrence of the true pulpal-periodontic combined lesion is exceedingly rare. More often than not, what may exist is a "concomitant lesion" in which both disease processes are present on a tooth but have different causes, do not communicate, and together require treatment for a good prognosis (see Fig. 12-8).

Is root or tooth resection a viable treatment for teeth with periodontal disease?

Root resection is a viable treatment for some periodontally involved roots as well as for root fractures, perforations, and some endodontic surgical failures (See Chapter 8). The question of selecting this treatment is contingent on the postoperative periodontal status and the structural integrity of the tooth. The first criterion to evaluate preoperatively is the relationship of the furcation to the level of crestal bone. If the furcation is well below the level of surrounding crestal bone, a deep periodontal pocket will remain in the resection site. Restoration and maintenance of this situation will be difficult or impossible. On the other hand, when the furcation is at the level of crestal bone, the postoperative probings will be virtually normal (that is, as though the root had never been there). This is the ideal in case management.

A second consideration is the difficulty of the root canal treatment. Severe calcification or root curvature might defeat the outcome, even if the root or tooth resection is ideal.

Finally, an evaluation should be made of the restorability or structural integrity of the tooth. If the root to be removed for periodontal reasons is located where the coronal tooth structure is abundant and strong, the removal of the root would leave a very weak tooth. Similarly, removal of a root supporting an area of the crown where occlusion is heavy would probably lead eventually to cracking of the remaining tooth structure.

Generally the best candidates for root resection are the buccal roots of the maxillary molars. Only

rarely is root resection of a premolar root reasonable. Resection of mandibular roots is possible, but tooth resection (hemisection) is preferable, since unfavorable occlusal forces on the remaining root are eliminated with the latter approach.[14]

Is vital root resection considered as a feasible treatment in the management of pulpal-periodontal problems?

The use of vital root resections is rare but can occur when the exact determination of osseous destruction cannot be made until the time of surgical intervention. If one is treatment planing this type of procedure, practical considerations should include the fact that long-term prognosis of pulpal viability and function should be considered a high-risk procedure. Secondly, teeth known to require resection should receive root canal treatment before resection. Third, teeth with a questionable need for resection should be thoroughly assessed at the time of surgery. This must include a pulpal assessment and

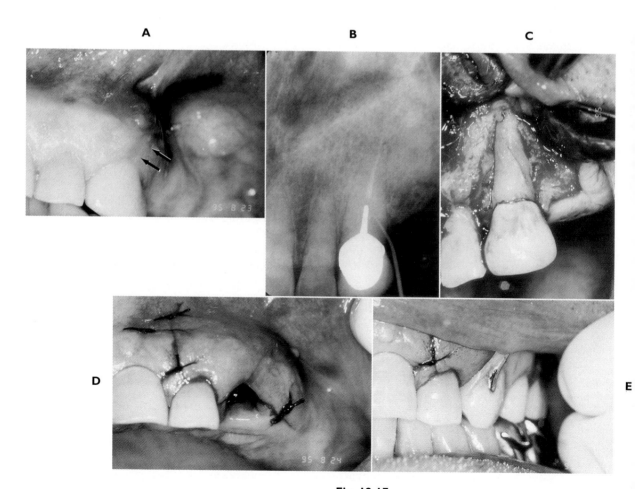

Fig. 12-17

determination of previous factors that may have initiated pulpal inflammation or degeneration. Even though teeth resected have received pulp caps over the exposed pulp stump, invariably tissue degeneration, calcification, or internal resorption may occur.

References

1. Belk CE, Gutmann JL: Perspectives, controversies and directives on pulpal-periodontal relationships, *Can Dent J* 56:1013-1017, 1990.
2. Bender IB, Seltzer S: The effect of periodontal disease on the pulp, *Oral Surg Oral Med Oral Pathol* 33:458-474, 1972.
3. Black GV: Amputation of the roots of teeth. In Litch WF, editor: *The American system of dentistry*, Philadelphia: 1886, Lea Brothers.
4. Bergenholtz G, Lindhe J: Effect of experimentally induced marginal periontitis and periodontal scaling on the dental pulp, *J Clin Periodontol* 5:59-73, 1978.
5. Blomlöf L, Lindskog S, Hammarström L: Influence of pulpal treatments on cell and tissue reactions in the marginal periodontium, *J Periodontol* 59:577-583, 1988.
6. Burch JG, Hulen S: A study of the presence of accessory foramina and the topography of molar furcations, *Oral Surg Oral Med Oral Pathol* 38:451-455, 1974.
7. Cahn LR: Pathology of pulps found in pyorrhetic teeth, *Dent Items Int* 49:598-617, 1927.
8. Clarke NG, Hirsch RS: Periodontitis and angular alveolar lesions: a critical distinction, *Oral Surg Oral Med Oral Pathol* 69:564-571, 1990.
9. Coolidge ED: Anatomy of the root apex in relation to treatment problems, *J Am Dent Assoc* 16:1456-1465, 1929.
10. Cutright DE, Bhaskar SN: Pulpal vasculature as demonstrated by a new method, *Oral Surg Oral Med Oral Pathol* 27:678-683, 1969.
11. Czarnecki RT, Schilder H: A histological evaluation of the human pulp in teeth with varying degrees of periodontal disease, *J Endod* 5:242-253, 1979.
12. Dongari A, Lambrianidis T: Periodontally derived pulpal lesions, *Endod Dent Traumatol* 4:49-54, 1988.
13. Gutmann JL: Prevalence, location, and patency of accessory canals in the furcation region of permanent molars, *J Periodontol* 49:21-26, 1978.
14. Gutmann JL, Harrison JW: *Surgical endodontics,* St. Louis, IEA [Ishiyaku EuroAmerica] Publishers, pp 420-439, 1994.
15. Harrington GW: The perio-endo question: differential diagnosis, *Dent Clin North Am* 23:673-690, 1979.
16. Hattler AB, Snyder DE, Listgarten MA, Kemp W: The lack of pulpal pathosis in rice rats with the periodontal syndrome, *Oral Surg Oral Med Oral Pathol* 44:939-948, 1977.
17. Hirsch RS, Clarke NG, Srikandi W: Pulpal pathosis and severe alveolar lesions: a clinical study, *Endod Dent Traumatol* 5:48-54, 1989.
18. Kipioti A, Nakou M, Legakis N, Mitsis F: Microbiological findings of infected root canals and adjacent periodontal pockets in teeth with advanced periodontitis, *Oral Surg Oral Med Oral Pathol* 58:213-220, 1984.
19. Koenigs JF, Brilliant JD, Foreman DW: Preliminary scanning electron microscope investigations of accessory foramina in the furcation areas of human molar teeth, *Oral Surg Oral Med Oral Pathol* 38:773-782, 1974.
20. Kramer IHR: The vascular architecture of the human dental pulp, *Arch Oral Biol* 2:177-189, 1960.
21. Langeland K, Rodrigues H, Dowden W: Periodontal disease, bacteria, and pulpal histopathology, *Oral Surg Oral Med Oral Pathol* 37:257-270, 1974.
22. Lowman JV, Burke RS, Pelleu GB: Patent accessory canals: incidence in molar furcation region, *Oral Surg Oral Med Oral Pathol* 36:580-584, 1973.
23. Mandi FA: Histological study of the pulp changes caused by periodontal disease, *J Br Endod Soc* 6:80-82, 1972.
24. Mazur B, Massler M: Influence of periodontol disease on the dental pulp, *Oral Surg Oral Med Oral Pathol* 17:592-603, 1964.
25. Rubach WC, Mitchell DF: Periodontal disease, accessory canals and pulp pathosis, *J Periodontol* 36:34-38, 1965.
26. Saunders RL: X-ray microscopy of the periodontal and dental pulp vessels in the monkey and in man, *Oral Surg Oral Med Oral Pathol* 22:503-518, 1966.
27. Seltzer S, Bender IB, Ziontz M: The inter-relationship of pulp and periodontal disease, *Oral Surg Oral Med Oral Pathol* 16:1474-1490, 1963.
28. Simon JHS, Glick DH, Frank AL: The relationship of endodontic-periodontic lesions, *J Periodontol* 43:202-208, 1972.
29. Simring M, Goldberg M: Pulpal pocket approach: retrograde periodontitis, *J Periodontol* 35:22-48, 1964.
30. Sinai I, Soltanoff W: The transmission of pathologic changes between the pulp and the periodontal structures, *Oral Surg Oral Med Oral Pathol* 36:558-568, 1973.
31. Stahl SS: Pulpal response to gingival injury in adult rats, *Oral Surg Oral Med Oral Pathol* 16:1116-1119, 1963.
32. Stahl SS: Pathogenesis of inflammatory lesions in pulp and periodontal tissues, *Periodontics* 4:190-195, 1966.
33. Stallard RE: Periodontic-endodontic relationships, *Oral Surg Oral Med Oral Pathol* 34:314-326, 1972.
34. Torabinejad M, Kiger RD: A histologic evaluation of dental pulp tissue of a patient with periodontal disease, *Oral Surg Oral Med Oral Pathol* 59:198-200, 1985.

Chapter 13

▼

Problems Encountered in Restoring Endodontically Treated Teeth

James L. Gutmann
Paul E. Lovdahl

"I have made a diligent search to find whether or not teeth from which the pulp had been removed, and the canals and pulp chamber filled without admitting the fluids of the mouth, were subject to a similar deterioration of strength. It is now well known that teeth treated in this way retain their color almost perfectly; and from my observation of the relation of color to strength of the teeth I am prepared to entertain the suppositions that they retain their strength also. Only one tooth came into my hands with a root-filling. It was a central incisor, and had not sufficient tissue for me to obtain a block; but it showed no undue percentage of water, and the color was good. Up to the present time I have been unable to obtain the history of the filling of this root."*

INTRODUCTION

Endodontically treated teeth are structurally compromised.[21,37,43,53,54] Whether caused by decay, previous restorations, fractures, or the wearing away of sound enamel and dentin, these teeth require careful and immediate attention to their reconstruction to ensure their maintenance as a functioning member of the dental arch.

For years there was little scientific rationale for the reconstructive technique chosen for these teeth. Textbooks were replete with directives to restore all endodontically treated teeth with a post-core and crown. This empirical dictate was based on years of successful clinical practice.[67] Coupled with the commonly held belief that endodontically treated were brittle, practitioners routinely treatment-planned extensive restorations after endodontic treatment. When the tooth had a

*From Black GV: *Dent Cosmos* 37:353-421, 1885.

periradicular lesion, it was also advisable to wait at least 6 months for radiographic evidence of healing before commencing the restorative procedure.

In the last 15 to 20 years, a plethora of scientific studies, clinical technique articles, and new materials and techniques have addressed the enigmatic issue of restoring an endodontically treated tooth. This creates a natural scenario for the application of the principles of "problem solving." Although scientific insights and technologic explosions have provided a clearer understanding of this issue, sound clinical judgment and experience must still enter into the decision-making process when one is restoring these teeth. This includes the choices of interim restorations before and during root canal treatment in addition to the final restoration.

In this chapter considerations in the restoration of endodontically treated teeth are approached through a discussion of commonly observed clinical concerns encountered during treatment planning and restoration. Techniques and materials designed to enhance clinical success and avoid the occurrence of endodontic or restorative failure are discussed.

PRETREATMENT AND INTERIM RESTORATIONS

Pretreatment and interim temporary restorations are just as important as the final permanent restoration after endodontic treatment. The most important functions of temporary restorations are to enhance tooth isolation and to prevent leakage during or between treatments. Occlusal function and aesthetics are of secondary concern.

Control of leakage of irrigating solutions and saliva during treatment are essential for patient comfort and to prevent canal contamination.[24,35] Salivary leakage through incompletely removed caries or poorly placed temporary materials is the primary cause of interappointment flare-ups.

Long-term leakage through inadequate posttreatment temporary restorations or permanent restorations has been identified as a primary cause of endodontic failure following root canal obturation.[59]

Tooth Isolation and Control of Coronal Leakage

Key aspects of tooth isolation are addressed in Chapter 3, and adjunctive periodontal and orthodontic considerations are addressed in Chapter 8. However, with coronal leakage contamination as the primary concern before, during, and after root canal treatment, the soundness of the remaining tooth structure, the restoration in place, if any, and the adequacy of a temporary placement and the material itself must be considered when one is trying to prevent problems (Fig. 13-1).

Caries must be removed from all teeth before root canal treatment is begun (Fig. 13-2). Cervical decay under crown margins must be excavated and the tooth adequately temporized. It is not unusual for such decay to be subgingival, since the crown margins are usually at the level of the gingival margin.

A major source of leakage is inadequate caries control either directly from a carious exposure or

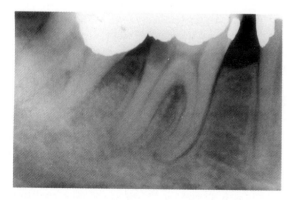

Fig. 13-2 *Deep distal caries that must be removed and the tooth effectively sealed along the distal wall before an endodontic access opening is begun. Because of the depth of the carious lesion, crown lengthening may also be indicated.*

indirectly as in the case of gross caries under a crown, through which a minimal access opening has been made. Leakage into root canals also occurs around defective or loose restorations and through cracks in the tooth structure. The potential avenues of contamination must be identified and removed as part of the root canal treatment.

CLINICAL PROBLEM: A 44-year-old female patient presents in your office with symptoms of an acute alveolar abscess (see Chapter 9). She attributes her frustration with the treatment she has been receiving from her previous dentist. The tooth in question (the mandibular right first molar) has been under treatment for 2 months, during which time she has had to return on an emergency basis five times. An endodontic access has been made through a large IRM [intermediate restorative material] temporary restoration and is filled with a satisfactory Cavit restoration. A radiograph is exposed (Fig. 13-3, *A*). Clinically there is no evidence of marginal leakage, but radiographically it is apparent that gross decay remains under the IRM. The cause of repeated flare-ups in this case is most likely bacterial leakage from the decay under the IRM.

Solution: Before root canal treatment can be continued, the entire IRM temporary must be removed and the remaining caries excavated. In this case the excavation was temporarily sealed with a glass-ionomer cement through which an endodontic access was remade, and treatment was completed uneventfully (Fig. 13-3, *B* and *C*).

Occasionally after caries has been excavated, it is very difficult to get adequate isolation under the rubber dam. Three strategies might be considered. First, a rubber dam seal or caulk is very effective if the rubber dam clamp is secure. Isolation using adjacent teeth is also quite popular (see Fig. 3-26). Secondly, where insufficient tooth structure remains to secure the rubber dam clamp, temporization with a bonded composite or glass-ionomer cement is appropriate. It does not seem reasonable to go to the extent of placing an extensive permanent pin-retained amalgam or composite buildup if followed by an endodontic access preparation. These buildups will not be useful for a permanent core under a crown and would likely have to be redone. Attempts to use bands or custom-shaped aluminum shell crowns often fail to address the need for a sound restorative margin and often lead to two major problems for the patient. The first is leakage under the band that cannot be properly adapted to the tooth cervically, and leakage ensues. Second is the opportunity for significant impinge-

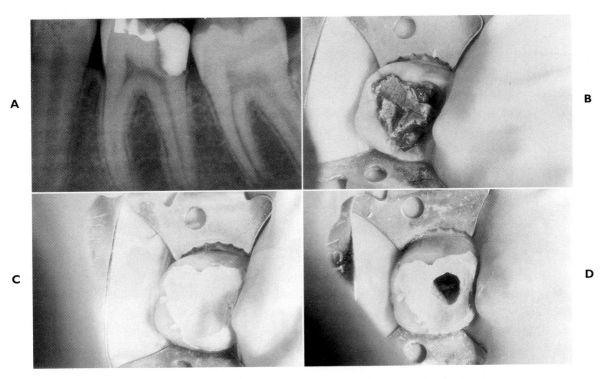

Fig. 13-1 *A, Radiograph taken at time of emergency examination. Previously placed temporary restoration is inadequate. Reexcavation and new temporary is necessary before initiating root canal treatment. B, Defective coronal restoration and recurrent decay that extended into the pulp chamber. C, Removal of caries and restoration and replacement with a glass ionomer as a temporary. D, Endodontic access opening prepared in the glass ionomer.*

ment of the cementing media on the periodontal attachment, which is discussed later in this section.

CLINICAL PROBLEM: A 35-year-old male patient presents with severe pain in the mandibular right quadrant. He cannot bite on his first molar, and the restoration on this tooth feels loose. A clinical examination reveals a fixed partial denture from the first molar to the first premolar. There is clinical evidence of decay around the margins of the crown on the molar, and the bridge is firmly secured to the premolar but is loose on the molar. Radiographically there is evidence of significant decay under the molar crown (Fig. 13-4, *A*). Percussion and palpation give an abnormal response on the first molar, with adjacent teeth responding normally to all sensibility tests.

Solution: The subjective and objective findings indicate a diagnosis of irreversible pulpitis with acute periradicular periodontitis. Caries under the crown is the primary cause. Proper treatment planning requires removal of the crown and all carious tooth structure. Removal of the pontic is also indicated to prevent undesirable occlusal forces on the premolar abutment (Fig. 13-4, *B*). Notice that there is no cement remaining in the crown. Once the prosthesis has been removed consideration must be given to proper tooth isolation (Fig. 13-4, *C*). An orthodontic band was placed, and a glass-ionomer core was built on the tooth. A routine access cavity was made through the core, and the working length was determined (Fig. 13-4, *D* and *E*). After obturation of the canals, the glass ionomer was removed and the band was used for a matrix in which a dentin-bonded amalgam core with extensions into the canals was placed (Fig. 13-4, *F*). (Case courtesy Dr. David E. Witherspoon.)

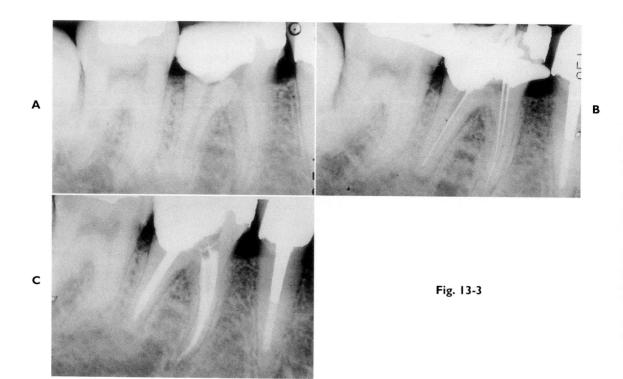

Fig. 13-3

Third, an alternative usually requiring no more time than a coronal buildup is a periodontal crown-lengthening procedure (see Chapter 8), which can be used solely to enhance isolation or in conjunction with a buildup. In those situations with deep carious or fractured tooth margins the crown lengthening is mandatory to ensure the proper placement of the coronal margin of the final restoration[67] (Fig. 13-5).

Coronal leakage may also be directly observed during treatment. Once identified, these defects can be sealed with Cavit (ESPE/Premier, Norristown, Penna.), IRM (LD Caulk, Milford, Del.) or glass ionomer. The sealing usually occurs from the inside of the tooth outward. Although this will prevent leakage during treatment at the first patient visit, it may also be a source of leakage between appointments if the coronal avenue of leakage is not properly sealed on the external surface of the tooth. During the placement of these types of seals, the pushing of restorative materials into the canal orifices must be prevented (see the discussion of blockage of the canal system in Chapter 5).

Another problem that often occurs when attempting to block a coronal avenue of leakage by placing restorative materials is the pushing of the filling deep into the gingival sulcus. If that filling is not removed, severe postoperative pain is often encountered because of the impingement of these materials on the tissue attachment deep in the sulcus. This situation is similar to that found in a localized periodontal abscess. This also occurs commonly when poorly fitting temporary crowns or bands are used as interim restorations and excessive cement is driven deep into the gingival sulcus. The best way to manage this problem and to ensure the integrity and health of the supporting periodontium is always to use processed, well-fitting, and contoured temporary crowns. This type of interim restoration can be retained on the tooth during root canal treatment, or removed at the discretion of the treating clinician. Either way a plethora of problems are prevented with this approach to coronal coverage and leakage prevention.

Coronal leakage between appointments may be observed as canal contamination upon reopening at subsequent patient visits. In these situations, calcium hydroxide in a commercial preparation, such as Calasept (JS Dental, Ridgefield, Conn.) or TempCanal (Pulp Dent Corp, Watertown, Mass.) may

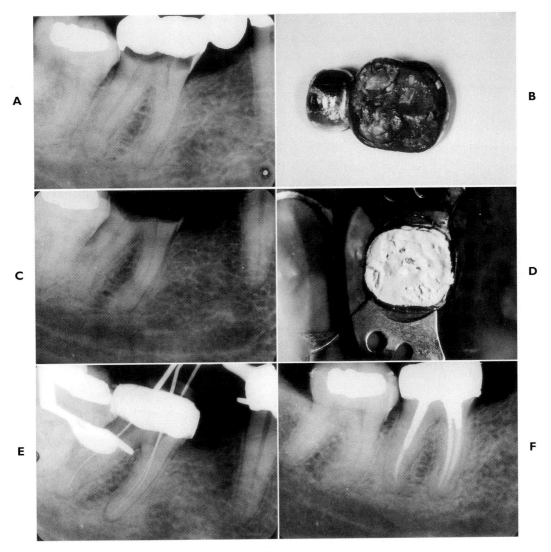

Fig. 13-4

be placed in the canal as an interappointment dressing to control bacterial influx. These materials are injected into the canal with a syringe. They will function as an excellent temporary physical barrier to leakage between appointment or postoperatively, should long-term temporization be required.

At times coronal leakage may be suspected, but the source cannot be confirmed. One option would be to remove all restorations completely. This approach will be the most reliable way to prevent leakage and eliminate the probability of interap-

pointment flare-up. However, complete removal of existing restorations is not always practical or desirable and the routine use of this approach is not recommended when clinically sound restorative dentistry is in place. Specific considerations for restoration removal are listed in Table 13-1.

A final point that cannot be overemphasized in the discussion of endodontic flare-ups and the use of proper temporization is the necessity of complete canal débridement.

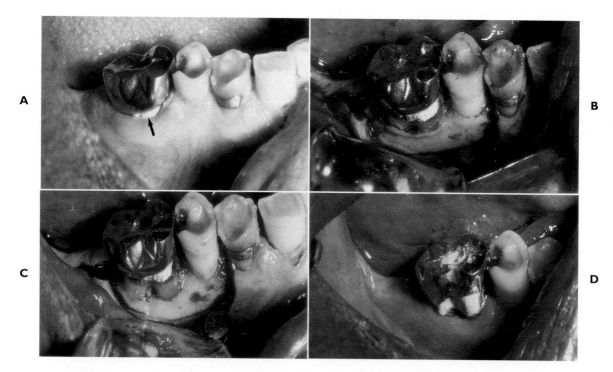

Fig. 13-5 *A, Mandibular right first molar referred for management of recurrent flare-ups during root canal treatment. Cervical caries had been minimally excavated and temporized with Cavit (arrow). B, Tissue reflected during crown lengthening revealing unexcavated caries and pathway for leakage. C, After osseous recontouring, the leaking margins are quite visible. D, Healing of periodontal tissues after crown lengthening. The caries was excavated, and a proper IRM temporary was placed. The restorability of the tooth has now been satisfactorily determined, and the leakage has been controlled.*

▼ Table 13-1 Specific considerations for restoration removal

COMPELLING REASONS TO REMOVE RESTORATIONS
- Evidence of continued leakage during treatment
- Unexpected carious invasion beneath restorations, especially full crowns
- Fractures uncovered during access preparation
- Loose, defective, or undermined restorations

REASONS OF CONVENIENCE TO REMOVE RESTORATIONS
- Malpositioned teeth or restorations that may impede direct access to the canals
- Need to search for calcified orifices
- Need to establish tooth restorability, especially with possible chamber perforations
- Need to enhance clinician orientation
- Treatment-planned restoration replacement

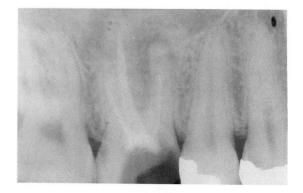

Fig. 13-6 *Failing root canal treatment secondary to exposure to salivary contamination for 14 months.*

If caries has been completely excavated and leakage potential has been completely controlled, a flare-up is still possible when infected necrotic material remains in the canal system (see Chapter 5).

PERMANENT RESTORATIONS

Until an endodontically treated tooth is fully restored to function, treatment is considered incomplete.[42] Therefore the ultimate success of endodontics is somewhat rooted in the overall and timely restorative management of the compromised tooth.[19,52,58] Many factors regarding the materials and techniques advocated to achieve these goals have been considered and their proper use and integration will be addressed using a problem-solving approach.

Postendodontic Timing of Tooth Restoration

It is no longer necessary to wait for extended periods of time after root canal treatment to restore the tooth.

If the root canal treatment has been performed at the standard of care, the periradicular tissues will heal. Consistent with this outcome, as previously discussed, is the need to carefully seal the coronal orifice of the root canal system from any contamination by oral fluids and microorganisms. Recent studies have confirmed that coronal leakage is a significant cause in the failure of root canal treatment[40,59] (see Fig. 1-12).

Failure to restore the endodontically treated tooth as soon as possible may also result in the fracture of tooth structure that could render the tooth unrestorable. If a final restoration cannot be placed within a few weeks after treatment, a strong, leak-resistant, protective provisional restoration is indicated. Common is a well-processed temporary crown or bridge; glass ionomers or acid-etched composite buildups may also be considered as well as properly fitted and cemented orthodontic bands.

Frequently, a tooth may present with a coronal fracture or caries that extends to the gingival margin and exposes the gutta-percha root filling (Fig. 13-6). Similarly, long-standing temporary fillings may have worn out of their cavities with exposure of the root filling. The patient is symptom free, and radiographically the supporting bone appears normal. A common question posed is, Is it appropriate to begin immediately the restoration of the tooth? Current information on coronal leakage patterns indicates that even a well-filled canal may show evidence of bacterial leakage to the apex in as little as 19 days of exposure to saliva.[71,73] Even in the presence of an IRM temporary, significant leakage has been shown to occur within 90 days.[73] Leakage may also occur when previously placed posts are exposed to oral fluid contamination.[15] Unless it is certain that the gutta-percha was only recently exposed to salivary contamination, or the temporary filling has been in place for only a short time, retreatment of the canal system is highly recommended in these cases before final restoration.[19] This dictate is of even greater importance in the presence of silver cones or paste root-canal fillings.

Factors Influencing the Choice of Restoration

Multiple factors must be considered in the choosing of a final restoration. Of importance are the amount of remaining sound tooth structure, occlusal function, opposing dentition, position of the tooth in the arch, length and width of the roots, and the curvature of the roots.[21] In addition to alterations in the tooth architecture caused by removal of the roof of the pulp chamber and the loss of cusps and marginal ridges, it is important to understand that changes occur in the dentin of endodontically treated teeth, and such changes also directly affect the ability of the tooth to function under stress. Recent studies indicate that the bonds between the collagen that makes up the dentin are weakened and subject to breakage under different types of forces.[57] Likewise, alterations in the tooth that result in the potential for brittleness are not attributable to changes in moisture content.[28,47] Rather these changes are attributable to architectural changes in the remaining compromised dentin, especially in the loss of the marginal ridges.[54] Recently it was shown that similarities in the biomechanical properties of endodontically treated teeth and their contralateral vital pairs indicated that teeth do not become brittle after endodontic treatment.[60]

However, the strongest tooth will always be the one in which sound dentin and enamel can be retained and used to rebuild the tooth.[44]

Coupled with the ability to bond contemporary restorations to the remaining tooth structure, multiple restorative options are available to best serve the patient's needs.[26,32] These options, however, must be carefully chosen for each particular situation.

In anterior teeth with intact marginal ridges, cingulum, and incisal edges, the placement of a lingual or palatal dentin-bonded composite resin is the treatment of choice.[38] Because most anterior teeth experience fewer functional forces than posterior teeth do, the routine removal of sound, intact tooth structure in favor of extensive post-core restorations is rarely warranted.[45,65] In this regard, many endodontically treated and discolored teeth may be bleached to an aesthetically acceptable color by use of a chemical or "walking bleach" technique,[39] without the necessity of removing sound tooth structure for the placement of a veneer or porcelain-fused-to-metal crown. Some anterior teeth may require complete coronal coverage along with posts and cores because of the presence of large or multiple restorations or because aesthetic conditions cannot be adequately addressed with more conservative forms of treatment.[18] This is common when large proximal restorations are present, decay has undermined the remaining marginal ridges, or the majority of the incisal edge has been lost because of trauma.

Posterior teeth present with a different set of restorative needs primarily because of the loss of structural integrity,[37,46] especially the marginal ridges,[53,53] and the amount of occlusal force placed on these teeth during function. Contemporary thought, in both research and clinical practice, supports the placement of a full cuspal protective restoration on these teeth.[37,65] This is easily accomplished with a crown or onlay when sufficient tooth structure remains. When significant destruction of tooth structure exists, dentin-bonded cores,[26] sometimes supported by intraradicular posts are indicated (see discussion of posts and dowels, p. 333). Restorations of this nature are essential to prevent fracture when occlusal forces tend to separate cusp tips during function. In cases of posterior teeth opposing a partial or complete denture, the forces of mastication and cuspal interdigitation may be significantly reduced and tooth restoration with complete coronal coverage may not be warranted.

The relative amount of tooth reduction in a full crown preparation, both anterior and posterior, also has significant endodontic implications. Considering the presence of the access cavity and any existing restorations, the bulk of remaining dentin used to retain the crown may be minimal. This situation invites complete fracture of the crown at the base of the preparation, one that is not readily seen radiographically and may go undetected until the patient experiences significant acute problems. Specifically the practice of preparing a shoulder circumferentially for a porcelain veneer crown must be questioned, relative to the preservation of sound dentin. Not only is the lingual or palatal shoulder unnecessary for the purposes of the veneer, but it also requires the removal of valuable, supportive dentin. It is difficult to make the case that the removal of sound tooth structure and placement of a reinforced buildup would provide equivalent structural integrity. From a problem-solving respect, enhanced restoration of endodontically treated teeth may warrant some significant changes in the philosophy and technique of tooth preparation.

Core Build-Ups and Restorative Materials

The purpose of the core restoration is to provide needed resistance, retention, and stable configuration to the compromised coronal aspect of the tooth. A variety of accepted materials can be used for the core superstructure. Dentin-bonded, reinforced composite resins and amalgams are the contemporary materials of choice.[30,69] However, when various methods of intradentinal retention, such as slots or grooves are being used, composite cores have been shown to have greater resistance to fracture than amalgam cores have.[70] The use of retentive pins with composite materials increased the resistance to fracture even further.[70] The use of poly(methylmethacrylate) enhanced bonded amalgams with pins has been shown to achieve very high levels of shear bond strength when complex amalgam restorations are used.[31] These types of core foundations would provide excellent strength for the overlying castings necessary for endodontically treated posterior teeth.

The use of glass ionomers as a core material in high stress-bearing situations is not recommended[9] because the adhesion of these materials is insufficient when used alone with pins or posts.[4] Even glass ionomers with reinforcing particles, such as amalgam, have lower flexural strength than composite resins and amalgams.[30,65,74] Although their use within sound dentinal walls or as cores under crowns has been advocated,[12,22] their long-term fatigue life is highly questionable.[33] This may not necessarily negate their usage in *selected* anterior and posterior teeth.

All core materials may or may not be used with a post (see following discussion of posts and dowels) (Fig. 13-7). The core material occupies the entire pulp chamber and replaces lost tooth structure at the circumferential margins of the crown. When used at the gingival tooth margins, core materials should be distinguishable from tooth structure to enhance visibility and preparation of a crown margin that is 1.5 to 2 mm on sound tooth structure gingival to the core material. Many reinforced composite materials are available in colors other than that of the tooth structure for this purpose. Crown cementation on tooth margins gingival to the core margins significantly enhances stability and prevents dislodgment, especially in the presence of a properly placed cervical bevel (ferrule).[2,36,63,67] Resistance to root fracture and to core fracture is also enhanced.

No matter how well the core materials are bonded to the tooth structure the potential for leakage exists.

Core-tooth structure margins at or below the free gingival margin that are not covered and sealed by an overlaying crown margin are predisposed to coronal leakage.

From a more practical viewpoint, patients have a very difficult time maintaining these margins in a plaque and bacterial-free state. When these restorative objectives cannot be readily achieved because of deep carious or fractured tooth margins, periodontal crown lengthening is indicated.[67] This adjunctive approach to management of the severely compromised endodontically treated tooth not only ensures a properly reinforced and restored tooth, but also establishes a sound biologic relationship of the attached periodontal tissues (see Chapter 8).

Intracoronal Posts and Dowels

Many key issues surround the use of posts in endodontically treated teeth. Although some may seem to be resolved, lingering questions regarding the following issues still abound:

- What is the philosophy and purpose of a post?
- What is the ideal design and shape of a post?
- What is the proper post size?
- What is the proper post length?
- What is the best way to create post space and when can it be safely done?
- What is the best cementing medium for posts?
- What are common problems associated with the use of intraradicular posts?

Although experience can answer some of these questions, integration with scientific assessments is necessary to provide a thorough understanding of

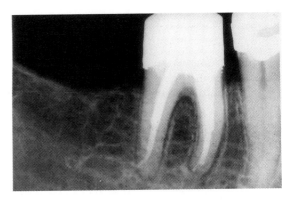

Fig. 13-7 *Newly placed amalgam core supported by cemented stainless steel posts. The core replaces lost coronal tooth structure and provides the configuration for crown retention.*

these issues. However, caution must be stressed when one is attempting to extrapolate fully the data secured in a laboratory setting. Likewise with the abundance of prefabricated post systems available, it is often difficult for the clinician to make well-informed decisions regarding their use.

Philosophy and purpose

The primary purpose of and the main indication for a post or dowel are to retain a core that can be used to support the definitive prosthesis.[18,43]

Posts do not reinforce endodontically treated teeth and are not necessary when substantial tooth structure is present after the teeth have been prepared.[18,21,38,42,43,67] Studies indicate that post placement may induce stresses in the tooth that ultimately may predispose to failure.[5,6,11,14,29,55] This is especially true when optimal bonding between the post and cementing media cannot be achieved.[49] With this contemporary change in philosophy regarding the role of a post, much effort has been expended in the assessment of post retention vis-à-vis its design, shape, size, and length. Because the research in this realm is primarily bench top in nature, clinical factors must also be considered.

Post design and shape

Threaded posts are the most retentive, followed by parallel-sided serrated posts[66,72] (Table 13-2). Tapered posts have also been successful in selected cases but are the least retentive and rely heavily on the integrity and strength of the cementing medium. Likewise, factors such as roughening the canal or post walls or notching the post also increase retention.[45,75] Although highly retentive, some threaded posts may predispose to root frac-

▼ **Table 13-2** Characteristics of generic post systems

Type	Retention	Installation stresses	Functional stresses
Tapered smooth	Low	Little or none	Wedging effect
Parallel serrated	Higher	Little or none	Uniformly distributed through the cement layer
Tapered self-threaded	Intermediate—affected by high installation stresses	Very high; wedging stresses	High stresses; accentuates installation wedging
Parallel threaded	Highest	Low after counterrotation	Relatively low; transmitted through individual threads
Parallel serrated tapered end	Similar to parallel serrated	Little or none	Wedging effect at apex
Cast post	Less retentive than parallel	Little or none	Wedging effect

ture. Based on design and shape, the overall effect of a post on the tooth structure will be greatly influenced by the root anatomy, choice of post, and its placement.[5]

The choice of a post system can also be greatly influenced by their installation and functional stresses and these factors must be considered in treatment planning the final restoration (Table 13-2).[29,62] The parallel-threaded post systems have relatively low installation and functional stresses compared to the tapered, self-threading systems. Other systems have similar characteristics depending on their usage.

Cast posts by their very nature cannot be given a specific design because they represent the shape of the prepared root canal in conjunction with a core buildup. In doing so, however, they are less retentive and may provide a wedging effect depending again on their usage. Retention is highly dependent on the cementing media or irregularities incorporated into the post design to enhance stability.

The use of bondable reinforcement fiber for post-and-core buildup has been recommended to both maximize strength and enhance aesthetics.[27] Advantages include minimal removal of tooth structure, placement of the materials in areas of excessively flared root canals, thinned roots, or curvatures, and the bonding of the dentin-root complex. Many previously thought unsalvageable teeth may possibly be retained using this or similar techniques that enhance the bonding of the compromised tooth into a stable unit.

Post size

Post size should not exceed one third of the root diameter (Fig. 13-8).

Large increases in post diameter do not increase post retention in the root.

On the contrary, the increased removal of tooth structure to accommodate a larger post is generally accompanied by a proportional increase in stresses placed on the root.[29] This can be especially harmful in the cervical portion of the tooth, where a reduction in the toughness and sheer strength of the dentin in endodontically treated teeth has been noted.[7] Additionally, at the apical extent of the posts, roots converge anatomically, resulting in thin dentinal walls that are subject to fracture during the initial post cementation or during the placement of functional stresses.

Post length

Post length has been clinically and scientifically controversial for decades and many formulas or recommended lengths are used. Although longer posts demonstrate increased retention, their position in the root may predispose the patient to clinical problems.[6,29] For example, in thin roots, mesiodistally, perforations or fractures may occur (Fig. 13-9, A), placement of posts into the curve of the root

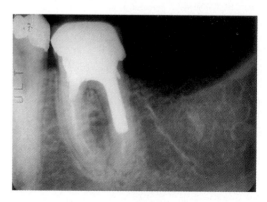

Fig. 13-8 *Post diameter is greater than one third of the root width, which minimizes the root support for force distribution during function.*

often leads to fracture (Fig. 13-9, B and C),[29] placement of long posts into short roots may result in the disruption of the apical root canal seal[76](Fig. 13-9, D), and placement of long posts in roots periodontally compromised and lacking proper bony support causes the concentration of forces on the tooth to be focused at the end of the post, which is in root structure unsupported by bone.[55]

Clinical success rates support the use of posts that are equal to or greater in length than the crown length of the tooth.

Coupled with the increase in retention commonly found with longer posts, especially under function, a widely held and scientifically supported formula for post length is one in which the post is approximately one half to three fourths the length of the root. These lengths may seem quite unreasonable and by themselves cannot be applied generically without compromising many roots anatomically and potentially altering the apical seal of the root canal filling.[76] Therefore, before applying this concept, the nature of the root morphology and the apical seal must be assessed.[48,77] Important root or tooth anatomic scenarios are listed in Table 13-3. Although generalities, they provide reasonable guidelines that must be considered when determining post length.

One of the goals of root canal treatment is to seal, three dimensionally, the apical extent of the root canal system. To achieve this, 4 to 5 mm of root canal filling material should be retained as the apical seal[23,41] (Fig. 13-10). Because of the irregular nature of many root apices, less than this amount may predispose to leakage from accessory communications, unidentified canal exits, or apical resorptive processes (Fig. 13-11). However, even this amount should not be considered as a clinically "safe" guideline[16] because both bacteria and their by-products can easily penetrate this thickness of remaining gutta-percha if the canal is not properly sealed coronally with the post, core, and crown. This numerical recommendation must also be modified, based on root length, width, and curvature.[48,76,77]

In the preparation of post space in the root with evidence of a lateral canal, it is important to prepare the post space short of the level of this aberrant opening (Fig. 13-12). Extension beyond the lateral canal may result in a lateral lesion, especially if the post space is improperly obturated. Since the presence of a lateral canal is often unknown at the time of post placement, the subsequent development of a draining sinus tract or lateral radiolucency should alert the clinician to consider this as an etiologic factor.

CLINICAL PROBLEM: A 70-year old female patient presents with a chief complaint of acute pain

---

▼ **Table 13-3** Specific anatomic root or tooth considerations relative to post usage

TOOTH GROUP	IMPORTANT ANATOMIC CONSIDERATIONS
Maxillary incisors	Sufficient root bulk for most post systems; tapering roots may negate long parallel posts; canines are wide buccopalatally; root invaginations most common in the canine; perforations common because of lack of orientation in the long axis of the root during post-space preparation, especially in the lateral incisor
Maxillary premolars	Thin root walls with rapid tapers or curves apically, especially in multiple dimensions; proximal invaginations and root splitting are common; roots easily weakened with large posts
Maxillary molars	Use of post should be limited to palatal root, which has a buccal curvature in 85% of cases; root invaginations on the buccal surface of the palatal root; long, thick posts are contraindicated
Mandibular incisors	Difficult to restore with posts; roots thin in proximal dimension with significant invaginations common; roots narrow rapidly in the apical half; canines similar to maxillary canines
Mandibular premolars	Sufficient root bulk for most post systems; multiple canals common but if not treated are obscured or blocked by a post; perforation common to the buccal of first premolar because of altered crown morphology
Mandibular molars	Thin root walls in a proximal dimension; root and canal anatomy not conducive to many prefabricated post systems; root invaginations often obscure post proximal perforations

From Gutmann JL: *J Prosthet Dent* 67:458-467, 1992.

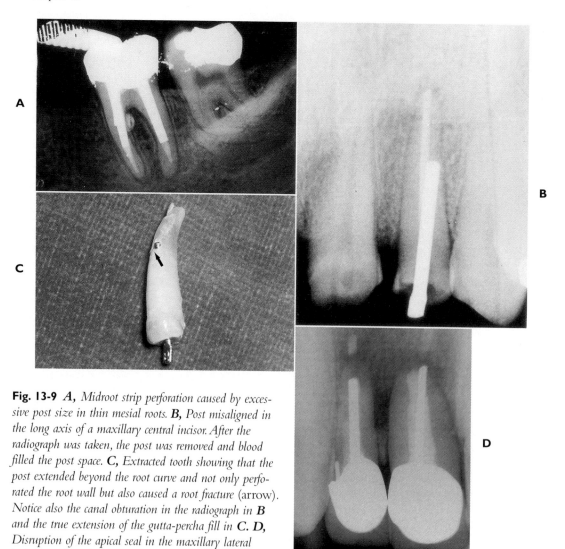

Fig. 13-9 **A,** *Midroot strip perforation caused by excessive post size in thin mesial roots.* **B,** *Post misaligned in the long axis of a maxillary central incisor. After the radiograph was taken, the post was removed and blood filled the post space.* **C,** *Extracted tooth showing that the post extended beyond the root curve and not only perforated the root wall but also caused a root fracture (arrow). Notice also the canal obturation in the radiograph in **B** and the true extension of the gutta-percha fill in **C**. **D,** Disruption of the apical seal in the maxillary lateral incisor resulting from excessive post length preparation.*

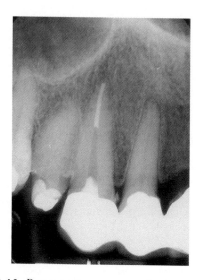

Fig. 13-10 *Proper post space preparation preserving 4 to 5 mm of the apical gutta-percha filling material.*

and swelling 3 weeks before this visit. Presently she is symptom free. Clinical exam revealed a draining sinus tract opening in the midroot of the maxillary left canine. Probings were normal on all teeth in this region, and there was no evidence of decay. Radiographically the tooth had had previous root canal treatment with a sectional silver cone, followed by a parallel-threaded post, core, and crown (Fig. 13-13). On the mesial aspect of the canine, a radiolucency was evident that paralleled an unfilled canal space between the silver cone and post.

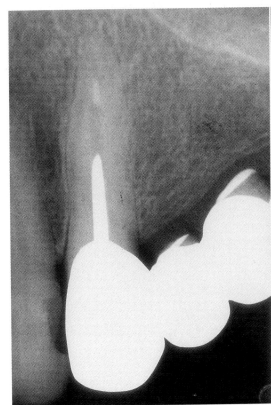

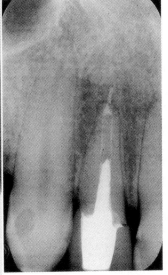

Fig. 13-11 *A and B, Two maxillary incisors with excessive post length preparation that compromises the apical seal.*

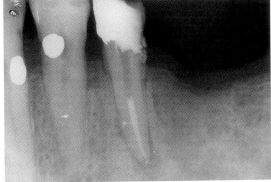

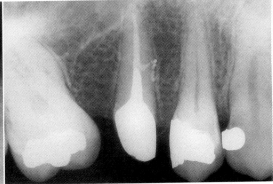

Fig. 13-12 *A, Proper post space preparation avoiding communication with a lateral canal. B, lateral canal at the midroot level may compromise the post length, but obturation of the lateral canal appears adequate.*

Solution: Because probings were normal, a root fracture was not considered. A tentative diagnosis of an endodontic restorative failure caused by a lateral canal was made. Upon surgical exposure it was confirmed that there was a lateral canal (Fig. 13-13, *B*) that was sealed with an amalgam that extruded into the main canal (Fig. 13-13, *C*).

Technique and timing of post-space preparation
Preparation of the post space can be accomplished immediately after obturation with gutta-percha and sealer by use of either a heated instrument or slow-speed rotary instruments, such as Peeso reamers, Gates-Glidden drills, or a GPX instrument (Brasseler, Savannah, Ga.).[3,10,16,23,41,50]

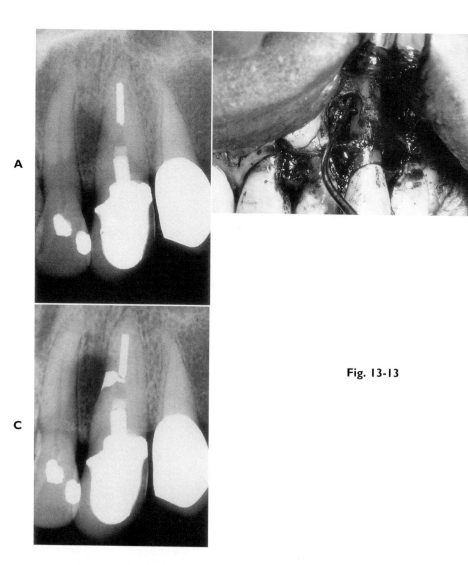

Fig. 13-13

Once the coronal filling is removed and the space prepared, the remaining material in the canal should be gently but firmly vertically condensed.

> With previously filled root canals, the practitioner must determine the acceptability of the treated case before creating a post space.

In all cases there should be no adverse clinical signs or symptoms. Radiographically there should be a dense, three-dimensional filling that extends as close as possible to the cementodentinal junction without gross overextension or underfilling in the presence of a patent canal[1] (Fig. 13-14). When a paste fill is present, retreatment of the canal is always indicated before post placement. If a silver cone is present and a post is necessary to accomplish the restorative treatment plan, it is always preferable to remove the silver cone and retreat the canal as opposed to removing the coronal portion of the silver cone with a bur. The latter approach often leads to root gouging or perforation and the significant possibility of breaking the apical seal provided by the silver cone.

Cementing media for posts

All posts, whether cast or prefabricated, are cemented inside the root canal. The cementing medium enhances retention, aids in stress distribution, and may seal any microgaps between the tooth and the post. Historically, zinc phosphate was the cement of choice, yielding high retentive values greater than those reported with polycarboxylate or standard resin cements. Recently, studies have advocated the use of a low-viscosity resin cement in combination with the gentle removal of the smear layer from the canal walls.[17] This permits a movement of the resin into the exposed, patent dentinal tubules. When using this

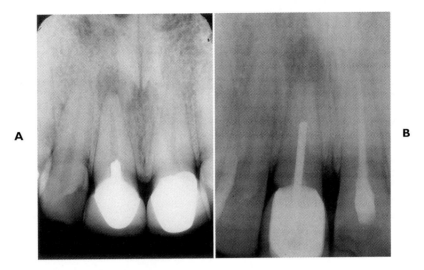

Fig. 13-14 *A* and *B, Two maxillary incisors restored using posts and crowns without previous root canal treatment.*

process for post cementation, a threefold increase in post retention has been noted when compared with zinc phosphate. Regardless, controversies still exist regarding the ideal cementing medium for a post because of the complexities that exist in trying to unite metal posts, cements, and dentin into a perfectly sealed unit. This is of considerable concern because the potential for coronal leakage around posts secured with contemporary cements has been shown to exist.[15] From a clinical perspective, however, the complete coronal seal is based on a combination of factors including the seal of the post, core, and overlying crown. It would seem reasonable to use a resin cement when posts are not fitted tightly to the prepared root canal space. Zinc phosphate should be selected when relatively tight-fitting posts are used.[8] None of the cements used, however, can overcome the inadequacies of a poorly designed post restoration.

Common problems with intraradicular posts

The most common problems with restorative posts can be considered in five major categories.

1. Inappropriate post-space preparation and selection of posts
2. Failure to properly restore the tooth over the post-core restoration
3. Effects of occlusal forces being transmitted to the post
4. Fracture of posts

5. Procedural errors in post-space preparation and post insertion

The first two problems have been dealt with previously in this chapter. Key to their prevention is to realize that a post does not strengthen the root; and, if a post is used, the coronal restoration must encompass sound dentin walls and be properly sealed at its margins.

One of the overall clinical goals of endodontic treatment is to retain teeth in a symptom-free, functional state (see Chapter 1).

Often overlooked is the need to ensure proper occlusal equilibration during and after both endodontic and restorative treatment.

During treatment occlusal refinement minimizes or prevents postoperative discomfort and a potential interappointment emergency visit. Attention to detail in this regard after restoration routinely provides the patient with immediate functional ability.

However, failure to adjust the occlusal patterns properly during function may very well lead to the transmission of excessive forces at the middle or apical portion of the post in the root, with fracture ultimately occurring. [6,49,55] Also identified in this realm is the loss of the integrity of endodontically treated abutment teeth for both fixed and removable partial dentures. Aberrant stresses to the

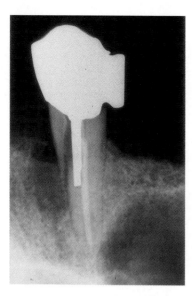

Fig. 13-15 *Root fracture resulting from excessive forces placed on the tooth by a precision-attachment removable partial denture.*

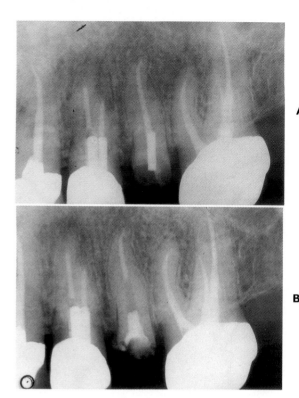

Fig. 13-16 *A,* *Fractured preformed stainless steel post.* *B,* *Post segment removed using techniques described in Chapter 7.*

improperly placed post-core complex may result in a coronal gingival fracture of the restoration[25,34,56,61,64] (Fig. 13-15).

Post fractures appear to be uniquely common to prefabricated posts because this is uncommonly seen with cast post-core buildups. Empirical observations would indicate that small-diameter metallic posts fracture more frequently than larger-diameter posts do. Secondly the fractures almost always occur in teeth with minimal coronal tooth structure. This is most likely at the core-root interface (Fig. 13-16). To minimize this occurrence, retention of coronal tooth structure, use of bonded posts and cores, and the creation of more tooth structure for coronal margins through crown lengthening are recommended. The removal of broken posts is discussed in Chapter 7.

The prevention of errors during post-space preparation and post cementation is fully within the realm of the clinician. First, as previously discussed, post-space preparation, both in length and in width, must be as conservative as possible.

Whenever possible the diameter of the post should not exceed a third of the diameter of the root in any dimension at any depth.

Second, if the radicular space is prepared, it should be filled completely with the post and the cementing medium (Fig. 13-17). Third, caution must always be exercised when one is preparing a post space in curved roots or roots with anticipated or demonstrated proximal invaginations (see Table 13-3). Also the placement of posts in small or irregularly shaped roots is contraindicated. Preparation of the post space, especially with specific rotary instruments commonly found with prefabricated post systems, must always follow the long axis of the root.[20] Removal of the gutta-percha with a heated instrument and initial preparation of the canal space to a size smaller than ideal is preferred, with subsequent enlargement done in a careful manner is recommended. Most root perforations during post-space preparation can be prevented (Fig. 13-18).

CLINICAL PROBLEM: A 38-year-old female patient presents with a chief complaint of a "gumboil" next to her tooth. It has been present for 2 months. At first it appeared and then was gone in a few days. Now it is present constantly. She has soreness in her gingival tissues, and occasionally the tooth hurts to biting. Clinical examination reveals a draining sinus tract opening on the attached gingiva adjacent to the mandibular right first molar. In addition there is probing in the sulcus (6 mm) to the midroot level (Fig. 13-19, *A*). There is active

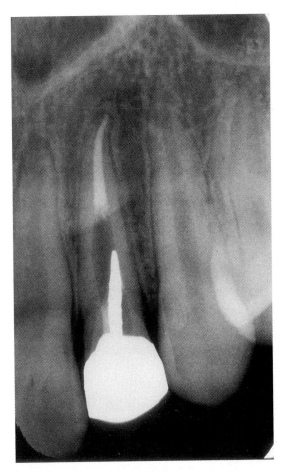

Fig. 13-17 *Post inadequately adapted to the prepared canal space. Likewise no effective cementing medium is apparent.*

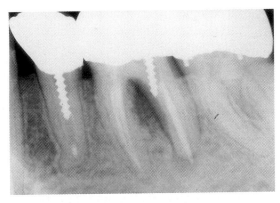

Fig. 13-18 *Preventable post perforation is present in the mandibular left first molar. Care must be taken to ensure that the post space preparation is in the long axis of the root and contained in the root canal. Notice the poor post space preparation and inadequate apical root canal filling in the adjacent premolar.*

drainage coming from the sulcus. A radiograph reveals a midroot radiolucency on the mesial aspect of the distal root. Root canal treatment had been performed and a post was present in the distal root (Fig. 13-19, *B*). Endodontic and restorative treatment appear adequate.

Solution: Based on the present findings it was not possible to make a definitive diagnosis, and surgical exploration was recommended as part of the diagnostic process. Tissue reflection and defect curettage revealed a probable post-strip perforation (Fig. 13-19, *C*). Subsequently the tooth was resected, and the distal root was removed (Fig. 13-19, *D*). Examination of the extracted root revealed deep external invagination, and a strip perforation with the post was clearly visible (Fig. 13-19, *E*).

Excessive forces encountered during post cementation can also be lessened if proper venting designs are used for the release of excess cement. Prefabricated systems come with these inherent designs,

whereas cast posts do not, unless they are incorporated during the fabrication. Likewise mixing the cementing medium to its proper consistency for post cementation is essential to allow for ease of post placement without undue installation stresses. These stresses will vary with cement type, post adaptation to the canal wall, and post design (see Table 13-2).

ENDODONTICALLY TREATED TEETH AS ABUTMENTS

Little information exists regarding the evaluation of endodontically treated teeth to serve as abutments for fixed or removable partial dentures or regarding any special requirements that these teeth may possess. Empirically it has been believed that these teeth always require a post to both reinforce the roots and to stabilize the tooth against the forces that may be encountered with a fixed or removable prosthesis. In this regard it has been shown that teeth that serve as fixed partial denture abutments bear greater stresses than single crown abutments do.[56] Likewise, teeth serving as abutments for removable partial dentures receive greater stress in function than nonabutment teeth do.[34] Distal-extension partial-denture abutment teeth withstand greater stresses than any other abutment tooth.[61]

The question then arises, Can endodontically treated teeth be used routinely as abutments for prostheses? Scientifically this question has not been resolved. From a retrospective, empirical standpoint, endodontically treated teeth have been

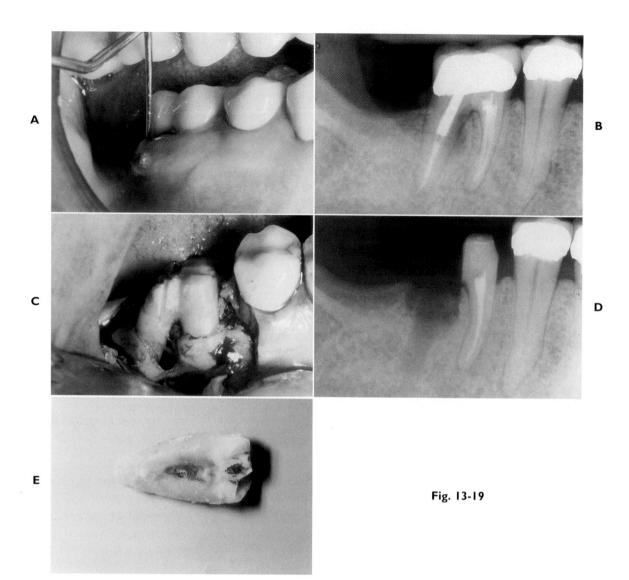

Fig. 13-19

shown to have a significantly higher failure rate when used as abutments for fixed or removable partial dentures as opposed to single crowns.[25,64] In an initial study, post placement had a limited influence on the success rate of fixed partial denture abutment teeth but did enhance success rates for removable partial abutment teeth.[64] In a recent study, the placement of a post core resulted in greater failure with fixed partial dentures as opposed to removable partial dentures.[25] Although these studies may provide a questionable outlook for endodontically treated teeth to serve as abutments, many factors must be considered, such as type of post used, method of post placement and cementation, undiagnosed root perforation during post-space preparation, proper distribution of

forces on the abutment teeth, intact sealed coronal margins on sound tooth structure, the use of the ferrule effect, unacceptable compaction forces during root canal treatment, misdiagnosis of vertical fractures before or during endodontic therapy, and restorative treatment (Fig. 13-20). Also the data in this study do not reflect modern concepts of tooth restoration, especially the ability to bond tooth restorative materials to tooth structure. Overlying all these concerns is the need for proper diagnosis and treatment planning for the patient. *Endodontically treated teeth can and do serve successfully as abutment teeth, and the clinician is strongly encouraged to treatment-plan these teeth for such.* Employment of the problem-solving approach when dealing with this clinical challenge will enhance this success.

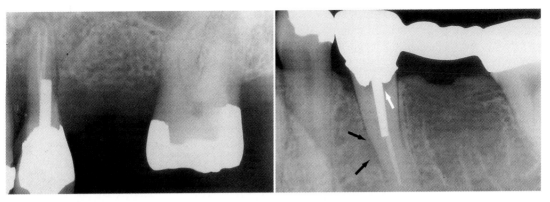

Fig. 13-20 *A, A 57-year-old male patient presents with a maxillary premolar removable partial denture abutment tooth that is very tender to percussion 6 months after completion of the root canal treatment and post, core, and crown placement. Post diameter relative to the root width and shape strongly indicates the presence of a perforation. A lateral radiolucency with periodontal probings confirms the diagnosis of post perforation in the furcation. B, Mandibular premolar fixed partial denture abutment tooth improperly restored resulted in an endodontic failure at the site of a probable lateral canal (black arrows). Restorative deficiencies include the placement of a crown margin on the core buildup material, which precludes the finishing of the crown margins on tooth structure and using a ferrule for crown stabilization and retention. The post is loose, but no fracture was identified. There is recurrent caries (white arrow) that probably accounts for the coronal leakage and ultimate lateral pathosis.*

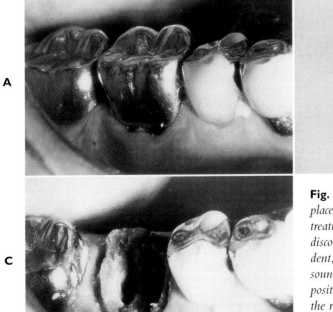

Fig. 13-21 *A, Apparent satisfactory full gold crown placed over a composite core build-up after root canal treatment. B, Patient's complaint of mobility led to the discovery of a loose post and crown. Leakage was evident, and there was the lack of coronal extension onto sound tooth structure. The crown margin is on the composite core on the mesial. C, Clinical examination of the remaining tooth structure confirms previous poor treatment planning for the restoration of this tooth. Crown lengthening was indicated to provide sufficient tooth structure for coronal retention and seal.*

RESTORING THE PREVIOUSLY RESTORED ENDODONTICALLY TREATED TOOTH

Frequently, root canal treatment is required on a tooth already restored with a satisfactory crown. Generally, replacement of the crown under these circumstances is not indicated unless significant destruction of the tooth structure or core material under the crown occurred during the endodontic access opening. Likewise, if decay was found under the crown when it was not readily detectable under the clinical crown margins, or if the seal of the crown has been altered by perforation under the crown margin, removal of the crown is recommended to enable the clinician to provide the best possible core buildup before the final restoration. In all cases of lost marginal integrity, crown removal is highly recommended before root canal treatment (see Table 13-1 and Chapter 3).

When the crown is going to be retained, there is little information regarding the best way to restore the endodontic access opening. Clinicians routinely use either amalgam, composite resin, or glass ionomer. Infrequently used is a gold inlay or gold foil. The placement of a post has been recommended to "reinforce" the crown,[13,51,68] but the achievement of this goal is highly suspect because the crown can be reinforced only by the nature and integrity of the core material beneath it. Initial evaluation of this latter approach to restoring endodontically treated teeth has indicated that there is a wide range of reasons for failure, including root fracture, radicular caries, crown dislodgment, and post and core dislodgment[25] (Fig. 13-21). Unfortunately, comparisons were not made with teeth that did not receive this mode of treatment. Therefore the routine placement of posts in access openings in crowns should be carefully considered because there is no documented support scientifically or clinically as to the efficacy of this technique. Often what does occur is the perforation of the root during the post space preparation or the initiation of the vertical root fracture attributable to post-installation stress—fractures that often go initially unnoticed because the coronal restoration holds the tooth together. Ultimately failure ensues only to be identified as an endodontic failure as opposed to a restorative one. Here again a cognizant problem-solving approach to treatment planning will prevent these unfortunate occurrences.

References

1. *Appropriateness of care and quality assurance guidelines:* Chicago 1994, American Association of Endodontists.
2. Barkhordar RA, Radke R, Abbasi J: Effect of metal collars on resistance of endodontically treated teeth to root fracture, *J Prosthet Dent* 61:676-678, 1989.
3. Bourgeois RS, Lemon RR: Dowel space preparation and apical leakage, *J Endod* 7:66-69, 1981.
4. Brandal JL, Nicholls JI, Harrington GW: A comparison of three restorative techniques for endodontically treated anterior teeth, *J Prosthet Dent* 58:161-165, 1987.
5. Bravin RV: Post reinforcement tested: The functional stress analysis of post reinforcement, *J Calif Dent Assoc* 4:66-71, 1976.
6. Cailleteau JG, Rieger MR, Akin JE: A comparison of intracanal stresses in a post-restored tooth utilizing the finite element method, *J Endod* 18:540-544, 1992.
7. Carter JM, Sorensen SE, Johnson RR, et al: Punch shear testing of extracted vital and endodontically treated teeth, *J Biomech* 16:841-848, 1983.
8. Christensen GJ: Posts, cores and patient care, *J Am Dent Assoc* 124:86-90, 1993.
9. Chung K-H: The properties of metal-reinforced glass ionomer materials, *J Oral Rehab* 20:79-87, 1993.
10. DeCleen MJH: The relationship between the root canal filling and post space preparation, *Int Endod J* 26:53-58, 1993.
11. Deutsch AS, Musikant BL, Cavallari J, et al: Root fracture during insertion of prefabricated posts related to root size, *J Prosthet Dent* 53:786-789, 1985.
12. DeWald JP, Arcoria CJ, Ferracane JL: Evaluation of glass-ionomer cores under cast crowns, *Dent Mater* 6:129-132, 1990.
13. Federick DR, Serene TP: Secondary intention dowel and core, *J Prosthet Dent* 34:41-47, 1975.
14. Felton DA, Webb EL, Kanoy BE, Dugoni J: Threaded endodontic dowels: effect of post design on incidence of root fracture, *J Prosthet Dent* 65:179-187, 1991.
15. Fogel HM: Microleakage of posts used to restore endodontically treated teeth, *J Endod* 21:376-379, 1995.
16. Gish SP, Drake DR, Walton RE, Wilcox L: Coronal leakage: bacterial penetration through obturated canals following post preparation, *J Am Dent Assoc* 125:1369-1372, 1994.
17. Goldman M, DeVitre R, White R, Nathanson D: An SEM study of posts cemented with an unfilled resin, *J Dent Res* 63:1003-1005, 1984.
18. Goodacre CJ, Spolnik KJ: The prosthodontic management of endodontically treated teeth: a literature review. Part I. Success and failure data, treatment concepts, *J Prosthodont* 3:243-250, 1994.
19. Goodacre CJ, Spolnik KJ: The prosthodontic management of endodontically treated teeth: a literature review, Part II. Maintaining the apical seal, *J Prosthodont* 4:51-53, 1995.
20. Gutmann JL. Preparation of endodontically treated teeth to receive post-core restoration, *J Prosthet Dent* 38:413-419, 1977.
21. Gutmann JL: The dentin-root complex: anatomic and biologic considerations in restoring endodontically treated teeth, *J Prosthet Dent* 67:458-467, 1992.
22. Gutmann JL, Rakusin H: Endodontic and restorative management of incompletely fractured molar teeth, *Int Endod J* 27:343-348, 1994.
23. Haddix JE, Mattison GD, Shulman CA, Pink FE: Post preparation techniques and their effect on the apical seal, *J Prosthet Dent* 64:515-519, 1990.

24. Hansen SR, Montgomery S: Effect of restoration thickness on the sealing ability of TERM, *J Endod* 19:448-452, 1993.

25. Hatzikyriakos AH, Reisis GI, Tsingos N: A 3-year post-operative clinical evaluation of post and cores beneath existing crowns, *J Prosthet Dent* 76:454-458, 1992.

26. Hernandez R, Bader S, Boston D, Trope M: Resistance of fracture of endodontically treated premolars restored with a new generation dentine bonding systems, *Int Endod J* 27:281-284, 1994.

27. Hornbrook DS, Hastings JH: Use of bondable reinforcement fiber for post and core build-up in an endodontically treated tooth: maximizing strength and aesthetics, *Pract Periodontics Aesthet Dent* 7(5):33-44, 1995.

28. Huang T-JG, Schilder H, Nathanson D: Effects of moisture content and endodontic treatment on some mechanical properties of human dentin, *J Endod* 18:209-215, 1992.

29. Hunter AJ, Feiglin B, Williams JF: Effects of post placement on endodontically treated teeth, *J Prosthet Dent* 62:166-172, 1989.

30. Huysmans M, Peters MCRB, Plasschaert AJM, van der Varst PGT. Failure characteristics of endodontically treated premolars restored with a post and direct restorative material, *Int Endod J* 25:121-129, 1992.

31. Imbery TA, Burgess JO, Batzer RC: Comparing the resistance of dentin bonding agents and pins in amalgam restorations, *J Am Dent Assoc* 126:753-759, 1995.

32. Kanca J: Conservative resin restoration of endodontically treated teeth, *Quintessence Int* 19:25-28, 1988.

33. Kovarik RE, Breeding LC, Caughman WF: Fatigue life of three core materials under simulated chewing conditions, *J Prosthet Dent* 68:584-590, 1992.

34. Kydd W, Dutton D, Smith D: Lateral forces exerted on abutment teeth by partial dentures, *J Am Dent Assoc* 68:859-863, 1964.

35. Lee Y-C, Yang S-F, Hwang Y-F et al: Microleakage of endodontic temporary restorative materials, *J Endod* 19:516-520, 1993.

36. Libman WJ, Nicholls JI: Load fatigue of teeth restored with cast posts and cores and complete crowns, *Int J Prosthodont* 8:155-161, 1995.

37. Linn J, Messer HH: Effect of restorative procedures on the strength of endodontically treated molars, *J Endod* 20:479-485, 1994.

38. Lovdahl PE, Nicholls JI: Pin-retained amalgam cores vs. cast-gold dowel-cores, *J Prosthet Dent* 38:507-514, 1977.

39. Madison S, Walton R. Cervical root resorption following bleaching of endodontically treated teeth, *J Endod* 16:570-574, 1990.

40. Magura ME, Kafrawy AH, Brown CE Jr et al: Human saliva coronal microleakage in obturated root canals: an in vitro study, *J Endod* 17:324-331, 1991.

41. Mattison GD, Delivanis PD, Thacker RW JR, Hassell KJ: Effect of post preparation on the apical seal, *J Prosthet Dent* 51:785-789, 1984.

42. Nathanson D, Ashayeri N: New aspects of restoring the endodontically treated tooth, *Alpha Omegan* 83:76-80, 1990.

43. Nathanson D, Dias KRHC, Ashayeri N: The significance of retention in post and core restorations, *Pract Periodontics Aesthet Dent* 5(3):82-90, 1993.

44. Nayyar A, Walton RE, Leonard LA: An amalgam coronal-radicular dowel and core technique for endodontically treated posterior teeth, *J Prosthet Dent* 43:511-515, 1980.

45. Nicholls JI: Rebuilding the treated tooth, *Calif Dent Assoc J* 16(11):34-38, 1988.

46. Panitvisai P, Messer HH: Cuspal deflection in molars in relation to endodontic and restorative procedures, *J Endod* 21:57-61, 1995.

47. Papa J, Cain C, Messer HH: Moisture content of vital vs endodontically treated teeth, *Endod Dent Traumatol* 10:91-93, 1994.

48. Perez E, Zillich R, Yaman P: Root curvature localizations as indicators of post length in various groups, *Endod Dent Traumatol* 2:58-61, 1986.

49. Peters MCRB, Poort HW, Farah JW, Craig RG: Stress analysis of a tooth restored with a post and core, *J Dent Res* 62:760-763, 1983.

50. Portell FR, Bernier WE, Lorton L, Peters D: The effect of immediate versus delayed dowel space preparation on the integrity of the apical seal, *J Endod* 8:154-160, 1982.

51. Priest G, Goerig A: Post and core fabrication beneath an existing crown, *J Prosthet Dent* 42:645-648, 1979.

52. Ray HA, Trope M: Periapical status of endodontically treated teeth in relation to the technical quality of the root filling and the coronal restoration, *Int Endod J* 28:12-18, 1995.

53. Reeh ES, Douglas WH, Messer HH: Stiffness of endodontically-treated teeth related to restoration technique, *J Dent Res* 68:1540-1544, 1989.

54. Reeh ES, Messer HH, Douglas WH: Reduction of tooth stiffness as a result of endodontic and restorative procedures, *J Endod* 15:512-516, 1989.

55. Reinhardt RA, Krejci RF, Pao YC, Stannard JG: Dentin stresses in post-reconstructed teeth with diminishing bone support, *J Dent Res* 62:1002-1008, 1983.

56. Reynolds JM: Abutment selection for fixed prosthodontics, *J Prosthet Dent* 19:483-488, 1968.

57. Rivera EM, Yamauchi M, Chandler G, Bergenholtz G: Dentin collagen cross-links of root-filled and normal teeth, *J Endod* 14:195, 1988.

58. Safavi KE, Dowden WE, Langeland K: Influence of delayed coronal permanent restoration on endodontic prognosis, *Endod Dent Traumatol* 3:187-191, 1987.

59. Saunders WP, Saunders EM: Coronal leakage as a cause of failure in root-canal therapy: a review, *Endod Dent Traumatol* 10:105-108, 1994.

60. Sedgley CM, Messer HH: Are endodontically treated teeth more brittle? *J Endod* 18:332-335, 1992.

61. Shohet H: Relative magnitudes of stress on abutment teeth with different retainers, *J Prosthet Dent* 21:267-282, 1969.

62. Sorensen JA, Engelman MJ: Effect of post adaptation on fracture resistance of endodontically treated teeth, *J Prosthet Dent* 64:419-424, 1990.

63. Sorensen JA, Engleman MJ: Ferrule design and fracture resistance of endodontically treated teeth, *J Prosthet Dent* 63:529-536, 1990.

64. Sorensen JA, Martinoff JT: Endodontically treated teeth as abutments, *J Prosthet Dent* 53:631-636, 1985.

65. Sorensen JA, Martinoff JT: Intracoronal reinforcement and coronal coverage: a study of endodontically treated teeth, *J Prosthet Dent* 51:780-784, 1984.

66. Sorensen JA, Martinoff JT: Clinically significant factors in dowel design, *J Prosthet Dent* 52:28-35, 1984.

67. Sorensen JA: Preservation of tooth structure, *Calif Dent Assoc J* 16(11):15-22, 1988.

68. Stackhouse JA: Reinforcement of nonvital crowned teeth, *J Am Dent Assoc* 104:859-861, 1982.

69. Taleghani M, Morgan RW: Reconstructive materials for endodontically treated teeth, *J Prosthet Dent* 57:446-449, 1987.

70. Tjan AHL, Dunn JR, Lee, JK-Y: Fracture resistance of amalgam and composite resin cores retained by various intradentinal retentive features, *Quintessence Int* 24:211-217, 1993.

71. Torabinejad M, Ung B, Kettering JD: *In vitro* bacterial penetration of coronally unsealed endodontically treated teeth, *J Endod* 16:566-569, 1990.

72. Torbjörner A, Karlsson S, Ödman PA: Survival rate and failure characteristics for two post designs, *J Prosthet Dent* 73:439-444, 1995.

73. Trope E, Chow E, Nissan R: *In vitro* endotoxin penetration of coronally unsealed endodontically treated teeth, *Endod Dent Traumatol* 11:90-94, 1991.

74. Walls AWG, Adamson J, McCabe JF, Murray JJ: The properties of a glass polykenoate (ionomer) cement incorporating sintered metallic particles, *Dent Mater* 3:113-116, 1987.

75. Young HM, Shen C, Maryniuk GA: Retention of cast posts relative to cement selection, *Quintessence Int* 16:357-360, 1985.

76. Zillich RM, Corcoran JF: Average maximum post lengths in endodontically treated teeth, *J Prosthet Dent* 52:489-491, 1984.

77. Zillich R Yaman P: Effect of root curvature on post length in the restoration of endodontically treated premolars, *Endod Dent Traumatol* 1:135-137, 1985.

Index

Q